THE METHODS AND FINDINGS OF QUALITY ASSESSMENT AND MONITORING:

AN ILLUSTRATED ANALYSIS

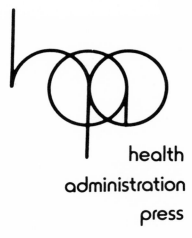

health administration press

*Health Administration Press was
established in 1972 with the support
of the W.K. Kellogg Foundation and
is a nonprofit endeavor of The
University of Michigan Program
and Bureau of Hospital
Administration.*

EXPLORATIONS IN QUALITY ASSESSMENT AND MONITORING

Volume III

THE METHODS AND FINDINGS OF QUALITY ASSESSMENT AND MONITORING:
AN ILLUSTRATED ANALYSIS

Avedis Donabedian, M.D., M.P.H.

The University of Michigan

Health Administration Press
Ann Arbor, Michigan
1985

Library of Congress Cataloging in Publication Data

Donabedian, Avedis.
  The methods and findings of quality assessment and monitoring: an illustrated analysis.

  (Explorations in quality assessment and monitoring/Avedis Donabedian ; 3)
  Bibliography: p.
  Includes index.
  1. Medical care—Evaluation. 2. Medical care—Quality control. 3. Medical care—Statistics. 4. Medical care—Charts, diagrams, etc. 5. Medical care—United States—Evaluation. 6. Medical care—United States—Quality control. 7. Medical care—United States—Statistics. 8. Medical care—United States—Charts, diagrams, etc. 9. United States—Statistics, Medical. I. Title. II. Series:
Donabedian, Avedis. Explorations in quality assessment and monitoring ; 3.
RA399.A1D65 vol. 3   362.1′068′5s   83-18397
ISBN 0-914904-89-2   [362.1′060′5]
ISBN 0-914904-88-4 (pbk.)

This volume is based on work supported by the National Center for Health Services Research, the Commonwealth Fund, the Carnegie Corporation of New York, the Milbank Memorial Fund, and the W. K. Kellogg Foundation. The views expressed in it are those of the author, and do not in any way represent his sponsors.

Health Administration Press
School of Public Health
The University of Michigan
1021 East Huron Street
Ann Arbor, Michigan 48109
(313) 764–1380

I have written this book

for my sister

MARGARET

and for my brothers

HOVHANNES and CHRISTOPHER

in remembrance of our happy growing up together

in a far away place, and in celebration

of the ties that still so lovingly bind us

though in this world we have walked

our too separate ways.

Table of Contents

PART IV   SOME PROBLEMS OF METHOD

Preface and Acknowledgments

This is most probably the last book that I shall ever write. What shall I say about it?

I shall say, first, that it was a labor of love. I, myself, have read every paper, monograph, or book upon which it is based, often many times over. I have collected and collated every bit of information, designed every chart, written every word, typed the manuscript, and verified every editorial amendment. In common with most of my other work, I have tried to make it a testament to individual craftsmanship. Insofar as possible, it is untouched by nonhuman hands.

Next, I shall say that this is the end of a road that I stumbled on as a student, almost thirty years ago, when I wrote a paper on the quality of care for my teacher Franz Goldmann. Without knowing it, I had set out on a journey that would continue, with occasional detours or interruptions, for the rest of my life.

During this time, quality assessment and monitoring have experienced many changes of fortune: ignored at first, then acclaimed, and now almost disdained. How quickly we have moved from unknowing indifference, to uncritical love, to misguided distrust! Yet, quality must remain, in spite of these inconstant moods, the one unchanging object of our commitment.

Even our current preoccupation with cost makes quality assessment more relevant, rather than less. First, it is our fondest hope that by improving efficiency we can reduce costs without damaging quality. How are we to know that our hopes are justified? Then, if we believe, as some unfortunately do, that costs must be cut still further, how are we to know what amount of quality we have relinquished for what savings in cost? If our institutions are to produce care at different levels of quality, so that clients may choose what best suits their purse, our assessments of quality must become more persevering and more precise, rather than less so. Otherwise, one could not escape the conclusion that our proposals to regulate quality and cost through "competition" are nothing more than a sham or a delusion. Without precise and publicly available information on the quality of care much of "cost containment" would inevitably be a means of withholding some quality from those less able to afford it, hoping that they will not perceive the magnitude of the loss.

The three volumes of these *Explorations in Quality Assessment and Monitoring* are a testament to these obdurate convictions. In the first volume, on *The Definition of Quality and Approaches to Its Assessment*, I tried to show how several legitimate views of quality, and of the ways it may be measured, are encompassed by a model that reveals the interrelations of these views, explains their differences, and identifies their particular applications. To some extent, the second volume, dealing with *The Criteria and Standards of Quality*, is an elaboration on these themes. This is because the criteria and standards are nothing more than the more precise, more concrete representations of the conceptual abstractions offered in the earlier volume. But there is also a great deal more on the classification, construction, and testing of the criteria as measurement tools. Finally, in this third volume, I try to show how the definition of quality, the approaches to its assessment, and the devices available to measure it, have been used to evaluate and monitor the quality of care, and with what results.

There is, I believe, a natural progression from one volume to the next. There is also a strong thread of continuity. Nevertheless, each volume can be read independently of the other, as well as an introduction either to a preceding or a subsequent volume.

The method of presentation in this, third, volume is illustrative and anecdotal. The book consists of a series of pictorial illustrations, each summarizing some key findings of a particular study. Facing each illustration, or chart, is a text that, to varying degrees, describes and comments on the methods of the study, summarizes the findings, and points out the more general significance of both methods and findings. In this way, the reader is familiarized with important milestones in the development of the field, gains a critical understanding of the several methods used, and learns about the factors that influence quality for better or worse. For though the presentation is pictorial and anecdotal, it is also highly systematic and firmly based on a clearly formulated conceptual foundation.

By referring to the Table of Contents, we see that the book is organized into four parts: one on the definition of quality; a second on the assessment of process; a third on the assessment of outcome, either alone or in conjunction with process; and a fourth on some problems of method. Each part is further subdivided into chapters which correspond to additional major categories of classification. Both the thematic unity and internal diversity of each chapter are indicated by an introduction that precedes the presentation of the charts in that chapter. Thereafter, the text facing each illustration, besides describing and assessing the methods and findings represented by the chart, carries the narrative forward from illustration to illustration, having regard to both continuity and further differentiation. Some, but not all, of that differentiation is also suggested by running heads to the charts; these notations identify similarities among shorter sequences of charts within each chapter.

Finally, the "Epilogue," which is the concluding section of text, pulls together the several themes of the preceding chapters into what one hopes is a reasonably coherent synthesis. I want to draw particular attention to the final pages which deal with the "epidemiology of quality," by which I mean its distribution among each of two "populations," one of providers and another of clients. Though still incomplete, this is perhaps the most comprehensive summary of its kind currently available. It has the added advantage of being a fresh reassessment that is uninfluenced by previous reviews, and one that is documented by reference to material readily available in preceding chapters of the book.

It is perilous, of course, to look for grand, unifying designs in a collection of largely unrelated empirical observations. One is easily suspected of including only what fits one's prejudices, and of only seeing what one wishes to see. The attempt to conduct a reasonably objective inquiry must, nevertheless, be made; the mind cannot accept or use a mere jumble of facts. In this case, by combining classification, description, and interpretation, I have tried to introduce order and meaning, while also allowing the reader to draw conclusions other than my own.

I believe that this collection of past work, done by many investigators, in various places, at different times, using diverse methods, offers us a treasure of experience to draw upon. It is certainly capable of illustrating the rich variety of methods available for our use. The recurrence of certain relationships under different circumstances can also suggest some enduring truths. But, though our view is panoramic, it is also too fragmented to give us a picture for the nation as a whole, either of the level of quality at any given time, or of the changes that level may have undergone over a period of time. We can only see how deplorably, and in how many ways, the quality of care has fallen short of our expectations.

To obtain this overview, I have selected the studies to be included with some care. First, I have tried to include as many variants of method as I could find, even though the representatives of particular methods may have been flawed. One can often learn more from the failures than the perfections of others. Next, I tried to offer a historical perspective of major developments as illustrated by substantial bodies of work done by our leading investigators. I wanted, in this way, to recognize our indebtedness to these pioneers, and to establish a scholarly tradition with a sense of history and continuity. Nothing betrays the moral and intellectual poverty of our field quite so much as our tendency either to plunder or reinvent, rather than build upon, the past.

In addition to their contributions to the methods of assessment, some

studies recommended themselves because they offered important findings pertinent to public policy or the design of systems to deliver health
care. Some others could not be used because, by only reporting measures
of association, they offered little opportunity for pictorial representation.
But when such work was particularly significant, it was referred to,
where appropriate, in the text. Occasionally, I have indulged myself by
including something of particular personal significance or interest, but
in general I have tried to be as fair and responsible as possible. Even
then, either through ignorance or inattention, I may have missed some
important work no earlier counterpart of which has been included. If so,
I ask that my readers write to me about the omission.

   Besides these inadvertent omissions, the book has some limitations
that I know about. I may have disappointed some colleagues by confin-
ing my attention almost exclusively to the care provided by physicians.
By doing so I have recognized the limits of my own competence. I do
hope, however, that the general principles that guide the assessment of
the physician's work will apply, of course with some modifications, to
other health care practitioners as well. The lack of attention to the quality
of the interpersonal process is not as easily remediable. Though I recognized the importance of the subject, I felt unable to do justice to the
extensive, seemingly tangled, body of literature on patient satisfaction.
Finally, if my time had permitted, I would have included much more
about the effectiveness of monitoring in bringing about changes in practitioner behavior. Someone else will have to undertake all these important, arduous tasks.

   And now, some comments about format.

   I consider the succession of text and charts, in face-to-face pairs, a
distinct advantage. The iron discipline imposed by this format required
me to identify clearly the main message in each chart, and to convey it
as simply and forcefully as I could. Sometimes, the narrative thread continues in the text to successive charts. But, even then, there is much that
the reader may wish to pursue in the original sources to which the text
alludes. When these citations give only a page number, the reference is
to the source for the chart itself. This source is briefly noted at the bottom
of each chart and cited in full in the bibliography.

   The construction of the charts has often required considerable re-
arrangement and manipulation of the data in the original sources. To
help the reader verify the charts, I have indicated as precisely as I could,
at the bottom of each chart, the location of the original data and the
nature of the computations I have performed. In order to keep the charts
as simple and uncluttered as possible, almost all other material that might
have appeared as footnotes (such as the meanings of asterisks and ab-

breviations) will be found in the text. When the source indicated the statistical significance of observed differences, this information is generally given in my text, but I have not done any additional tests of significance myself. What these charts have to say depends not so much on the detailed verification of each finding as on the directions in which the cumulative succession of findings seems to point.

The succession of charts is designed to lead the reader along carefully prepared paths to a discovery of such dominant themes. And yet, there is an unknowable number of additional paths that one might take in the pursuit of sequences and clusterings that correspond to some particular question that the reader may wish to ask. Much attention has been lavished on the subject index so it can permit, even encourage, such explorations. In using it for this purpose, it will be useful to know that the primary references in the index are to the pages of the relevant charts. The text pages are indexed only if they contain information not depicted on the charts themselves.

And now it is time for me to bring my own wanderings to an end. But, first, there is a happy obligation to discharge. Because this last volume of my *Explorations* has been so long in the making, there are many who, at one time or another, have lent me a helping hand. What a pleasure to recognize so many friends assembled so conveniently together.

The thought of preparing an annotated chartbook of health care administration has occupied me for over twenty years, but I never seemed to find the money or the time. In 1976, after *Benefits in Medical Care Programs* had been completed, I discovered that because of my habitual parsimoniousness some modest sums of money were left over. The Carnegie Corporation of New York and the Milbank Memorial Fund, who had sponsored the writing of the book, allowed me to keep this balance in return for a promise to prepare an annotated chartbook on quality assessment and utilization review. For almost ten years they have waited for me to make good on that promise. How can I thank them enough, not only for their financial support, but also for their unquestioning faith that I would, in the end, come through. After so many years, I place this book as a garland at their feet.

In some ways, this book can be seen as a by-product of the effort to prepare the preceding two volumes in this series. As I reviewed the literature, I took time to note the materials and prepare the charts that would be the candidates for inclusion in this volume. The National Center for Health Services Research and the Commonwealth Fund, the two organizations, one public and the other private, that sponsored the preparation of the earlier volumes have, in this way, contributed significantly to the final volume as well. Later, the Commonwealth Fund, through the good offices of Margaret Mahoney, its current president, provided additional direct support for the preparation of the charts and text so they could serve as "instructional modules" for the education of administrators and practitioners. In this way, Margaret Mahoney made a second propitious appearance in my professional life. It was she, while still at the Carnegie Corporation, who assembled the support necessary for my work on *Benefits in Medical Care Programs*. Now, again, when I was in direst need, she stepped in to smooth the way. How does one thank a fairy godmother? Not in words, I think; perhaps by living up to her expectations.

In recent years, my professional work has benefited considerably from support by the W. K. Kellogg Foundation for doctoral training at The University of Michigan's School of Public Health. This book, in common with my other scholarly work, owes a great deal to this support, and to the wise way in which it has been administered by Sylvester Berki, the chairman of my department. I deeply appreciate his unwavering commitment to scholarship and research.

As in all my previous work, I owe much to the Reference Collection of materials in health care organization at the School of Public Health. As always, Lillian Fagin and Jack Tobias, who staff and administer the Collection, have been responsive to my every request.

Yet once again, Barbara Black has kept her watchful eye over my financial affairs, deftly coordinating the several accounts that have contributed to this protracted work. After almost ten years of so much attention to so many small accounts, she richly deserves the relief she no doubt will feel when the final "bottom lines" are drawn, and the files are forever put away.

The production of a book that requires very close matching of visual materials and text has called for a great deal of additional effort by all concerned. I have been fortunate in enjoying the friendship, support, and expert help of my collaborators at Health Administration Press. I am indebted to Jacqueline Sharp for her precise and beautiful renderings of my original drawings, and for her exemplary patience with the seemingly endless adjustments that I kept calling for. I thank Mary Matthews for her expert, but restrained, editing of almost all the text.

The subject index, which I consider to be one of the most important features of this book, is the product of a happy collaboration with Jean Thorby, a colleague of many years' standing. Using her considerable knowledge of the subject matter, and her expertise in classification and index construction, Ms. Thorby completed the difficult task of integrating my detailed suggestions with her own judgments of what should be indexed and how. Both my readers and I have much to thank her for.

In addition to guiding and coordinating the tediously complicated production process, Robyn Fritz was responsible for repeatedly verifying the charts. I am indebted to her for detecting countless errors, and making many valuable suggestions.

I am particularly indebted to Daphne Grew, the director of the Press, who, throughout a decade of collaboration, has remained unwavering in her support, even when the ledgers should have prompted despair. We have comforted ourselves by thoughts of building for the ages. Only time will show the magnitude of our prescience or delusion.

Meanwhile, for all these years, my wife and children suffered the inevitable deprivations caused by my constant labors. There are no words to say what I owe these loved ones, and little I can do to make up for the losses they have suffered.

Home is the aged wanderer they scarcely know, sitting by the domestic hearth, dozing into sleep.

Avedis Donabedian
Ann Arbor
A cold day in March

PART I

The Definition of Quality

Perspectives on the Quality of Health Care

ONE

Before attempting to assess "the quality of health care" one should first define the term and explain the concept. But the concept is so elusive, and the term has been used by so many in such different ways, that one is reluctant even to ask for an explanation in advance. Some might prefer, rather, to arrive at an answer circuitously, perhaps by saying that "quality" is whatever the methods of its assessment assess.

This third volume of my *Explorations* may seem to be taking this roundabout road, relying on the examples of assessment encountered on the way to prompt the insights that, little by little, will illuminate the subject. Thus, empirical observations will contribute inductively to our knowledge. It is important, however, to be prepared for the encounters of a journey, to know what to look for, so as not only to appreciate what one finds, but also to be aware of what should be there, but is not.

I tried in the first volume of these *Explorations* to construct the formulation from which the major attributes of the methods of quality assessment could be deduced. The definition of quality that has guided this entire enterprise is presented there in full. In the first part of this volume I will deal with only two aspects of that definition. This chapter will be concerned with different viewpoints of quality, and the next with the influence of monetary cost on the way quality is defined.

The process of health care is meant to achieve certain objectives. These are generally related to the promotion, preservation, and restoration of health. Moreover, health care ought to be conducted in a way that is acceptable, pleasing, even rewarding, to clients; and it should be provided in settings that take account of the patient's comfort, sensitivities, and other needs. In summary, a judgment of quality can be made relative to technical care, to the management of the interpersonal relationship between the patient and the practitioner, and to the amenities of care.

All judgments involve valuation, and because individuals and groups differ in their values, they also differ in their judgments of the same thing; this is true also of judgments of the quality of health care. Differences of a most fundamental kind can arise from the many ways in which "health" may be conceived of and defined. There are also differences of opinion as to what aspects of health a practitioner may legitimately assume responsibility for. Expectations concerning the amenities of care and the conduct of the more personal relationship between practitioners and patients can also vary a great deal.

Physicians and other health care practitioners can be expected to be aware of the range of considerations that contribute to the clients' definition of quality. But the practitioners are trained to be expert in the details of technical care; this is their distinctive contribution and their consuming preoccupation. How practitioners define quality will become more apparent when, in later chapters, we examine the criteria which they recommend or use to assess their own performance and that of their colleagues. In this chapter I shall touch only briefly on the correspondence between the practitioners' and the clients' views of quality.

Clients know very little about the details of technical care, though they can be expected to appreciate its importance, especially in situations that pose a clear threat to their health and well-being. Most of the time, clients are reduced to judging the quality of technical care indirectly, by evidence of the practitioner's personal interest in, and concern for, the patient's health and welfare. Clients can also derive direct satisfactions or dissatisfactions from the conditions under which care is provided, and from the manner in which they are treated by the practitioner and by those who surround him. One must never forget that, as far as these nontechnical matters are concerned, the clients are the ultimate authority on the criteria of good care.

This chapter will include some studies that document the breadth and variety of technical and nontechnical concerns, and that attempt to weigh their relative importance to clients and practitioners. In this regard, we shall find that clients differ from each other; that, as a group, they are both similar to and different from the practitioners; and that the similarities and differences vary according to the situation in which the clients find themselves. The hypothesis that seems best to explain these rather complicated findings is that clients want technical expertise and personal concern in equal degree because neither is efficacious without the other, but that either the one or the other may receive greater attention depending on which is seen to be more lacking, and more critical to the patient's welfare, in any particular situation.

Chart 1–1

People are seldom asked to define "the quality of medical care." The question is put indirectly. What is a good doctor, nurse, or clinic? What is a bad one? What does the respondent like or dislike? What kind of doctor or clinic would the respondent choose, if a choice were possible? From the answers to such questions about the attributes of providers, inferences must be drawn about the ingredients of "goodness" in the care they give.

This chart is based on a study of this kind. The respondents are adults, one to each household or subunit of a household, among those in the Yorkville Welfare District of Manhattan, which were found to be newly eligible for public assistance during the period between July 1, 1961 and June 30, 1962. As part of an extensive survey, in preparation for a controlled experiment designed to study the effects of comprehensive care, each respondent was given a list of 13 attributes and asked: "Would you pick out three or four which describe the kind of doctor *you yourself* like best?" (p. 270).

The chart shows the most frequently selected attributes. Not shown are the following additional ones: "Doesn't ask unnecessary questions," included among their choices by 16 percent of respondents; "Tries not to give me too much medicine," selected by nine percent; and "Is my own religion," selected by six percent. We are also told that "respondents picked old rather than young doctors in a ratio of four to one and men rather than women doctors by more than two to one," but we are not told how often these attributes were included among the three or four selected by each respondent (p. 48).

These answers are, of course, shaped primarily by the list of choices; in this case it contained very little about the technical aspects of care. The answers also reflect the viewpoints of a rather distinctive population group: poor urban dwellers, over half of whom were of Puerto Rican descent and about a fifth of whom were black. But while the attachment of this group to a more traditional cultural heritage may prompt us to question the general applicability of their preference for older male physicians, it makes their evident desire for more information about their illnesses even more compelling than it otherwise would have been. I believe it is safe to say that people want to be participants in medical care, not merely the objects of it.

Chart 1–1

Percent of Respondents Who Select Specified Attributes To Describe the Doctor They Themselves Would Like Best. Adults in Households or Units of Households Newly Eligible for Public Assistance, Yorkville Welfare District, New York City, July, 1961–June, 1962.

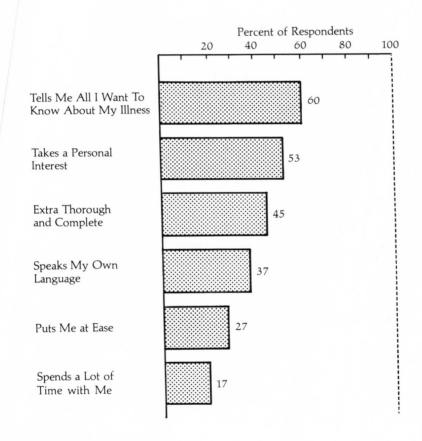

Source: Goodrich et al. 1970, Table 18, p. 50.

Chart 1–2

We have here some findings of a study that appears to have overcome the troubling limitations of the preceding one. It reports opinions unconstrained by a preconceived listing of attributes, and the respondents are a representative sample of an entire population, though it is one in another country, with a system of health care rather different from ours.

"What are the qualities, the things about your G. P., that you appreciate?" each adult respondent was asked during an interview at home. The most frequent answers are shown in the chart, as classified by the investigator herself. The most frequently mentioned attributes indicated appreciation of something about the doctor's "manner or personality." Also very often, though somewhat less frequently, the respondents mentioned attributes that pertained to the way their doctors "looked after them." A small percentage of respondents mentioned attributes that could have belonged under either of the two categories used to classify the answers.

It is easy to see a correspondence between the first of Cartwright's categories and that aspect of quality pertaining to the management of the interpersonal relationship between patient and practitioner. The second of Cartwright's categories corresponds to the quality of "technical care," but less perfectly, since it includes some attributes, such as "visits promptly or without grumbling," that I would have included under the management of the interpersonal process.

Cartwright points out that it is "in many ways inappropriate to separate" the two classes of attributes, as she has done (p. 7). Nevertheless, classifications more or less similar to hers appear frequently in studies of client preferences, often leading to speculation as to which of the two categories of attributes is the more important to people. Our next chart addresses this very issue.

Chart 1–2

Percent of Respondents Who Appreciated Specified Attributes of Their General Practitioners. England and Wales, Summer 1964.

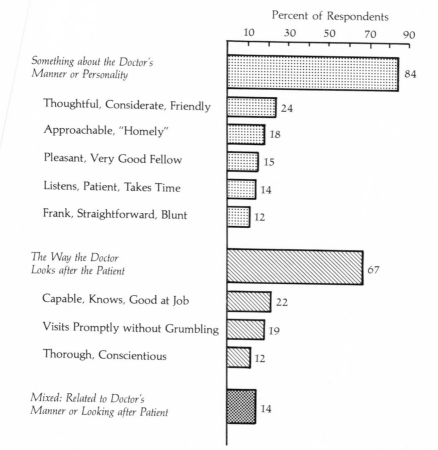

Source: Cartwright 1967, pp. 5–7.

Chart 1–3

This chart comes from a remarkable study of ambulatory care provided in the outpatient clinics of the hospitals affiliated with Western Reserve (now Case Western Reserve) University. During each of 1960, 1961, and 1962, a random sample was drawn from the medical records of patients who frequented the outpatient clinics that mainly treated long-term patients. The chart shows what the patients in these three samples said when asked to describe the "good doctor."

In response to this question, 26 percent of patients mentioned only attributes that the investigators judged to pertain to "technical skills," 49 percent mentioned only attributes judged to describe "interpersonal and communication skills," and 24 percent mentioned some attributes pertinent to each of the two categories of skills. When the three categories of patients are combined, one finds that 73 percent mentioned at least some attributes assigned to "interpersonal and communication skills," and 50 percent at least some attributes assigned to "technical skills."

These findings may not be generally applicable, since the respondents are not only chronically ill, but also more likely than the general population to be black, female, over 65, unemployed, poor, and divorced, widowed, or separated. The findings do, nevertheless, illustrate two questions that have been asked in studies of client preferences. First, are there two categories of persons, one comprising those who mainly want care of high technical quality, and another including those who mainly want a satisfying and congenial interpersonal relationship? Second, irrespective of whether people can be so neatly categorized, which of the two aspects of care, technical excellence or interpersonal affinity, is the one more often wanted, or desired more intensely?

The nature of the questions, and the evidence bearing on them, are discussed in some detail in the first volume of these *Explorations* (pp. 36–46). I tend to agree with Freidson that people can differentiate the attributes that respectively signify "personal interest" and "competence," but that they want them both, and in equal degree (Freidson 1961, pp. 50–56). This is because "personal interest" does not cure organic illness, nor does mere "competence," unless it is put to work for the patient by virtue of the physician's personal interest and commitment. But in any given situation, the one of the two which is more likely to be wanting, or to be critical to health, is the one more likely to be emphasized.

Chart 1-3

Percent of Patients Who Mention Attributes in Specified Categories When Asked To Describe the "Good Doctor." Patients in Outpatient Clinics that Mainly Serve Long-term Patients, Hospitals of Western Reserve University, Cleveland, Ohio, 1960-1962.

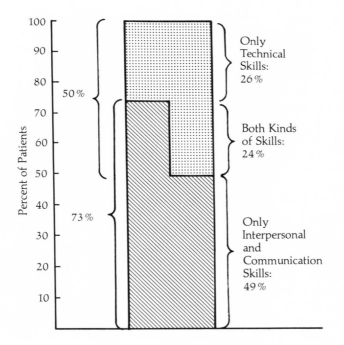

Source: Sussman et al. 1967, Table 3, p. 50.

Chart 1–4

In another part of the study illustrated by the preceding chart, patients in the clinics that treated mainly long-term illness were shown a list of ten items and asked to select the "three things most important for a good clinic." The chart shows the most frequently chosen attributes.

The findings demonstrate the high and equal importance given to a well-trained doctor and a doctor with whom the patient has a stable relationship. The importance of some other aspects of the interpersonal relationship, such as "personal interest" and "information," is also evident. Of the amenities of care, "privacy" and a "short wait for the doctor" stand rather high among the most important preferred attributes of a good clinic, whereas others, not shown in the chart, rank rather low. The three other attributes of the ten offered to each respondent were "pleasant staff," "good rest rooms," and "comfortable waiting rooms." These are not shown in the table from which the chart was drawn, but we are told that each was selected by less than 20 percent of patients.

The great attention paid to aspects of the interpersonal relationship is in keeping with the findings of many other studies. But one wonders why not everyone chose "well-trained doctors" among the three most important attributes of the ten on the list. Perhaps the patients believed that in a university-affiliated clinic, technical competence could be assumed. Finally, it is useful to call attention to the importance of monetary cost, an attribute I have not mentioned so far, but which will concern us in the next chapter and repeatedly thereafter.

The investigators also report the choices made by a sample of patients with acute illnesses who were asked the same question about the attributes of a good clinic. Despite small differences between their responses and those of patients with chronic illness, the similarities between the two sets of answers were rather striking.

We do not know to what extent any or all of the findings described above were influenced by the restrictions imposed by the list from which the choices had to be made.

Chart 1–4

Percent of Patients Who Select Specified Attributes To Be Among the Three "Most Important for a Good Clinic." Patients in Outpatient Clinics that Mainly Serve Long-term Patients, Hospitals of Western Reserve University, Cleveland, Ohio, 1961.

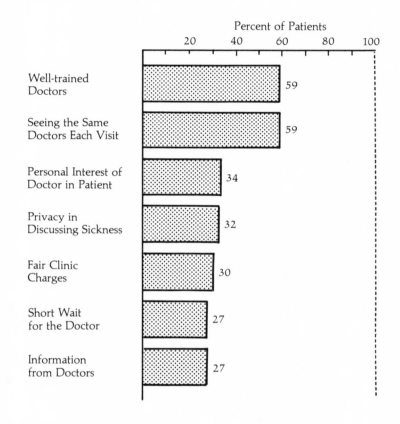

Source: Sussman et al. 1967, Table 21, p. 92.

Chart 1–5

This chart offers a rough impression of the relative importance of different aspects of care as viewed by at least some physicians under some circumstances.

The information comes from a study designed to develop a classification of physician "actions" (which I equate to "process"), and of "end results" (which I have called "outcomes"). To obtain the information, the investigators first selected 14 states to represent all regions in the United States, and then asked the medical schools in these states to recommend physicians, in each of four specialties, who actually taught in these schools, but who were also engaged in full-time private practice. Each of the nominated physicians who agreed to participate was asked to describe three episodes of "effective" and three episodes of "ineffective" care that either had occurred in the physician's own practice, or had been observed in the work of a colleague, during the preceding year. The investigators used these descriptions to develop their classifications of "actions" and "end results." This chart is based on the classification of "actions" which the investigators derived from the reports of the internists in their sample.

To construct the chart, I reclassified the more detailed categories reported by the investigators, my purpose being to separate the interpersonal and the technical aspects of care. One sees as a result that only 20 percent of actions reported were clearly pertinent to the management of the interpersonal relationship. Included under this heading are the original categories of "professional responsibility," "professional manner," "psychological perception," "psychological support," and "patient education." My second grouping, that of access, continuity, and coordination, comprises categories that I found difficult to classify. It contains "availability of the physician," "use of health team," "use of community resources," "review of problem," "review of treatment," and "follow-up." These perhaps represent a second level in the organization of the simpler elements in the "process" of care. The third grouping, that of technical care, is by far the largest, accounting for 70 percent of the reported actions.

These results are, of course, heavily conditioned by the peculiarities of the method used to obtain them. They do, however, correspond to the general impression that physicians are preoccupied with the details of technical care and tend to define "quality" largely in these terms. Much of this book can be offered as evidence.

Chart 1-5

Percent Distribution of Actions Taken by Physicians, Classified According to Whether They Belong to Specified Types of Care. Actions Reported by Selected Internists as Examples of "Effective" or "Ineffective" Care, U.S.A., circa 1965.

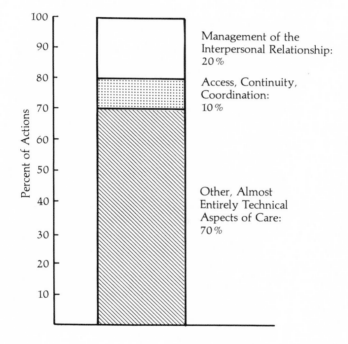

Management of the Interpersonal Relationship: 20%

Access, Continuity, Coordination: 10%

Other, Almost Entirely Technical Aspects of Care: 70%

Source: Sanazaro and Williamson 1968, Table 2, p. 394.

Chart 1–6

This chart, the first of three that show how the views of clients and physicians compare, draws on the study of outpatient care used in two earlier charts in this chapter. In this part of the study, a list of clinic features was submitted to physicians and others who worked in the clinics that mainly served long-term patients. Each member of the staff was asked to rate each clinic attribute according to its importance to patient care in the respondent's opinion, and also according to what each respondent thought the importance of the attribute to the clinics' patients might be. A sample of patients in the same clinics also rated each listed attribute according to its importance.

The chart shows only part of the findings: that comparing the percentage of physicians who said a clinic attribute was "very important to patient care," with the percentage of patients who said that attribute was "important to a good clinic." I have divided the attributes into two groups. The first, shown in the upper section of the chart, I thought to be part of, or closely related to, the management of the interpersonal relationship between patient and practitioner. The second group includes attributes more pertinent to access, convenience, and the physical amenities of the clinic. Within each of these groupings, the attributes are arranged in descending order of their importance to the physicians.

One gets the impression that physicians, as a group, are very discriminating in their assessments, large majorities agreeing that some features are very important, but others are not. Patients are more likely to accord roughly equal importance to many of the same features. The two groups of respondents agree on the importance of some features, notably "pleasant staff," "privacy in discussing illness," and "same physician on each visit." They disagree on many others, in particular on the importance of the clinics' amenities.

Additional findings, not included in the chart, show that physicians have a reasonably good understanding of the importance of the several attributes to patients, though the physicians tend to overestimate the importance of some (such as seeing "the same physician on each visit"), and underestimate the importance of others (such as "patient's knowledge of his condition"). This suggests that physicians may fail to meet the patient's expectations partly out of miscalculation but also partly out of an unwillingness or inability to do so.

Chart 1–6

Percent of Patients and Physicians Who Select Specified Attributes of Clinics To Be "Important to a Good Clinic" or "Very Important to Patient Care," Respectively. Outpatient Clinics that Mainly Serve Long-term Patients, Hospitals of Western Reserve University, Cleveland, Ohio, 1960.

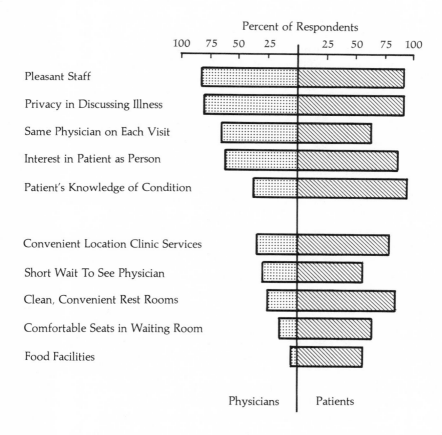

Source: Sussman et al. 1967, Table 40, p. 129.

Chart 1–7

Another set of comparisons between the viewpoints of physicians and clients comes from one part of a long series of studies devoted to the measurement and prediction of physician performance, conducted by a group of investigators at the University of Utah. In order to identify the determinants of good performance, it was necessary to first define what good performance meant. Accordingly, the investigators began by asking a group of selected physicians to answer the following question: "With regard to your field of specialty, what do you consider to be the basic factors of success?" Based on the answers, and on additional comments from over a hundred other "thoughtful individuals," the investigators developed two lists, one of 87 "desirable" attributes and another of 29 "undesirable" ones. These lists were then submitted to selections of various categories of people; each respondent was asked to rank each attribute from "one" to "five," depending on "importance to superior physician performance" if the attribute was a "desirable" one, or on "detrimentality to superior physician performance" if the item was on the list of "undesirable" attributes. The mean of these rankings was taken to represent the judgment of each group of respondents on each attribute (pp. 48–49).

The chart shows the distribution of the "desirable" attributes by the mean of the ranks assigned by a selection of practicing physicians and by a selection of members of the "general public." The two are obviously associated in a positive manner. The Spearman rank correlation coefficient is 0.83. The coefficient for the "undesirable" attributes, the distribution of which is not shown, was 0.88.

The configuration of points on the chart suggests a closer concordance of rankings at both ends of the scale, with a greater disparity of views in between. In any event, a comparison of the top ten attributes as ranked by the physicians with the top ten as ranked by the general public shows that seven were shared and that the discrepancy in ranks is small for another two. Both groups of respondents agree on the preeminent importance of knowledge, judgment, thorough examination, and an appropriate recognition by the physician of his own limitations, as shown by a readiness to refer patients when this is needed. I consider all these to be aspects of the responsible exercise of a high level of clinical competence. But it is a pity that, rather than asking about the quality of care, the investigators used words like "success" and "superior performance."

Chart 1-7

Desirable Attributes of Physicians Distributed According to the Mean of the Ranks Assigned to the Attributes by Selected Groups of Physicians and of Members of the General Public. Utah, circa 1969.

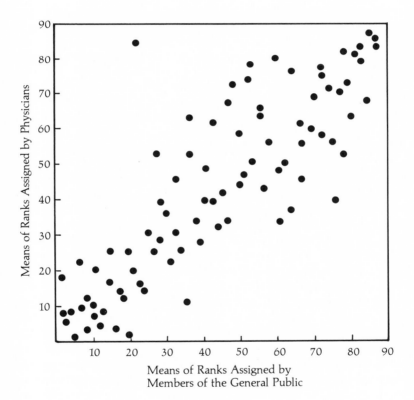

Means of Ranks Assigned by
Members of the General Public

Source: Price et al. 1972, Table 10, pp. 51-53.

Chart 1–8

The study illustrated by this chart provides additional information about different views of quality, including a comparison of the importance attached to the technical and interpersonal aspects of care.

The site was a hospital-based prepaid group practice. The subjects were members of the medical and nursing staff, and two samples of male patients between 21 and 65 years of age, one sample drawn from among those who came to the walk-in clinic not suffering from an emergency, and the other drawn from among those who had been in hospital for more than five days. Each patient was given two lists of three attributes and asked to rank each set of three in order of importance. The members of the staff ranked the same attributes twice: once having in mind a group of walk-in patients, and again having hospitalized patients in mind.

The chart shows part of the findings: the percentage of physicians and patients who ranked each attribute in a set of three to be the most important of the three. The attributes are identified in somewhat abridged versions of the original descriptions.

An examination of the findings for ambulatory care for walk-in patients shows that both patients and physicians attach high importance to "personal interest," which meant "explaining things and showing personal concern for the patient." "Scientific knowledge: the specific knowledge needed" is given equal importance by both groups, but is in second place. Both parties also agree on the rather low level of importance given to "having pleasant surroundings and services that add to the patient's comfort." We may infer a rough identity of views concerning the relative importance of the three aspects of care that I have called the management of the interpersonal relationship, technical care, and amenities of care.

The findings for hospital care are different, but mainly because the physicians have reordered their priorities, moving scientific knowledge and technical skill to first place, presumably because these are more critical to hospital care. The order of preferences for patients remains roughly the same, but there is now a disparity between patients and physicians in the importance attached to patient comfort; the hospitalized patients value this more than do the physicians.

This partial description of the findings suggests that the relative importance given to the several attributes of care may vary according to the respondent's role, and according to the nature of the patient's condition.

Chart 1–8

Percent of Physicians and of Patients Who Assign First Rank to Specified Attributes of Care, by Site of Care. A Prepaid Group Practice Plan, Detroit, Michigan, circa 1968.

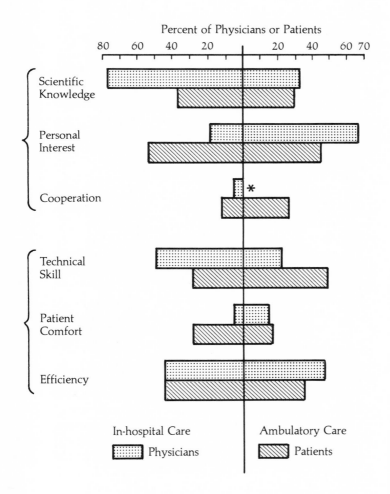

Source and Note: Smith and Metzner 1970, Table 8–11, pp. 271–74. The asterisk indicates a value of zero percent.

TWO

**Monetary Cost as a
Component of Quality**

TWO

The relationship between monetary cost and quality can be more easily understood if we begin with a patient who, if care were not given, would experience a specified loss of function for a specified duration. The task of the health care practitioner is to select, sequence, and implement a variety of services which are expected to bring about a change for the better in the functional disability which is expected in the absence of such services, the improvement being in shortening the duration of disability, in reducing its magnitude, or in both. Such improvements are perhaps the most precise indicators of the quality of care. It follows that the more services that are marshaled, and the more skillfully they are used, the larger their expected ameliorative effect, and the higher the quality of care which they signify. Thus, increments in the quality of care call for additional "inputs" of services and skills, but the precise relationship between the inputs and the benefits is not clear. It is likely, however, that as more and more services are added to the total amount of care, the increments of health achieved, and the corresponding increments in quality, become smaller and smaller, so that, eventually, further additions in services produce no additional increments in health or quality. The highest achievable level of quality has been achieved.

This formulation allows us to identify a number of relationships between monetary cost and quality. To begin with, it is obvious that improvements in quality require increases in appropriate services and, therefore, corresponding increases in monetary cost. By contrast to the justified increases in cost which come with improvements in quality, lack of skill in implementing care is responsible for unjustified monetary cost. This happens in two ways. First, whenever the practitioner uses services that are more likely to injure than to benefit health, there are added monetary costs associated with *reductions*, rather than increases, in quality. Second, if a practitioner uses services that, on the average, are neither harmful nor useful, there are added costs without corresponding increases in quality. This, too, means that the quality of care is poor, since wasteful care diminishes the funds available for useful care; it also suggests that the practitioner may be ill informed, careless, or unwise.

All of these relationships between quality and monetary cost will be repeatedly illustrated in subsequent chapters of this book. The high incidence of "unnecessary" or unjustified diagnostic tests, therapeutic interventions, surgical procedures, hospital admissions, and hospital stays suggests that there is a large potential for cost reductions that would leave the quality of care certainly unimpaired, and very probably much improved. By contrast, the many studies which show that the standards of good care are often not met suggest that any improvements in this regard would require further expenditures. Unfortunately, we know very little about the relative magnitudes of the financial consequences of the two kinds of error, so we cannot say whether more appropriate care for all would, on the whole, require more money or less. There is no doubt, however, that we shall get the most for our money by avoiding inappropriate care while providing what is appropriate.

The clarity of this mandate for action is lost when monetary cost is allowed to enter the definition of what appropriate care is. And yet, this is what inevitably must happen, since as the practitioner adds to the care of any one patient, there comes a time when the additional improvements in health are not worth the monetary cost of added services, the values being assigned either by the individual or by society. In other words, either the individual or society may have to call a halt to further care before the very best that health care can achieve has been attained. Thus, there is a "trade-off" between quality and monetary cost, the precise magnitude of which cannot be determined unless one not only knows the cost of added care, but is also willing and able to put a monetary value on increments in the duration and the quality of life itself.

I have described this "trade-off' and discussed its consequences in the first chapter of the first volume of these *Explorations,* and in some more recent publications to which the reader is referred (Donabedian et al. 1982; Donabedian 1983). In this chapter I shall only provide an illustration, to be followed by additional preliminary examples of some of the other relationships between quality and cost described in this introduction. Many other illustrations will be encountered later on; this chapter only introduces a subject that remains relevant throughout this book.

Chart 2–1

Neuhauser and Lewicki used a hypothetical, though lifelike, situation to determine the added costs of added quality and to demonstrate the consequences of the relationship. To do so they employed existing information to compute the probabilities and costs of finding a case of cancer of the colon in 10,000 persons over 40, of whom 72 were expected to have the tumor.

Cancer of the colon tends to bleed in small amounts. This inapparent ("occult") bleeding can be detected in the feces by a guaiac test. Any one test on a specimen of stools may be negative though cancer is present ("false negative"); it is also quite often positive when there is no cancer ("false positive"). When a test is positive, confirmation of the presence or absence of cancer is sought by X-ray studies after the patient receives a barium enema, a relatively unpleasant and costly procedure. The question addressed by this chart is this: How many negative guaiac tests should be obtained for each participant in a screening program before the search is stopped? In other words: How many tests constitute sufficiently good quality?

The chart shows that if only one test is used and all "positives" are X-rayed, while all "negatives" are dismissed, each case of cancer found costs an average of $1,175. If two tests are used, and all who are "positive" are X-rayed, more cases of cancer will be found, at a cost of $5,492 per *additional* case. Because the number of additional cases is small, and becomes progressively smaller as the number of tests in the sequence increases, while the cost of the many additional tests and X-ray examinations mounts, the cost of finding a case additional to those found by the preceding sequence increases at a remarkable rate. The average cost does not rise so rapidly because the additional cost of the additional tests is assigned to all the cases already found.

Policy makers may decide that the cost of finding an additional case may not be worth, for example, as much as $4,724,695, and accordingly recommend a sequence of only four tests. A more informed decision would require information about the costs and benefits of early treatment as compared to the cost and benefits of waiting until the cancer is found later.

An individual, if he had a choice, would presumably have the situation presented to him in the form of the added cost and added probability of having a present cancer discovered, and make his decision accordingly.

Chart 2–1

Illustrative Probabilities and Costs of Discovering Cancer of the Colon by Specified Sequences of Stool Guaiac Tests Followed by X-ray Examinations of Those Who Have at Least One Positive Test. Based on Findings in a Study of Asymptomatic Patients Mostly Over 40 Years Old.

Number of Tests in a Sequence	Cost of Finding a Case of Cancer Additional to those Found by the Preceding Sequence	Average Cost of Finding a Case of Cancer by Each Sequence	Probability that a Sequence of Tests Will Find Cancer if Present
1	$ 1,175	$1,175	0.916667
2	5,492	1,507	0.993056
3	49,150	1,810	0.999421
4	469,534	2,059	0.999952
5	4,724,695	2,268	0.999996
6	47,107,214	2,451	0.999999

Source: Neuhauser and Lewicki 1975, Tables 1 and 2, p. 227, Reprinted by permission of the *New England Journal of Medicine.* The basic data were reported by Greegor in 1969.

Chart 2–2

The information in this chart, and in the four that follow it, does not tell us whether or not cost is related to quality, but it does raise disquieting questions about the possible relationship.

The findings shown in this chart are one instance of the frequent observation of wide variations (often unexplained) in the patterns of practice among physicians. In this instance, seven physicians, all internists who practice in the same group and use the same hospital, are seen to differ considerably in the average yearly charges that their decisions generate for clients of the group practice who used the physicians' services at least once during the preceding two years. Differences of age, sex, and diagnosis in the case load of each physician did not explain the differences in the charges. Rather, these differences seem to be inherent in the modes of practice of each physician. And judging by the correspondence in the two rankings of the physicians, one according to office charges and the other according to hospital charges, the physicians' behavior has similar consequences to cost, whether in the hospital or office practice of each physician. The one physician (G) for whom this observation does not hold was different from the others in a number of ways; conceivably, he could be substituting office care for hospital services.

Such variations could, of course, represent different responses to financial incentives. In this group, patients pay on a fee-for-service basis, and the physicians' income depends largely on the gross revenue they generate for the group. The investigators report, however, that "physicians who had the highest cost figures did not necessarily have the highest income. . . . Many of the high costs were for services from which the physicians derived no income" (pp. 4–5).

Are the differences observed related directly to the quality of care? That, obviously, is the fundamental question, which the study does not answer beyond implying that all the physicians were highly qualified and practiced good medicine.

Chart 2-2

Office and Hospital Charges per Active Patient under the Care of Each Physician in a Group Practice. U.S.A., 1972.

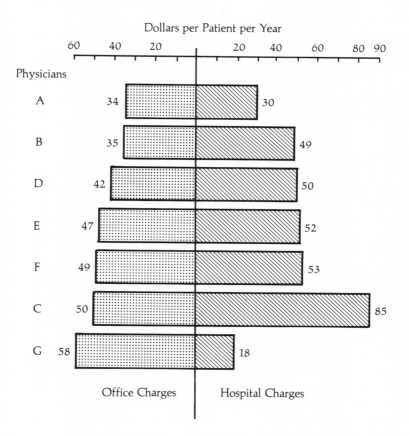

Source: Lyle et al. 1974, Tables 3 and 4, pp. 3 and 4, with some additional computations.

Chart 2–3

This chart is similar to the one immediately preceding in showing variability of practice among physicians, even though, in this case, there is no obvious financial incentive to provide more care, since the physicians are either salaried employees of, or partners in, a prepaid group practice. In addition to differences among physicians in the number of laboratory tests requested at each visit, the chart also documents a shift in utilization, so that in 1970 a larger proportion of physicians asked for more tests, as compared to 1967.

Although no data are given on the subject, the investigators assume that the patients seen by the internists are similar. They note, however, that any one physician tended to remain either a high user or a low user of laboratory services. Furthermore, physicians who were low users were more likely to be older, to be board certified, to have been with the group practice longer, and to have a "leadership role" in it. None of these relationships was, however, statistically significant. The investigators also report that there was no relationship between the use of laboratory services and the number of patients seen by a physician on each day, which suggests that laboratory services were not a substitute for more time with the patient.

The investigators attribute part of the increase in the use of laboratory services between 1967 and 1970 to a rise in the use of preventive services. Another small part of the increase is attributed to a reduction in the share paid by the patient for laboratory tests, suggesting that physicians are responsive to changes in the patients' ability to pay. But much of the increase in laboratory use remains unexplained.

The implications of these findings to quality are, obviously, unclear. If experience and board certification are evidence of expertise, better quality seems to be associated with lower use of the laboratory. On the other hand, an emphasis on prevention, which seems to generate more laboratory tests, would also be positively associated with quality. The more striking finding, however, is that there is so much variability in the use of laboratory services among physicians who are mostly board certified or board eligible in internal medicine, and who are believed to provide reasonably good care.

Chart 2–3

Percent Distribution of Physicians According to Number of Laboratory Tests per Office Visit. Department of Internal Medicine, Kaiser-Permanente Group Practice Plan, Portland, Oregon, January through June, 1967 and 1970.

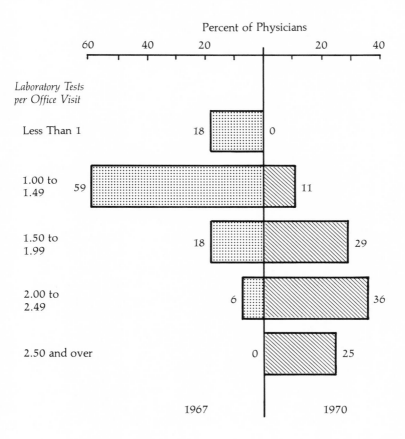

Source: Freeborn et al. 1972, Table 2, p. 848.

Chart 2–4

In this chart we get a glimpse of one factor, years since graduation from medical school, that accounts for some of the variation in the patterns of practice among physicians. Obviously, the more recent the year of graduation, the greater the resort to testing, and the gradient is quite steep for both laboratory and X-ray examinations, though it is somewhat less steep for the latter. The relationship between years since graduation and the use of diagnostic services is statistically significant for each of laboratory tests and roentgenograms, and it remains so after corrections are made for other factors that were found to influence the use of diagnostic services.

The cost implications of these findings are obvious, but their interpretation is less clear. The diagnostic practices observed may represent habits that were established during training and that may, therefore, mirror the temporal progression of medical technology. It may be, at least in part, that the older graduates are somewhat more skilled or self assured, and find it less necessary to resort to diagnostic investigations. If so, these physicians might be providing care of comparable quality at less cost.

Although the findings of this study strike one as generally applicable, one should remember that Medicaid beneficiaries and the physicians who care for them are not typical. The findings are more credible because of the attention given to achieving comparability in case mix. This was done by selecting a subset of patients who were hospitalized during the study period for one of three groups of diagnoses: cardiac disease, pulmonary disease, and diabetes. We do not know, however, to what extent the diagnostic services provided on an outpatient footing were restricted to the management of these conditions, and to what extent physicians differ systematically in their readiness to hospitalize patients and to use inpatient workups as a substitute for outpatient management. An additional bias of undetermined direction and magnitude may have been introduced by the necessity to count tests conducted as a battery as one procedure.

The paper contains information on the influence of additional physician attributes (medical school attended, specialty, board certification, urban or rural location) and a careful discussion of several questions of method. Particularly interesting are the observations on the use of Medicaid claims as a source of information, and the discussion of the statistical procedures used.

Chart 2–4

Relative Rates of Outpatient Roentgenograms and Laboratory Tests per Visit, Billed for by Physicians Categorized by Years since Graduation. Recipients of Medicaid, in Three Diagnostic Categories, in Three Counties of Northern Pennsylvania, March 1, 1974 through May 1, 1977.

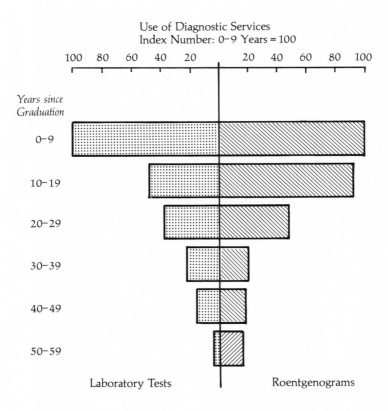

Use of Diagnostic Services
Index Number: 0–9 Years = 100

Years since Graduation

Laboratory Tests   Roentgenograms

Source: Eisenberg and Nicklin 1981, Figures 5 and 6, pp. 304 and 305.

Chart 2–5

The findings in this chart illustrate the complexity of the factors that influence the use of services and, therefore, the quality and cost of care. The chart is based on a study of radiological services provided in an old age assistance program, one that serves poor persons 65 years old or older and pays for a wide variety of services, including radiological examinations irrespective of who provides them. The findings are presented in two parts.

The top part of the chart shows that physicians who own their own X-ray equipment, performing at least some of the X-ray examinations themselves, are about twice as likely to use such examinations as are physicians who must refer their patients to a radiologist. The difference occurs even though the patients of both groups of physicians are roughly comparable in age and sex. Moreover, the difference holds irrespective of whether the physician is a generalist or an internist, and whether he graduated before or after 1946.

The physician characteristics mentioned above do, however, influence the kinds of X-ray examinations done by physicians. This is illustrated in the lower part of the chart, which pertains to the subset of chest X-rays. In particular, older internists (those who graduated before 1946) often relied on fluoroscopy of the chest as an independent procedure, a practice that radiologists decry. General practitioners and younger internists often relied on a single anteroposterior view of the chest, whereas radiologists usually employed multiple views. These significant differences in how radiological examinations are conducted are not due to differences in the age, sex, or race of the patients of the different categories of physicians.

The investigators conclude that physicians who own X-ray equipment were more likely to provide X-ray services because the equipment was readily available, and also because the physicians had a financial incentive to use the equipment they had purchased. Unfortunately, X-ray equipment was most likely to be owned by the older internists, the category of physicians who were most likely to use it improperly, partly because they continued to adhere to a pattern which may have represented good care when they received their training. Younger physicians used X-ray equipment more appropriately when they had it, and because they were less likely to have such equipment, obtained even more appropriate use through referral to a radiologist.

Chart 2-5

Percent of Patients Who Received Diagnostic X-ray Examinations, and the Percent Distribution of Chest X-rays by Kind of Procedure, Each According to the Category of Physicians Caring for the Patient or Doing the Examination. Recipients of Old Age Assistance, Alameda County, California, September 1965-January 1966, Inclusive.

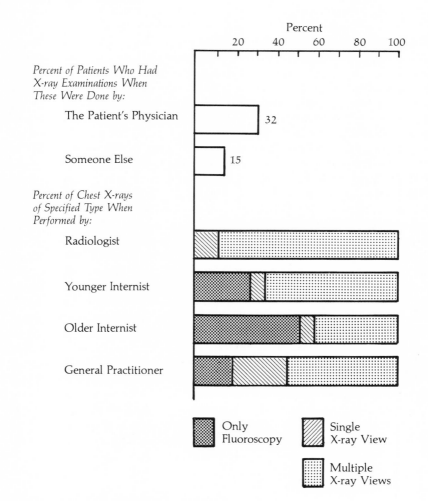

Source: Childs et al. 1972, Tables 1 and 4, pp. 327-30.

Chart 2–6

This chart illustrates, on a small scale and through the experience of only one hospital, a trend of great general importance: the proliferation of technology, with the attendant rise in the cost of care.

We observe "a single, medium-sized, voluntary community hospital with an excellent reputation among local physicians . . ." (p. 290). We find there, during the period under study, a large increase in the number of tests done for each case of myocardial infarction admitted to the hospital. In the panel on the left-hand side of the chart we see that after an initial drop in case fatality there were no further reductions during this period. In the panel on the right-hand side we find that the number of tests per case, and the pattern of increase in that number, are very similar for cases of infarction in two categories of severity.

The investigators write, "In clinical medicine, the question may be asked, Are there routines that are used because of habit and that overweigh the data available on the natural history of the illness and the individual patient's progress? . . . One might suggest the existence of a predetermined treatment and diagnostic pattern for many patients without reference to their diagnostic status, severity of illness, or clinical course of the episode. Frequently, these routines were placed in the patient order sheet on the day of admission" (p. 292).

In a study such as this, the selection of cases and their grading by severity is, of course, critical. This study included only cases admitted alive within two days of the infarction. Cases were classified according to an index of severity devised by Burgess (1970). Because there were so few of them, the most severe cases (Groups Five and Six) were excluded from the chart. I also adjusted for the slightly different incidences of cases in Groups One and Two combined, as compared to Groups Three and Four combined, during the four time periods studied. The tests counted (chemistry tests, X-ray procedures, bacteriological examinations, and the electrocardiogram) are a subset that I chose to roughly represent total diagnostic effort.

I do not, of course, intend to generalize *from* the findings shown in this chart. Rather, the chart particularizes a more general question which challenges the bases of clinical practice itself, calling attention to the relationship between quality and cost at this fundamental level.

Chart 2-6

Relationships Between the Severity-adjusted Case Fatality Rate for Myocardial Infarction and the Number of Diagnostic Tests per Case, and the Relationship Between Case Severity and the Number of Diagnostic Tests per Case. Selected Years, One Community Hospital, Massachusetts, 1939–1969.

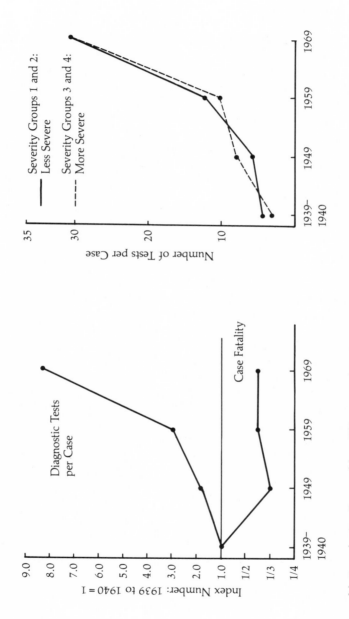

Source: Martin et al. 1974. Computed from Tables 3, 4, and 5, pp. 291–92.

Chart 2–7

This chart provides more direct evidence of unjustifiable costs as a result of unnecessary care. The method used to identify unnecessary care is also of great interest, since it represents an application of algorithmic criteria, an important development in auditing quality. The algorithm or protocol is a set of instructions that describes how a patient who comes with a given set of signs or symptoms should be managed, step by step, so that the findings at each step influence which next step is to be taken, until the patient is successfully diagnosed and treated.

The investigators formulated a protocol that specified the optimum progression of procedures for establishing the stage of the disease, and selecting the appropriate method of treatment, for patients with Hodgkin lymphoma. The sequence of diagnostic investigations was meant to begin with the procedures that were least hazardous and yet capable of leading to a speedy decision.

Using this protocol as their standard of care, the investigators reviewed the records of 50 cases of Hodgkin lymphoma. The charges for all procedures in accord with the protocol were considered "necessary," while those that contravened it represented "perceived excess." Some charges were placed in an intermediate category, called "justifiable," for one of two reasons. Hospitalization was considered justifiable if the patient lived 50 miles or more from the hospital, with one additional day allowed for each additional 50 miles. In this way, social considerations were permitted to enter the definition of technical quality. The charges for all care attributable to illnesses other than Hodgkin lymphoma were also considered "justifiable," even though more careful assessment might have shown some of this care also to have been unnecessary.

The first bar of the chart shows that 30 percent of the total charges were unnecessary ("perceived excess"). The rest were either "necessary" or "justifiable," the former accounting for 59 percent of the total and the latter for 11 percent. As the second bar of the chart shows, the unnecessary charges were largely due to hospital stays that the investigators did not consider justified, but almost a third (32 percent) were due to tests and procedures that the protocol did not endorse.

There are no estimates either of the indirect costs of care or of the added hazards that may have been incurred due to unnecessary services.

Chart 2–7

Percent of Total Charges Judged To Be Unnecessary, Justifiable, or Necessary, and Percent Distribution of Unnecessary Charges According to the Type of Service Responsible for Them. Fifty Patients with Hodgkin Lymphoma, University of Iowa Medical Center, July 1975–September 1978.

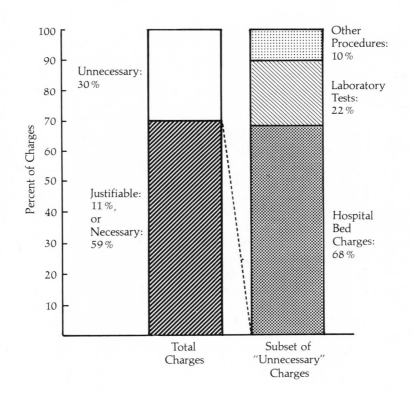

Source: Corder et al. 1981. Text on p. 377.

Chart 2–8

In this chart and the next, there are actual ratings of quality that can be compared, more or less directly, to observations about costs or expenditures.

This chart shows the positions of 21 interns in two sets of ranks, one of clinical competence, and another of the costs of laboratory tests requested by each intern for patients with uncomplicated chest pain or uncomplicated myocardial infarction during the first three days of their stay in a coronary care unit. The investigators assumed that the cases seen by the several interns were comparable. Tests done daily as a routine were not counted, since the object was to study variability in performance. The investigators also collected information on what they considered to be redundant tests, as well as on needed tests that were omitted. At the end of their internship year, the interns were ranked as to "overall clinical capacity" by each of five faculty members. Kendall's coefficient of concordance (W) for these ratings was 0.71, a level the investigators regard as "high."

The investigators' interest in the relationship between quality and cost was reinforced by a previous observation of "a 17-fold variation in the costs of laboratory (including X-ray) use among similarly trained faculty internists caring for similar groups of ambulatory patients" (Schroeder et al. 1973). As they pondered the possible relation to clinical competence, several hypotheses seemed equally likely: (1) that the ordering of more tests meant a more thorough, more conscientious physician, (2) that this behavior denoted lesser clinical competence which was compensated for by excessive reliance on the laboratory, and (3) that the behavior was related not to competence but to personality traits.

The findings of this more recent study tend to support the third of these hypotheses. There was no significant relationship between the clinical competence ratings of the interns and (1) the use of redundant tests, or (2) the non-use of needed tests, or (3) the overall costs of tests, this last being the information plotted in this chart. However, when one aberrant finding (the point next to the tenth position on the ordinate) is omitted, the resulting pattern suggests a "V" lying on its side with its angle to the right. If so, one would agree with the authors when they suggest that "there was a tendency for the poorer interns to be at either the cheap or expensive end of the cost spectrum. By contrast, . . . the best interns clustered about the mean" (pp. 711–12).

Chart 2–8

Interns Ranked According to "Overall Clinical Capacity" and According to the Cost of Laboratory Tests Requested by Them During the First Three Days of Care for Uncomplicated, Acute Myocardial Infarction. Coronary Care Unit, George Washington University Hospital, Washington, D.C., 1971–1972.

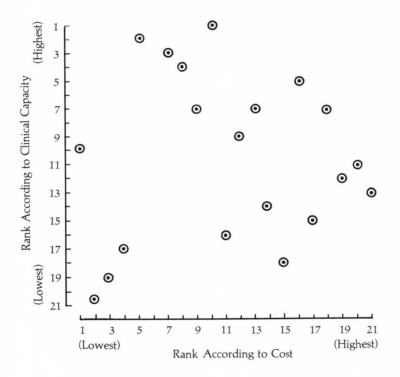

Source: Schroeder et al. 1974, and additional information provided by Professor Schroeder.

Chart 2–9

This chart shows 45 community pharmacies in northern Mississippi distributed by charge per prescription and by a score of the quality of pharmaceutical services given in filling these prescriptions.

The data were obtained by two trained "shoppers," who presented prescriptions to be filled at each pharmacy and asked preformulated questions pertaining to drug use. Based on their experience with each pharmacist, the shopper completed checklists which the investigators, with the help of explicit criteria, used to score each of five areas of performance: dispensing fundamentals, prescription usage control, over-the-counter-drug usage control, drug monitoring, and health information. The total score of quality (which is the one used in the chart) is an unweighted sum of the subscores for each area of performance.

It is quite clear from the chart that quality and prescription charges are unrelated. (The value of r, which was -0.2002, did not differ significantly from zero.)

The investigators also report a lack of correlation between charges and the weekly volume of prescriptions, and between weekly volume and the quality score.

In the immediately preceding chart, costs were related to a subjective estimate of overall competence. In this chart there is a gain in specificity through relating specific charges to an assessment of specific instances of performance that correspond precisely to these charges. The chart is additionally interesting because it illustrates quality assessment of professionals other than physicians, an application that is not recognized frequently enough in this book.

The absence of a clear relationship between quality and cost, either in this study or in the one illustrated by the immediately preceding chart, is rather disconcerting. One wonders, for example, what those who patronize the more expensive pharmacies get for the additional money they pay, if it is not higher technical quality. The investigators are unable to identify any particular benefit, even after taking into account the problems of interpretation that result from the pricing practices of pharmacists or from some of the other features of the particular study and of its locale.

Chart 2–9

Community Pharmacies Distributed According to a Score of the Quality of Professional Performance, and to the Average Charge per Prescription. Northern Mississippi, circa 1973.

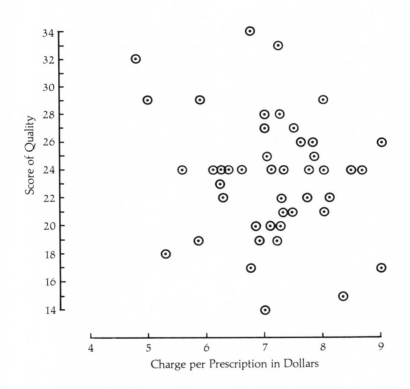

Chart 2–10

By providing information about the outcomes of care, this chart takes us to somewhere near the end of the road in our exploration of the relationship between quality and cost.

The data pertain to the costs and outcomes of care provided for patients with an acute illness by staff members with varying qualifications in an ambulatory care clinic. The "costs" were computed using charges that were uniform for all members of the staff, irrespective of differences in their salaries. A seven-level index of functional performance was used to characterize the patients' health status approximately six months before the clinic visit and again after the visit, at a time when the maximum benefit from treatment was predicted by each patient's physician. A "good outcome" was said to have occurred if the functional status at this later time was equal to or better than the status previous to the illness.

The chart shows the members of the clinic staff distributed by the charges generated by their care, and by the percent of their patients who attained "good" outcomes. Happily, there is a moderate positive relationship ($r = 0.39$; $p < 0.05$). This occurs even though, for the patients as a whole, without regard to who cared for them, there is an inverse relationship between good outcomes and cost. While the presence of a positive relationship is a reassuring finding, we do not know whether or not the most efficient strategies of care have been used so as to obtain the maximum attainable improvement in health at the lowest possible cost.

The chart distinguishes the types of attending practitioners because the investigators also examined the relationship between the qualifications of staff members, on the one hand, and the cost and outcomes of care on the other. The findings were complicated, but it is safe to say that higher qualifications were not clearly related to either lower cost or better outcomes.

In studies of this kind, a great deal hinges on the specificity and sensitivity of the measures of health status, and on the ability to assure comparability in type and severity of cases. When the diseases studied are often self-limiting, one needs to give particular attention to factors other than medical care that influence the speed and extent of recovery.

Chart 2–10

Practitioners in Specified Categories, Distributed According to the Charges Attributable to the Care They Provided, and to the Percent of Their Patients Who Had "Good Outcomes." Two Model Clinics of the Family Practice Residency Program, the University of Utah College of Medicine, Salt Lake City, circa 1973.

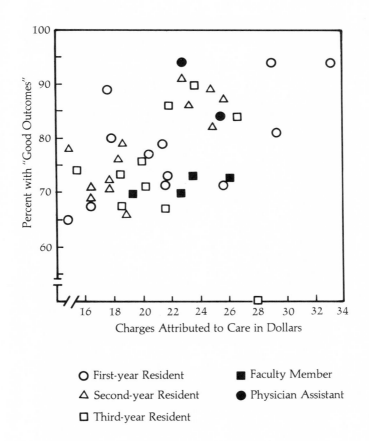

O First-year Resident   ■ Faculty Member

△ Second-year Resident   ● Physician Assistant

□ Third-year Resident

Source: Wright et al. 1977, Figure 3, p. 48. Used with permission; copyright 1956–77, American Medical Association.

PART II

The Assessment of Process

THREE

The Justification
of Resource Use

THREE

Almost every approach to assessing the process of care may be interpreted to involve the justification of resource use. In fact, the entirety of process assessment can be encompassed by only two questions: why certain things were done when they should *not* have been; and why other things were not done when they *should* have been. This chapter deals with the first of the two questions, but so do many other parts of this book as well. For instance, questions about the justifiability of resource use were repeatedly asked, either explicitly or implicitly, in the preceding chapter on quality and cost. The next chapter, on justification of surgery, deals exclusively with the same question, and the subject comes up again and again in later chapters as well. Having a separate chapter on the justification of resource use is, therefore, a somewhat arbitrary device which I use to accommodate the activities usually referred to as "utilization control."

Because hospital care is so expensive, and because hospitals are amenable to organizational restraints, much of utilization control has focused on these institutions. Accordingly this chapter pays greatest attention to the justification of hospital use. Many of the same principles and methods, with some modifications, would apply also to other facilities, including nursing homes. Increasingly, the uses of some specific costly or hazardous services, whether in the hospital or outside it, are also being questioned. I have, therefore, included some information on the use of drugs and injections as examples of these. The use of surgical procedures, which is studied in the next chapter, could easily have been included as well, but I judged that subject important and different enough to deserve separate consideration.

There are certain diagnostic and therapeutic interventions that are either obsolete or so rarely indicated that their mere use is reason enough to question the quality of care. This chapter begins with two studies of the use of one such therapeutic agent, chloramphenicol. The use of other procedures is open to question only if it departs from usual patterns, either in quantity or in some other characteristic. To represent this category, I have drawn on a study of the use of injections in treating Medicaid beneficiaries.

To assess the appropriateness of hospital use one needs a system of norms that specifies the proper place of the hospital, and of all other alternative sites, in the entire spectrum of care. This general perspective must next be translated to the more specific criteria and standards used to assign a patient to the most appropriate site. Different conceptions of the health care system lead to different criteria and standards of appropriateness. Even when the criteria and standards are agreed upon, many additional obstacles arise. First, one must be allowed access to the necessary information; then, one must have the ability to bring about compliance; and, finally, the spectrum of alternative facilities must be present in the community, and must function as envisaged by the criteria.

My objective in this chapter is to marshal some of the important information about the nature of hospital misutilization so that it may be used to design an effective and efficient system of monitoring and control. At the same time, some alternative methods for studying the phenomenon of improper use are described and assessed.

I draw first (and extensively) on a study of hospital care in Michigan which, though completed many years ago, remains the standard by which all subsequent work must be judged (McNerney et al. 1962). The study illustrates the use of preformulated explicit criteria and standards for hospital admission and length of stay, based on information in the medical record supplemented by an interview with the responsible physician. The findings offer a view of the incidence of inappropriate hospital use and of the factors that influence it. Among the latter are diagnosis (Charts 3–10 and 3–11), length of stay (Chart 3–12), day of the week on which the discharge takes place (Chart 3–19), and the method of paying the hospital (Chart 3–20).

Besides reviewing the medical record after the hospitalization ends, it is possible to review the care of a sample of hospitalized patients on a given day in order to determine whether a patient's being in the hospital is justified or not. I have drawn on two studies of this kind to illustrate differences in method, to show the incidence of inappropriate stay as hospitalization progresses, and to demonstrate the relevance of the findings to the design of a method for interrupting the hospital stay (Charts 3–13 to 3–18). The chapter ends with an introduction to a study by Morehead et al. (1964), the methods and other findings of which will be more fully explored in Chapter 6.

Chart 3–1

Because the antibiotic chloramphenicol can cause life-threatening anemia due to a depression of bone marrow activity, its legitimate use is restricted to a few conditions, usually in hospitalized patients. "Thus, only very rarely is it appropriate to treat an ambulatory patient with chloramphenicol" (p. 266).

In this study, pharmacy claims for Medicaid beneficiaries were used to identify physicians who had prescribed chloramphenicol for ambulatory patients. State licensure files were used to obtain information on physician characteristics, but without divulging the identity of individual physicians.

The chart shows that of the physicians who were considered likely to treat Medicaid patients, six percent prescribed chloramphenicol at least once during the study year. There is, however, a subset of chloramphenicol prescribers, amounting to nine percent of such prescribers, who use the drug so frequently that they account for 55 percent of all chloramphenicol prescriptions. The worst offender was a physician who alone was responsibile for 13 percent of all chloramphenicol prescriptions! Almost always, this antibiotic was used for infections that did not require it; and often it was used in amounts that were insufficient to treat the infection adequately, though they probably were sufficient to cause bone marrow injury.

The study is a fine illustration of monitoring certain aspects of physician performance through the use of claims for reimbursement. It also illustrates the general phenomenon of "error concentration." Quite often there is a subset of practitioners who are much more prone to error than the generality of their colleagues. Identification of these physicians may simplify the task of quality enhancement through education or through other means if education is not sufficient.

(Also see Ray et al. 1977 for a brief report on the "mal-prescribing of liquid tetracycline preparations," which, the authors say, have been "contraindicated among children less than eight years of age since 1970.")

Chart 3–1

Incidence of Chloramphenicol Prescribing for Ambulatory Patients Among Physicians Who Treated Medicaid Patients. Tennessee, July 1, 1973–June 30, 1974.

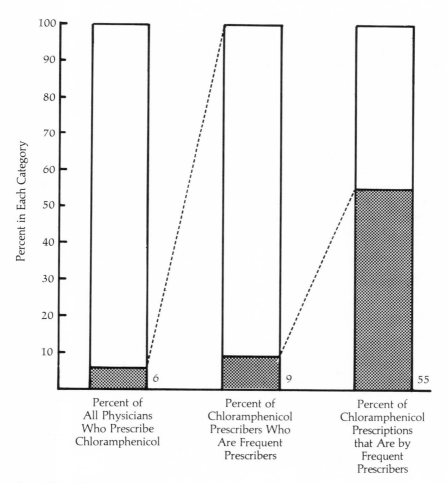

Source: Ray et al. 1976, p. 268.

Chart 3–2

The study by Ray et al., described in connection with the preceding chart, also looked into the factors associated with prescribing chloramphenicol for Medicaid beneficiaries.

This chart shows that the likelihood that a physician was a prescriber of chloramphenicol was greater for physicians in general or family practice, as compared to other specialists, and greater for physicians who practiced in rural areas as compared to those who practiced in cities. Year of graduation (classified in the wide intervals of 1935–1944, 1945–1954, and 1955–1972) was not related to prescribing chloramphenicol, even after controlling for specialty and location.

These findings do not explain precisely why some physicians prescribe chloramphenicol and others do not. They do, however, introduce us to the fascinating study of what might be called the "epidemiology of quality," which is its distribution in time, place, and person. Besides showing us under what circumstances care is more likely to be poor, an examination of the distribution of quality (which includes a study of the "structural" factors related to performance) can lead to hypotheses regarding the causal factors that influence professional performance, as well as to action intended to reduce error and to enhance quality.

Chart 3–2

Of Physicians Considered Likely to Treat Medicaid Beneficiaries, the Percent
Who Prescribed Chloramphenicol for Such Patients, by Location and Specialty
Status of Physician. Tennessee Medicaid Program, July 1, 1973 – June 30, 1974.

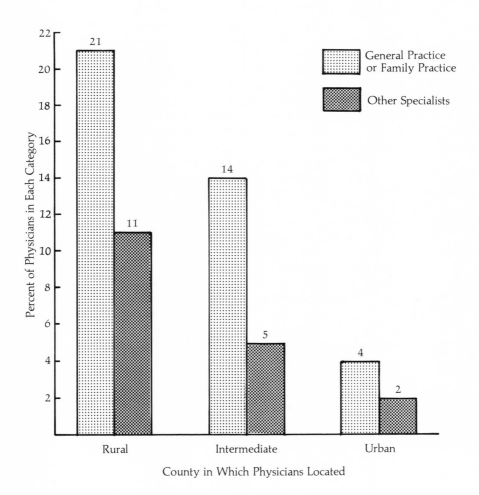

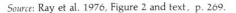

Source: Ray et al. 1976, Figure 2 and text, p. 269.

Chart 3–3

This chart describes some aspects of drug use by members of a federally funded program that paid for primary care, including prescribed drugs, for low income, nonhospitalized patients in a rural county of southern Appalachia. The drugs prescribed were classified as "recommended" or "not recommended" by the Council on Drugs of the American Medical Association (1971). Drugs were rated "not recommended" because they were ineffective, hazardous, or occurred in combinations which prevented adjustments of dosage or ingredients to the needs of the patient.

Since this was a study of a population of patients and the care that they received (rather than of the entire practice of each of a group of physicians), patients were classified according to whether at least 90 percent of their prescriptions were for recommended drugs, and whether they received at least 90 percent of their prescriptions from specialists or generalists, respectively.

Two kinds of relationships are shown in the chart. Patients of general practitioners are more likely to receive drugs classified as "not recommended"; and those who receive more prescriptions per visit are more likely to receive "not recommended" drugs. This is true for patients of specialists as well as generalists, though perhaps more so for the latter. One can also see that for some subgroups of patients exposure to the hazard of using "not recommended" drugs is very high.

In their discussion the authors point out that the indiscriminate use of antibiotics (sometimes in combination) can be harmful, not only to the patients who receive them, but also to the community at large, through contributing to the emergence of resistant strains of microorganisms. This is an excellent example of one component in the "social definition" of the quality of care (Donabedian 1980, pp. 15–16).

Chart 3-3

Percent of Patients Ten Percent or More of Whose Prescriptions Were for "Not Recommended" Drugs, by Preponderant Source of Care and by Number of Prescriptions per Visit. A Federally Funded Primary Care Program in a Rural County in Southern Appalachia, 1973 and 1974.

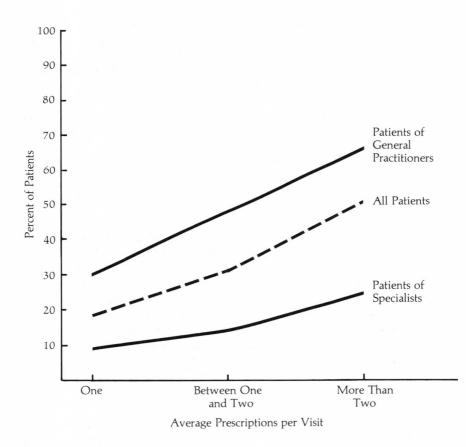

Average Prescriptions per Visit

Source: Miles 1977. Computed from Table 4, p. 8.

Chart 3–4

This chart and the two that follow it (as well as some others used in subsequent sections of this book) are based on the experience of a highly developed system of utilization control that monitors the use of inpatient admissions and stays for hospitals as well as nursing homes, outpatient visits, and a variety of services that include laboratory tests, X-rays, prescriptions, and injections. This system deserves the careful study it has received because it was developed by organizations regarded to be the precursors of the PSROs, and its activities exemplify those that can be undertaken by a local PSRO (Brook and Williams 1976; Lohr et al. 1980).

The charts selected for this section deal with the use of injections for Medicaid beneficiaries because this procedure was found to be very often inappropriate by medical criteria (in 30 percent of cases) and it was most sensitive to control measures.

The first chart provides another illustration of the phenomenon of "concentration" which was referred to earlier in this section. First, Brook et al. found that only 360 of 1342 physicians (M.D. and D.O.) in the state provided 100 or more visits to Medicare patients during the study period. These 360 were responsible for 95 percent of all ambulatory visits and 89 percent of all injections received by Medicaid beneficiaries during the two years of the study. Thus, for some programs there is what might be called "service concentration." This is in addition to the other kind of concentration which I earlier referred to as "error concentration."

The chart shows the joint effects of these two phenomena. One finds that a very small percentage of physicians accounts for a disproportionately large number of ambulatory visits, a larger proportion of injections, and a still larger proportion of injections that are judged to be inappropriate and, therefore, are not paid for by the program. Described in more detail, 4.6 percent of all physicians were responsible for 32 percent of ambulatory visits, 36 percent of injections billed, and 46 percent of disapproved injections. A subset of 22 physicians amounting to only 1.6 percent of all physicians was responsible for 12 percent of ambulatory visits, a remarkable 22 percent of injections billed, and an astounding 31 percent of disapproved injections.

It is clear which physicians deserve watching.

Chart 3-4

Percent in Each of Specified Categories Accounted for by 22 and 39 Physicians (M.D. or D.O.) Who Are in the Highest and Next Highest Ranks as Ordered by Percent of Injections Not Approved by Medical Peer Review. Medicaid Program, New Mexico, September 1971- August 1973, Inclusive.

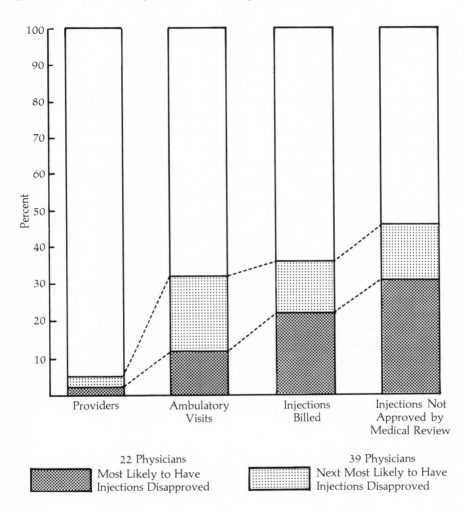

Source: Brook and Williams 1976, text p. 63, and Tables 3.6, 6.1 and 6.26, pp. 29, 64 and 92.

Chart 3–5

In this companion to the preceding chart, the subset of physicians who provided 100 or more ambulatory care visits to Medicaid beneficiaries during the study period are further studied in order to see whether training and specialization are related to (1) the frequency with which injections are used, and (2) the frequency with which the injections that are used are judged on medical review to be inappropriate.

On examining the right-hand portion of the chart one can clearly see that both professional identification (M.D., D.O.) and specialization have a role in creating a gradient of increasing propensity to use injections. By contrast, the proportion of injections judged to be inappropriate seems to depend mainly on specialization, being about equally lower among specialists when compared to generalists, regardless of professional identification. However, because the doctors of osteopathy (D.O.) use more injections, irrespective of their specialization, they have a larger number of disapproved injections per 100 visits when compared to physicians in the corresponding category of specialization. (All differences between provider types and certification status groups were significant at $p = 0.05$ or less, by the chi square test.)

The investigators also found that the particular specialty of the medical practitioner was a factor related to the use of injections, both overall and inappropriately. For example, pediatricians were least likely to give injections inappropriately, and obstetricians–gynecologists were most likely to do so. Graduates of foreign medical schools (except Canadian schools) were more likely to have injections disapproved when compared to graduates of U.S. schools, but the difference was small, though statistically significant. Degree of urbanization was not consistently related to the proportion of injections disapproved, though this was highest for physicians in rural counties.

The association with age is shown in the next chart.

Chart 3–5

Percent Distribution of Billed Injections, and Injections per 100 visits, by Whether or Not Approved for Payment on Medical Peer Review, by Type of Physician. Medicaid Program, New Mexico, September 1971–August 1973, Inclusive.

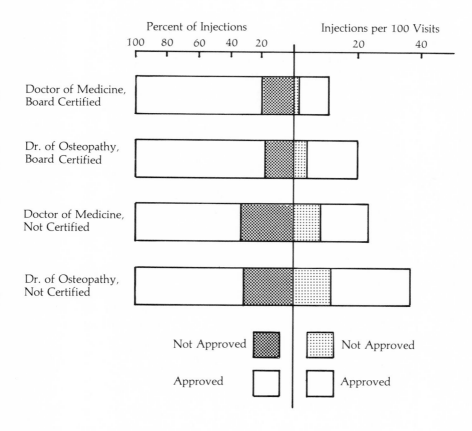

Source: Brook and Williams 1976, Table 6.10, p. 71. I computed the percentages.

Chart 3–6

This last chart in this series from the New Mexico program of utilization review shows the relationship between age and the proportion of disapproved injections separately for doctors of medicine and doctors of osteopathy. For the latter, the proportion of injections judged to be inappropriate increases regularly with age. For doctors of medicine there are two groups particularly likely to use injections inappropriately: those who are 34 or younger (only six in number) and those who are 65 or older.

Obviously, these findings are not corrected for possibly age-related differences in specialization. Furthermore, because this is a "cross-sectional" sample, it would be inappropriate to infer that the observed relationships occur as a cohort of practitioners ages.

Chart 3–6

Percent of Injections Not Approved for Payment as a Consequence of Peer Review, by Age and Type of Physician. Medicaid Program, New Mexico, September 1971 – August 1973, Inclusive.

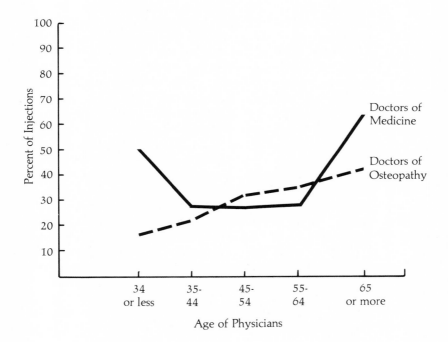

Source: Brook and Williams 1976, Table 6.8, p. 69.

Chart 3–7

With this chart we begin looking at the methods and findings of a landmark study that profoundly influenced subsequent work in this field. Among other things, the study attempted to measure the amount of unnecessary use of short-term, nonfederal, general and special hospitals in Michigan. To do so, it was thought necessary to convene panels of expert physicians who specified the criteria of appropriate care for each of a selected set of eighteen diagnoses. The criteria specified the conditions under which a case was considered to need admission, the number of days of hospitalization required for each case, and the conditions under which the patient would be considered ready to leave the hospital. These criteria were used to review abstracts of the medical records of a representative sample of discharges with each specified primary diagnosis. All cases provisionally judged not to have complied with the criteria, as well as samples of cases that seemed to have been either compliant or of questionable compliance, were checked further by interviews with the managing physicians, whose reports contributed to the final judgment on the appropriateness of use.

Admission was judged to have been inappropriate in 2.9 percent of cases (including appropriate admissions for diagnostic purposes in 0.6 percent of cases). Overstay following appropriate admission occurred in 6.7 percent and understay in 6.8 percent of patients discharged alive. Not shown in the chart is the 0.1 percent of patients who experienced both overstay and understay because of different judgments on the preoperative and postoperative components of stay in surgical cases.

About a decade later, a group of investigators led by Payne, who was one of the principals in the earlier Michigan project, used many of the same diagnoses, and roughly similar criteria, to study the appropriateness of stay and other aspects of the quality of hospital care in Hawaii, except that physicians were not interviewed to obtain additional information about the appropriateness of hospital use. The findings of this more recent study are also shown in this chart. More detailed comparisons are reported by Payne et al. (1976, pp. 11–13). There will be a great deal more concerning the methods and findings of the Hawaii studies in later sections of this book.

Chart 3-7

Percent Distribution of Hospital Discharges, by Appropriateness of Admission and Length of Stay. Patients with Selected Primary Discharge Diagnoses, Short-term, Nonfederal Hospitals, Michigan, 1958, and Hawaii, 1968.

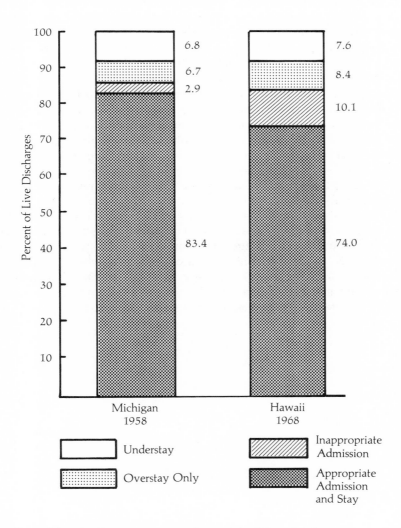

Source: Fitzpatrick et al. 1962, pp. 471–72, 474; Payne et al. 1976, pp. 11–13.

Chart 3–8

In order to assess the potential usefulness of a utilization control procedure, it is important not only to know how often cases are admitted to the hospital inappropriately, or stay too long, but also to draw a balance sheet of *days* of overstay and understay. Such a balance sheet is shown in the facing chart, based on the findings of the Michigan study briefly described in the preceding chart. In this chart all days of hospital stay due to inappropriate admissions are added to the days of overstay produced by inappropriately delayed discharges.

In the unlikely event of a fully effective utilization control procedure, we could eliminate the 6.8 percent of days judged to be unnecessary, and add the 2.3 percent judged to be missing, so as to achieve a net reduction of 4.5 percent in total hospital days for the care of the conditions sampled in this study. For reasons to be described later, this estimate of net reduction is very probably an unreliable estimate of what a fully effective procedure could accomplish. On the other hand, this balance sheet does not take account of the possible presence of cases in the community who need hospital care but do not get it.

It is interesting that the data reported by the more recent Hawaii study (also referred to in the preceding chart) do not allow us to draw a balance sheet of this kind. As the authors say, "understay days were not counted, because there was no rational method of predicting when discharge criteria would have been met" (Payne et al. 1976, p. 13). This change of heart should make us realize how heavily all such findings depend on the criteria, standards, and assumptions that are used.

Chart 3–8

Percent Change in Days of Hospital Care Currently Used that Is Expected To Occur as a Result of the Elimination of Overstay, Understay, or Both. A Sample of Cases with One of 18 Primary Discharge Diagnoses from a Sample of Short-term, Nonfederal Hospitals, Michigan, 1958.

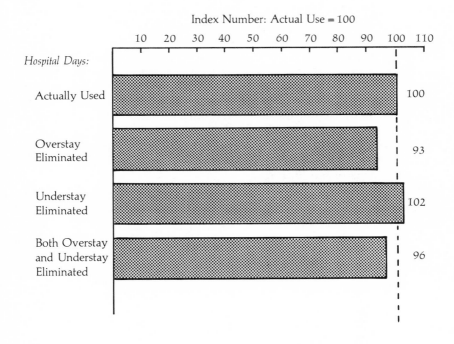

Index Number: Actual Use = 100

Source: Fitzpatrick et al. 1962, Table 219, p. 488.

Chart 3–9

The design of a system to monitor and control hospital admissions and stays requires a thorough understanding of the characteristics of these phenomena.

This chart, drawn from the study of Michigan hospitals which was described in connection with the preceding chart, shows the frequency distribution of only those cases that were judged to suffer from either overstay or understay, according to the number of days by which the cases deviated from the standard. It is clear that in a large majority of cases the deviation is small, amounting to no more than one or two days to either side of the standard embodied in the criteria. It would require a sensitive and expeditious method of control to deal with these small aberrations. On the other hand, the prevention of the fewer but more extreme deviations from the standard could be expected to yield larger returns relative to effort.

In subsequent charts we shall examine the effect of diagnosis, of length of stay, and of other factors on inappropriate hospital use, and point out the implications of the findings.

Chart 3–9

Percent Distribution of Discharges Judged To Be Characterized by Understay
and Overstay, Respectively, by Days of Understay and Overstay in Each Case.
A Sample of Cases with One of 18 Primary Discharge Diagnoses, from a Sample
of Short-term, Nonfederal Hospitals, Michigan, 1958.

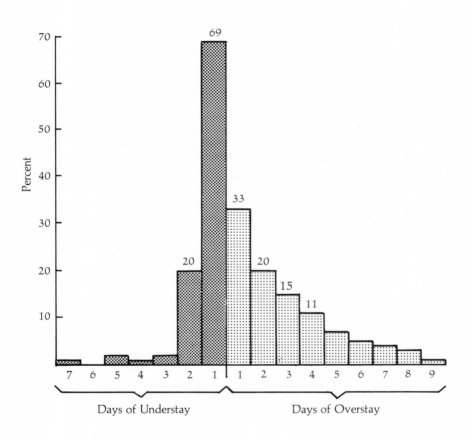

Source: Fitzpatrick et al. 1962 , Table 216, p. 486.

Chart 3–10

Continuing with the Michigan study of hospital use, one finds that diagnosis is a major correlate of inappropriate use.

In order to draw samples and classify their cases, the investigators used the discharge diagnosis that was primarily responsible for admission to the hospital. In the facing chart, the 18 diagnoses are arranged in ascending order of the percent of cases that were judged to have had a totally or partially inappropriate stay. The range is from a low of 4.1 percent for hypertrophied tonsils and adenoids to a high of 43.4 percent for fibromyoma of the uterus. Inappropriate admissions range from zero percent to 22.8 percent.

It follows that the efficiency and effectiveness of a system of utilization control can be improved by a judicious selection of cases so as to take account of the frequency of the cases and the likelihood of the occurrence of inappropriate use, and by a knowledge of whether the deviation from standards occurs mainly at admission or later during the hospital stay.

It also follows that any given selection of cases may not represent hospital care as a whole unless corrections are made for differences in diagnostic mix, among other things. In this particular study, the magnitude of inappropriate use was probably underestimated, because admission was justified in all the cases within several diagnostic categories, which are marked in the chart with an asterisk. Several features of the criteria and standards also added to the underestimate. For example, all cases who were operated on were considered to have been appropriately admitted, without checking whether the operation itself was justified.

The diagnoses listed in the chart are, going down the list, hypertrophy of tonsils and adenoids (HTA); fracture of radius and ulna (FRU); conditions of pregnancy, other (CPO); appendicitis (Ap); delivery (Del); abortion (Ab); bronchial asthma (BA); prematurity (Pr); diarrhea, infants (DI); broncho-pneumonia (BP); urinary tract calculus (UTC); acute myocardial infarction (AMI); diabetes mellitus (DM); cholecystitis, cholelithiasis (CC); inguinal hernia (IH); urinary tract infection (UTI); fracture of the neck of the femur (FNF); and fibromyoma of the uterus (FU).

Chart 3-10

Percent of Discharges Judged To Have Been Admitted Inappropriately, and Percent Judged To Have Had Stays of Inappropriate Duration, by Primary Discharge Diagnosis. Short-term, Nonfederal Hospitals, Michigan, 1958.

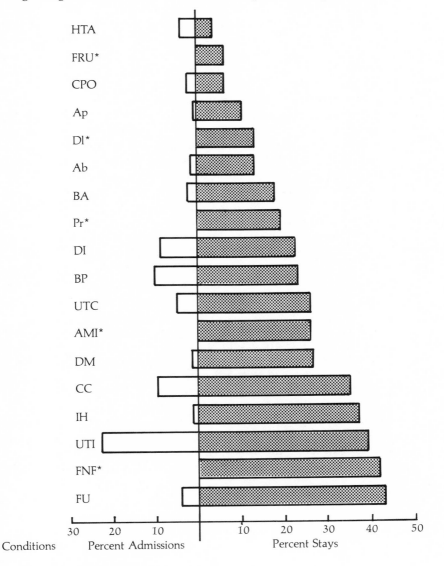

Source: Fitzpatrick et al. 1962, Table 212, p. 484.

Chart 3–11

In this chart, another one drawn from the study of Michigan hospitals, we continue the examination of the relationship between diagnosis and the appropriateness of hospital use which began in the preceding chart.

The new features of this chart are that it shows the percentage of inappropriate days (rather than cases) and the subdivision of inappropriate use into its two components, "understay" and "overstay," the latter including all days of care for unnecessary admissions. The chart also shows the net change that would result if a hypothetical fully effective control mechanism were to abolish all inappropriate use.

The diagnoses are arranged beginning with the one that has the largest net understay, and ending with the one that has the largest net overstay. The diagnostic categories are fewer than those in the preceding chart, because estimates of understay were not made for the five categories in which the number of cases was smaller than ten. The diagnostic abbreviations are explained in the text of the preceding chart.

Once again we observe a strong relationship between diagnosis and inappropriate use, but in addition we see a further differentiation between diagnoses in which the preponderant error is understay and others in which there is a greater likelihood of overstay, which is very marked in some categories. To take the two extremes, there would be a net *addition* of 3 percent to the days currently used to care for acute myocardial infarction, and a net *reduction* of 25 percent in the days attributed to urinary tract infection. An earlier chart in this section (Chart 3-8) shows the consequences for all the 18 diagnoses combined.

There are interesting implications to the relationship between quality and cost. If the findings are accepted at face value, an improvement of quality for some diagnoses would mean higher cost, whereas for others the costs could be reduced without damage to quality, assuming that equally appropriate care can be provided at an alternative site. The net effect in this instance is at least equal quality at lower cost.

It is important to keep in mind how heavily these findings depend on the "conventional wisdom" embodied in the criteria and standards which are used to judge the appropriateness of stay. The characteristics of this particular set are discussed in more detail in Donabedian 1982, pp. 31–37.

Chart 3–11

Percent of Hospital Days Actually Used that Were Judged To Be Inappropriate, and Percent Change in Days Currently Used that Is Needed To Correct Inappropriate Stay, by Primary Discharge Diagnoses, Short-term, Nonfederal Hospitals, Michigan, 1958.

Conditions

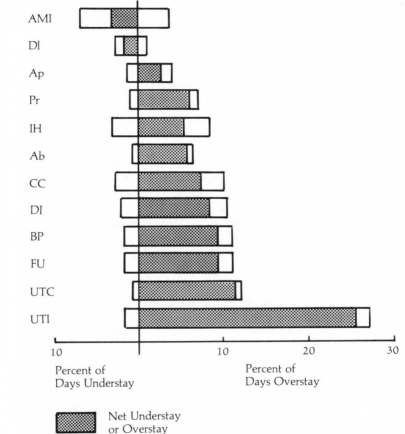

Source: Fitzpatrick et al. 1962, Table 219, p. 488.

Chart 3–12

Continuing our exploration of the factors that are related to the appropriateness of hospital use and that consequently influence the procedures of utilization control, we come to length of stay, which may be the most important component of hospital misuse.

This chart is drawn from a more detailed analysis of the data from the study of Michigan hospitals. To illustrate some important relationships, the chart uses data for only one diagnosis, urinary tract infection, which, as shown in the preceding chart, is characterized by a great deal of overstay and a fair amount of understay.

The chart shows the percent of cases in each category of length of stay that were judged to show understay, overstay, or inappropriate admission. As one might expect, understay is clearly confined to cases with short stays. Overstays, however, can be found in cases spread across the entire range of stays, though they are infrequent among cases who stay in the hospital for less than a week. For cases of longer duration there is only a gradual increase in the percentage of cases with overstay as the length of stay increases. Inappropriate admissions seem to occur equally among cases that range in length of stay from one day to 14–16 days. Only in cases with unusually long stays can it be said that the admission is almost always appropriate.

Judging by these findings, one might conclude that, for urinary tract infections, one would have to review cases with short stays in order to find understays and that there is some justification for the older practice of reviewing cases with stays of longer than 21 days in order to control overstay. There is, however, no one length of stay which both conveniently *and* effectively separates cases with a high likelihood of overstay from those with a low likelihood.

Once again, the reader is warned that the findings are heavily influenced by the criteria used. In this case, stay was considered appropriate if it fell anywhere between seven and 14 days for children, or between three and five days for all others under age 65. Only for cases of longer stays was health status used as a criterion of readiness for discharge, and even then an extra day was granted, presumably in order to prepare the patient to leave.

Chart 3–12

Percentage Distribution of Cases Discharged Alive at Specified Lengths of Stay with a Diagnosis of Urinary Tract Infection, by Appropriateness of Admission and Stay. Short-term, Nonfederal Hospitals, Michigan, 1958.

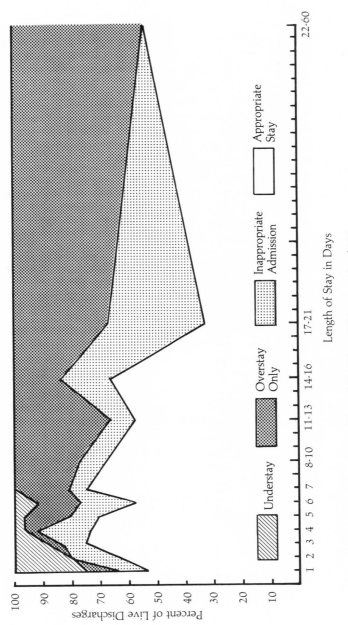

Source: Riedel and Fitzpatrick 1964, computed from Tables IV-6 and IV-8, pp. 146 and 148.

Chart 3–13

The data in the preceding chart came from a sample of discharges. An-other approach to the study of hospital misutilization is to sample days during the week, and patients who are in the hospital on these days, and to judge whether the stay on that particular day for each particular patient is or is not appropriate. This chart is based on a study (one of several by Zimmer) that uses this method. This investigation also differs from the study of Michigan hospitals used earlier in this section in al-lowing the physicians who reviewed the days of care to use their own judgments, without the imposition of explicit criteria.

Because most days of stay were rated independently by two physi-cians, it is also possible to measure the reliability of judgments. In this case, there was complete agreement in 89.5 percent of these observations, and complete disagreement in 6.1 percent. But of the cases in which there was some question as to appropriateness in the opinion of at least one observer, the other observer agreed completely in only 15.6 percent of cases. The accuracy of measurement is, therefore, a major problem in studies of this kind (Donabedian 1969a, pp. 85–92; 1973, pp. 386–87). It is a problem that must necessarily have important implications for any system of control that uses such judgments.

The data in this chart relate not to days of care but to observations, which include the many duplicate reviews described above. What is shown is the percent of these observations that judge the day of hospital care as inappropriate or of doubtful appropriateness. For all the units of the hospital combined, there is an increase in such judgments as the day on which the observation is made is more distant from the time of ad-mission. This pattern is more marked for patients on the medical service, and particularly marked on the neurological service (the findings for which are shown only in part so as not to clutter the chart). Other ser-vices, for example surgery and pediatrics, show somewhat different pat-terns. In addition, the several service units of the hospital are markedly different in their susceptibility to harboring inappropriate use.

Chart 3–13

Percent of Judgments Concerning Individual Days of Hospital Stay at Specified Intervals since Admission that Rated the Day of Stay To Be Inappropriate or of Doubtful Appropriateness. Strong Memorial Hospital, Rochester, N.Y., January 1968–August 1970.

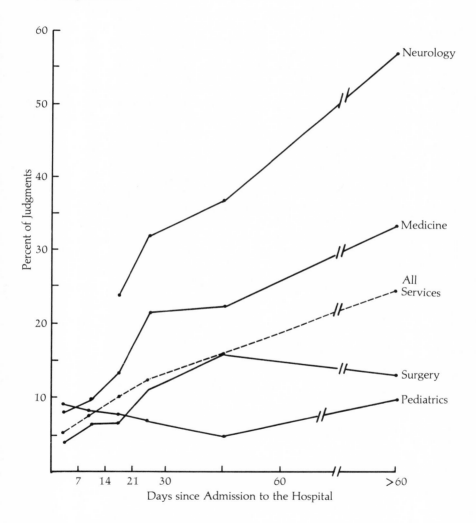

Source: Zimmer 1974. Computed from Table 1, p. 456.

Chart 3–14

As part of the study used to prepare the preceding chart, Zimmer also reports on the reasons why the physician reviewers made a judgment of inappropriate or doubtfully appropriate care. These reasons are reported as "admission unnecessary," "delay in hospital procedure," and "delay in discharge." The chart shows the percentage distribution of these explanations for the negative or doubtful judgments concerning the days of care, these latter being grouped by interval since admission.

As one would expect, unnecessary admission is much more likely to account for an unfavorable judgment early in a hospital stay. When the stay was beyond 60 days in length, the only errors found by this study were delays in discharge. Earlier in the patients' stays, however, there were significant proportions of cases which were not ready for discharge, but were still not receiving appropriate care because of a delay in performing needed hospital procedures. The patients were in the hospital, as it were, marking time. For more on this kind of inefficiency in hospital operations see Donabedian 1973, pp. 389–90.

The findings depicted in this chart are generally in keeping with those shown in chart 3-12, p. 75, drawn from the study of Michigan hospitals. The reader should note, however, that the data in this chart (and in the one immediately preceding this) pertain neither to discharges nor to hospital days, but to judgments. Since some cases were judged twice and others only once, there is no way of converting judgments to days judged without resorting to unpublished information.

Chart 3–14

Percent Distribution of Judgments of Inappropriate or Doubtfully Appropriate
Care for each Category of Days since Admission to the Hospital, by Reasons for
the Judgments. Strong Memorial Hospital, Rochester, N.Y., January 1968–
August 1970.

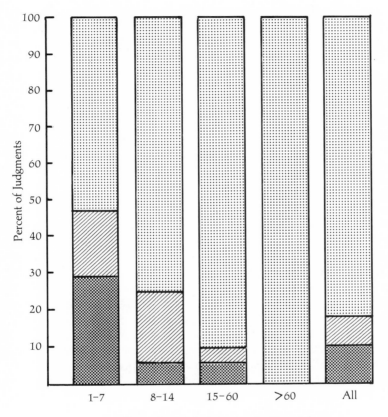

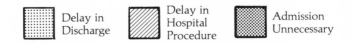

Source: Zimmer 1974. Computed from Tables 1 and 4, pp. 456 and 458.

Chart 3–15

So far we have encountered two methods for studying the appropriateness of hospital care. One reviews the discharges after care is completed, possibly supplementing the information in the record with an interview with the patients' physicians. The other assesses a sample of patients who are in the hospital on a given day using information in the record, supplemented by interviews and, sometimes, even a direct examination of the patient. Data from such a study could be used to construct an "artificial" cohort of patients who are seemingly followed from admission to discharge. A third method is to study an actual cohort of admissions by assessing the need for care on every day until each patient leaves. If this is done unobtrusively, so as not to influence the usual practices of the hospital, one gets information of vital importance to the design and implementation of utilization control systems.

This chart and the two that follow are drawn from a study of this third kind. Because it deals only with the beneficiaries of Medicare and Medicaid, and that only in one medium-sized, community hospital, the magnitudes of the findings may not be generally applicable, but the fundamental phenomena depicted are of general significance. The first of these is a confirmation of the observation, shown or suggested in earlier charts, that with every day of stay after admission, the percent of inappropriate days tends to increase. In this particular case, the relationship (shown by the solid line in the chart) has large irregularities which may be due to the rather small numbers of days (between 28 and 48 for the last four groups) under observation. Nevertheless, one should consider the possibility of a cyclical acceleration of discharges, perhaps at weekly intervals, which in this instance may also be compounded by the presence of a very heterogeneous assemblage of diagnoses.

There is a second phenomenon of fundamental importance. Although inappropriate days as a *proportion* of all days increases with the lapse of time since admission, there are so many more days of stay during the earlier period that the *number* of inappropriate days is largest within a few days of admission. This is illustrated in the chart by the percentage distribution of inappropriate days, by day since admission.

The implications of these two phenomena are that to be efficient one should intervene later on in the hospital stay, but to have the largest yield one should intervene earlier.

Chart 3-15

Percent of Days of Hospital Care (Each Representing a Patient in the Hospital) on Each Day since Admission that Were Judged Not To Require Acute Hospital Care; and Percent Distribution of All Inappropriate Days, by Day since Admission. Medicare and Medicaid Patients Only, Herrick Memorial Hospital, Berkeley, California, October 1, 1973–August 15, 1974.

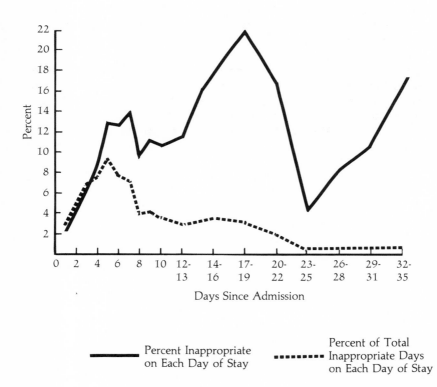

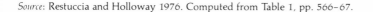

Source: Restuccia and Holloway 1976. Computed from Table 1, pp. 566–67.

Chart 3–16

This chart uses a different format to show the relationship between the frequency of inappropriate days and the days since discharge that was depicted (in dashed lines) in the preceding chart. By plotting the cumulative percentage distribution, one can read off the chart the percent of inappropriate days that have already occurred by, or prior to, any given day since admission. For example, if one uses the eighth day, which is close to the mean length of stay for these cases, as the first "checkpoint" in a utilization control procedure, one finds that 50 percent of inappropriate days will have already occurred. Needless to say, the specific findings shown in the chart are only true for these particular patients who, one should remember, are recipients of Medicare and Medicaid benefits, and who have not been further subclassified, for example by diagnosis.

Further subclassification of patients by diagnosis, or by "diagnosis-related groups" (DRG), is a necessary prelude to the selection of the appropriate checkpoints for concurrent utilization review. But the general phenomena illustrated in the preceding chart, this chart, and the two that follow remain broadly applicable and important.

Chart 3–16

Cumulative Percentage Distribution of Days of Hospital Care that Were Judged Not To Require the Services of an Acute Care Hospital, by Day since Admission. Medicare and Medicaid Patients Only, Herrick Memorial Hospital, Berkeley, California, October 15, 1973–August 15, 1974.

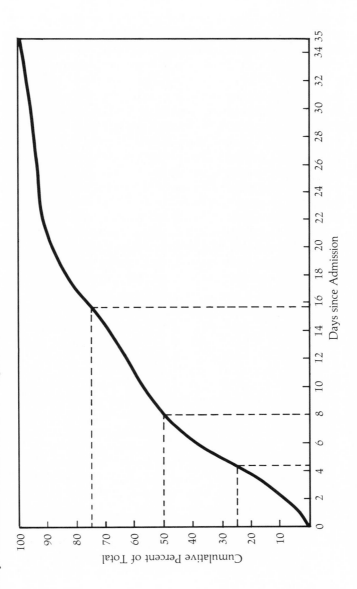

Days since Admission

Cumulative Percent of Total

Source: Restuccia and Holloway 1976. Computed from Table 1, pp. 566–67.

Chart 3–17

In this chart I continue to draw on the work of Restuccia and Holloway in order to depict another important phenomenon, the distribution of inappropriate days *within* each stay. This is illustrated by the experience of the 31 patients with the shortest stays, arranged in order of length of stay.

Three patterns emerge. Some cases are inappropriate at admission and continue so throughout the stay. In others, the stay becomes inappropriate later on, remaining so until discharge. In still others, there are one or more inappropriate days during the stay, occurring singly or in short sequences, preceded and followed by appropriate days. For the entire sample of cases, approximately ten percent of inappropriate days were of the first kind, 65 percent of the second kind, and 25 percent of the third kind. The authors call these "initial-stage," "end-stage," and "mid-stage" misutilization, respectively. The reason for mid-stage misutilization is, most probably, a delay in providing needed services.

This configuration of inappropriate use is critical to an understanding of some of the consequences of concurrent review. In this instance, the chart shows five admissions (numbers 1–4 and 21), consuming 16 days of care, that are potentially preventable by precertification. But a review on the day *after* admission would be much less effective, because it takes time to get patients discharged, and four out of the five unnecessary admissions result in stays of very short duration.

To take another example, a review on the fifth day of stay would intercept seven patients (numbers 9–15) about ready to leave, and an additional nine (number 16, 17, 19–23, 26, and 27) who do not merit hospitalization on that day. But 27 inappropriate days of stay would already have occurred, of which only eight would have been preventable by percertification of admissions. Excluding the day on which discharge would occur in any case, there are 19 preventable days of inappropriate stay after the fifth day but only nine are in the sequences interrupted by a review on that day. What proportion of these can actually be prevented depends on how speedily action can be taken and how remediable are the causes of inappropriate care.

In this particular study, the barriers to appropriate use were classified as attributable to the physician, the hospital, the patient or his family, or the environment. By far the most frequent barriers were the unavailability of suitable nursing home care, and certain characteristics of the physicians' style of practice.

Chart 3–17

Occurrence of Inappropriate Days within a Stay, by Day since Admission. Patients Who Remained in the Hospital Ten Days or Less in a Sample of Medicare and Medicaid Patients, Herrick Memorial Hospital, Berkeley, California, October 15, 1973–August 15, 1974.

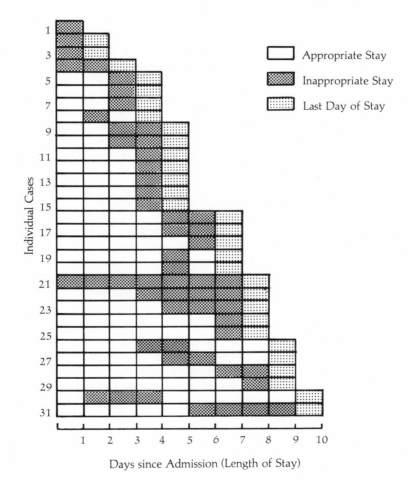

Days since Admission (Length of Stay)

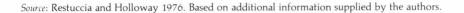

Source: Restuccia and Holloway 1976. Based on additional information supplied by the authors.

Chart 3–18

This chart is constructed from a display similar to the preceding chart, but which gives the findings in full. First, this chart shows the number of patients who are in the hospital on each day after admission. This is the number of cases that will be assessed when any given day after admission is selected as a checkpoint for review. The chart also shows how many days are *potentially* preventable by a review on each day after admission. These are estimated under the following assumptions: (1) only patients found to be inappropriately placed on the day of review are subject to action, (2) action becomes effective only on the day following the identification of an inappropriate day, (3) only subsequent days of inappropriate stay in an uninterrupted sequence are preventable, and (4) the day on which discharge occurs without benefit of the concurrent review procedure is not credited to that procedure. For example, one can determine by inspection of the chart that a check conducted on the tenth day will review 55 cases and prevent 15 days of future inappropriate stay, under the assumptions already cited.

Whether this is worth doing or not depends on the cost of review as compared to the savings from hospital days prevented. Accordingly, the chart also shows the savings, expressed in hospital-day equivalents, assuming the cost of the review procedure is that of 0.10 hospital day, and the cost of alternative care is 0.25 times each unnecessary hospital day eliminated. Thus, the chart shows that on certain days, mainly early in the stay, intervention is more costly than beneficial. The chart also shows when intervention has the greatest net benefit. Unfortunately, the distribution of inappropriate days is such that more than one intervention is needed to prevent a large proportion of inappropriate days. Because there is temporal overlap in sequences of inappropriate days for the several admissions, the effect of review on more than one day cannot be determined from this chart, but it can be estimated, under appropriate assumptions, from a display similar to that in the preceding chart. The assumption concerning the lag time between discovery and discharge is particularly critical, as shown by Averill and McMahon 1977. It is also possible that the presence of a review mechanism will have a deterrent effect. Finally, prior classification of cases into categories that are more homogeneous with respect to length of stay can be expected to improve cost effectiveness.

Chart 3-18

The Consequences of Instituting Review on Each Day after Admission, as Days Reviewed, Days of Inappropriate Stay Potentially Prevented, and Net Savings in Hospital-day Equivalents. Medicare and Medicaid Patients, Herrick Memorial Hospital, Berkeley, California, October 15, 1973–August 15, 1974.

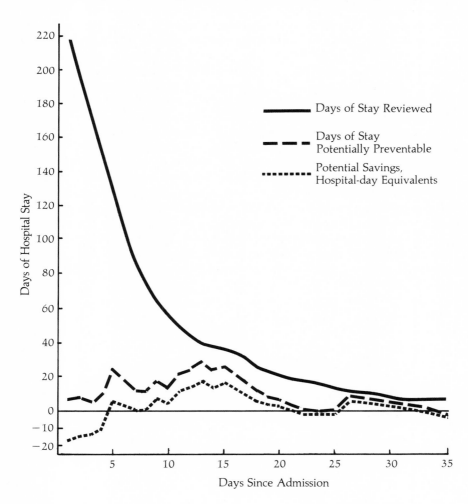

Source: Restuccia and Holloway 1976. Based on additional information supplied by the authors.

Chart 3–19

So far, we have looked at diagnosis, length of stay, and day since admission as factors that influence the occurrence of hospital misutilization. We have also examined some of the implications of these influences to the design and potential effectiveness of the concurrent review of hospital use. In the next three charts we see the effects of some additional factors, and there will be more in subsequent sections of the book.

The first of these three charts draws on the study of Michigan hospitals to show the effects of the day of the week on which discharge takes place. The authors speculate that the relatively large proportion of overstays among those who are discharged on weekends means that the patients were allowed to stay in the hospital until it was more convenient for them to leave, whereas the relatively large proportion of overstays among those discharged on Mondays and Tuesdays means that patients were kept over the weekend so that the steps preparatory to discharge could be made when the hospital was more fully staffed. On the other hand, the relatively high frequency of understays on weekends and Mondays may represent the determination of some patients to resume their usual activities even if they are not completely well enough to do so.

Unfortunately, there is no direct evidence to substantiate these views. Nor is there an analysis by day of admission, a factor that is often said to be related to hospital occupancy and length of stay. I have briefly reviewed some of the literature on this subject in Donabedian 1973, pp. 360–62.

Chart 3–19

Percent of Hospital Discharges on Each Day of the Week that Were Judged To
Have Stayed Fewer or More Days than Is Appropriate. A Sample of Cases with
One of 18 Primary Diagnoses, Short-term, Nonfederal Hospitals, Michigan,
1958.

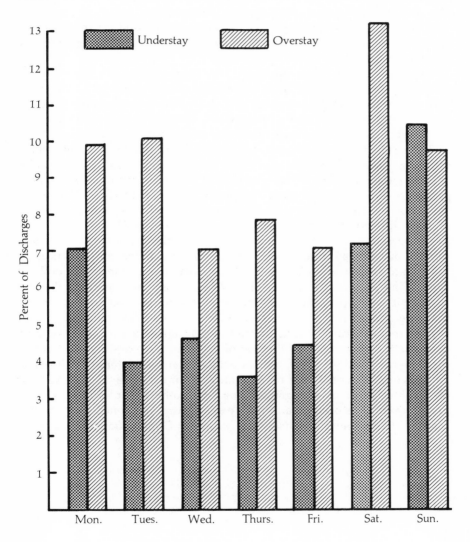

Source: Fitzpatrick et al. 1962, Table 228, p. 494.

Chart 3–20

In this chart we see the relationship between the appropriateness of hospital stay and the source of payment for the hospital bill, as revealed by the study of Michigan hospitals. The several categories of payment distinguished in the study are consolidated into two: the one in which the patient paid the entire bill, and all the other forms of payment, including those by "third parties." The chart is based on the findings for 17 out of the 18 diagnoses, because the cases with "hypertrophy of tonsils and adenoids" have been excluded.

When the patient pays the entire bill, there is a greater likelihood of understay, whereas when third parties pay at least part of the bill, there is a greater likelihood of overstay. These effects are presumably brought about partly by the wishes of the patient and partly by decisions made by physicians who are aware of the patient's financial situation.

The relationship between use of service and insurance status has attracted a great deal of study which, in turn, has generated a voluminous literature (Donabedian 1976, pp. 41–200). But information on the *appropriateness* of use is rather meager (Donabedian 1976, pp. 82–85). Later in this book we shall observe the relationship between source of payment and the appropriateness of appendectomies (Chart 4-21).

In assessing the influence of any factor on the tilt toward either understay or overstay, one needs to consider the relative consequences of the two to health as well as to monetary resources. One might end up concluding that the reduction of understay associated with health insurance is well worth the added overstay. Of course, this does not mean that one should not try to reduce *both* understay and overstay. Some believe that this can be done through the design of the health insurance plan itself, for example by the use of copayments, possibly adjusted to the patients' ability to pay. Others believe that the system of delivering and paying for care should be reorganized, for example through the use of "health maintenance organizations." Still others emphasize the need for direct controls on utilization, for example through concurrent review. Many of these issues are discussed further in Donabedian 1976.

Chart 3–20

Percent of Hospital Patients Who Were Judged To Have Stayed More or Fewer Days than Appropriate, by Source of Payment for the Hospital Bill. Patients with One of 17 Primary Discharge Diagnoses, Short-term, Nonfederal Hospitals, Michigan, 1958.

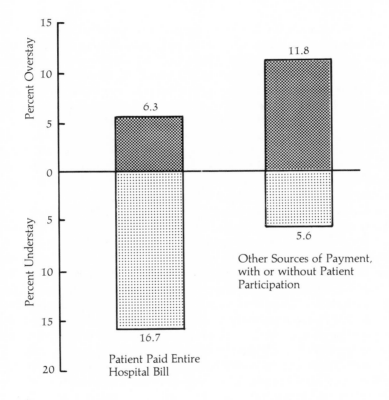

Source: Fitzpatrick et al. 1962, Table 221, p. 490.

Chart 3–21

This final chart introduces us to still another school of quality assessment about which we shall learn a great deal more in a subsequent section. It is distinctive in not using explicit criteria. Instead, it asks expert physicians to be guided in their judgments by how they, themselves, would have managed each case. For this reason, I have made a basic distinction between methods that use "implicit" and "explicit" criteria (Donabedian 1969a, p. 70ff.).

The chart shows the appropriateness of hospital admissions for this particular group of patients, in this particular locale, as influenced by several factors. We are already familiar with the relevance of hospital service units, which perhaps reflect the effects of diagnostic peculiarities, the training of medical practitioners, and possibly other factors as well. The chart illustrates this by showing how far pediatric cases exceed the average for all cases in the proportion of unnecessary admissions.

The nature of the hospital is another important factor, unnecessary admissions being most frequent in proprietary hospitals and least frequent in the hospitals that are affiliated with a medical school. In the proprietary hospitals one finds, moreover, a marked difference between the patients of "Class I" physicians, who are diplomates of an American Speciality Board or fellows of an American College, and "Class III" physicians, who are not diplomates or fellows, and who do not have staff appointments in either a voluntary or a municipal hosptial. In fact, the former physicians are no more likely to be responsible for unnecessary admissions than is the average physician in a hospital affiliated with a medical school. As we shall see in a subsequent section, the "Class III" physicians, who have privileges to practice only in a proprietary hospital, are also most frequently faulted for the quality of the care that they provide. They are, therefore, a clearly defined group of physicians whose patients are doubly at risk: first of being admitted to the hospital unnecessarily, and then of receiving care of "less than optimal" quality.

The more general significance of hospital and physician characteristics as correlates of professional performance will receive a great deal of attention in succeeding sections of this book.

Chart 3–21

Percent of Hospital Admissions Judged To Be Unnecessary, by Hospital Service Unit, by Type of Hospital, and by Physician Characteristics. Teamsters Union Members and Their Families, New York City, 1962.

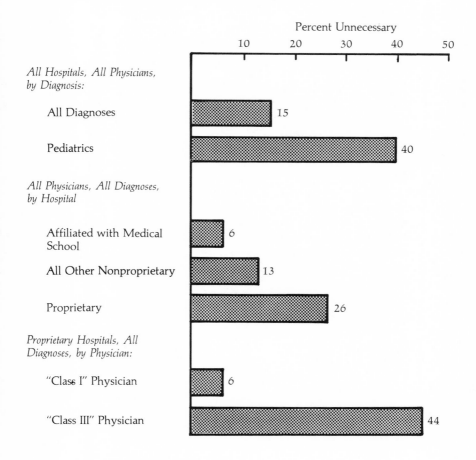

Source: Morehead et al. 1964, Tables 8 and 9, pp. 53 and 54.

The Justification
of Surgery

FOUR

Because surgical procedures involve resource use, the question of whether they are justified or not could easily have been included in the preceding chapter. The separation is largely a matter of convenience, though one could make some weak arguments to justify it on conceptual grounds.

A distinction is often made between resource use that is only wasteful, and resource use that is potentially harmful as well as wasteful. On these grounds, an unnecessarily lengthy hospital stay would not be as reprehensible as an unnecessary surgical intervention. Preventing the former would be a contribution to "cost containment," whereas avoiding the latter would contribute to quality in addition to reducing costs. But I do not believe that the distinction holds as a general principle. Most diagnostic and therapeutic measures, even seemingly simple ones, carry some risk. Moreover, purely wasteful use also damages quality, though indirectly, by leaving fewer resources available for more appropriate use. Finally, the provision of unnecessary services suggests that the practitioner responsible for them is careless, unwise, or uninformed—all these being traits that indicate at least a potential for more substantial breaches of good practice.

This chapter begins with some selections from the considerable body of epidemiological studies of the incidence of surgery. Besides the information which they convey, these studies demonstrate the ways in which epidemiological methods and observations can contribute to our understanding of health care problems in general and of the quality of care in particular. Other health care procedures can be studied in the same way. There is, then, an epidemiology of health care; and when judgments are made concerning the appropriateness of that health care, we have an "epidemiology of quality." An interesting feature of this epidemiology is that it has two categories of populations within which any given phenomenon is distributed: one of potential providers and another of potential clients. There will be many examples of this duality, in this chapter and later.

In the first part of this chapter there is information about (1) the secular trend for the incidence of all surgery, and of specific surgical procedures, (2) geographic variations in that incidence, and (3) variations in incidence that are related to some socioeconomic characteristics of clients. A study of the factors associated with these variations suggests hypotheses about their pertinence to quality. It is important, for example, to know (1) to what extent the variations are explained by population characteristics that represent the need for surgery; (2) to what extent they derive from differences in provider characteristics that represent the ability of providers to meet or to exceed the need; and (3) to what extent they can be shown to have an effect on health, as indicated by mortality or morbidity. Several of the charts in this part of the chapter address these questions. The concluding charts lead to inferences about the quality of surgery, based on differences correlated with client characteristics.

I have not considered the relationship between the incidence of surgery and methods of paying for care or of organizing the delivery of health care, because this would open up a subject of great breadth and complexity. Readers can get an overview of the pertinent literature, at several stages of its development, by referring to Klarman 1963, Donabedian 1969b, Roemer and Shonick 1973, and Luft 1980a.

Epidemiological studies, no matter how elegantly designed and how meticulously executed, yield only indirect evidence about the justifiability of surgical interventions. For more direct evidence we need to examine individual cases of surgery in greater detail. By showing us how to do so, the remainder of this chapter leads us into the more traditional domain of quality assessment, taking us through it in steps. First, we consider whether surgery already done should have been done. We shall see that in many cases the answer is tentative because it hinges merely on whether or not the tissue removed is diseased. In other more definitive studies, the evidence is supplemented by additional information that helps to decide whether the surgeon was justified in operating even though the tissue was later found to be normal. Either way, this is a "retrospective" method of assessment, since it studies a procedure only after the event.

From studies of surgery already done we can learn a great deal that helps improve future performance. But it may be better to use a "prospective" method of assessment, one which prevents unjustified surgery from being done at all. "Second opinion" programs, which are illustrated in the concluding part of this chapter, are designed to do precisely this, in the hope of thereby reducing both cost and unnecessary risk. In such programs, the insurer will either require (if the program is "mandatory") or urge (if the program is "voluntary") that when an "elective nonemergency" operation is recommended by the patient's surgeon or physician, a second opinion be sought from another surgeon, usually one chosen from a panel of expert consultants. The surgical consultant examines the patient and does whatever additional tests are needed. He then judges whether the operation is required as originally recommended, in some modified form, or not at all. According to McCarthy, Finkel, and Ruchlin

(1981) the consultant "must have no doubt that surgery should be performed," and "that it is in the best interest of the patient" (p. 34).

The purpose of the consultation is to help the patient to make the judgment based upon more complete information. If he continues to be in doubt, the patient is allowed still another consultation. The cost of these consultations is borne by the insurer. Most mandatory programs will not pay all or part of the costs of surgery unless a second opinion is obtained; once that is done, however, the patient can accept or reject the second opinion without loss of benefits. Some voluntary programs have offered incentives, such as forgiveness of coinsurance payments, if the patient obtains a second opinion and follows the recommendation of the consultant.

The effectiveness of second opinion programs depends partly on the incidence of insufficiently justified recommendations for "elective" surgery in a given community. It is also influenced by the way in which patients respond when they weigh the original recommendation against the judgment of the consultant. While a negative second opinion may persuade the patient to forgo surgery, a confirming second opinion may convince the patient to accept surgery. Though these two responses have contrary effects on the frequency of surgery, it is expected that the net effect will be a reduction. It is also possible that these programs will have what has been called a "sentinel effect," which means that physicians and surgeons in the community will be more careful in making their recommendations when they know that these are subject to review (McCarthy, Finkel, and Ruchlin 1981, pp. 160–61).

Besides the question of how effective second opinion programs are, and whether their costs justify the savings they may bring about, there is the even more important question of their impact on the quality of care. It is reasonable to assume that when a consultant confirms the initial recommendation for surgery, the operation is very likely to be justified. If patients are influenced by this concurrence of opinions to accept surgery, the frequency of justified surgery and its presumed benefits to health should increase. When the second opinion does not confirm the initial recommendation, surgery is more likely to be unjustified, and a rejection of surgery by the patient should, on the average, reduce the incidence of inappropriate surgery, with all the financial losses and dangers to health that it entails. However, harm could also be done if the opinion of the second surgeon is not as good as that of the first one, at least in some cases. This likelihood is reduced by choosing expert consultants and by eliminating any financial incentives for them to recommend surgery. But, as we shall see in Chapter 10, the likelihood of error could be increased by demanding that the consultant not recommend surgery unless he has no doubt that it is needed. Fortunately, in nonurgent cases, this error can almost always be rectified by a strategy of further observation, which is the one that the consultant is likely to recommend. Finally, there may be missed opportunities, since even when two surgeons agree that an operation is needed, this may not be the best course of action.

The final portion of this chapter deals with these questions, using data only from mandatory programs, since in voluntary programs only between two and five percent of persons ask for a second opinion.

Two important aspects of surgical care will not be considered in this chapter. The first is that of surgical interventions that should have been done, but were not. It is true that epidemiological evidence can suggest an excess of surgery in some populations and a deficit in others, but this is far from conclusive. As we shall see in later chapters, particularly in Chapter 10, more direct evidence can be obtained only by studying patients whose condition offers a choice between operating or not, when either decision could be wrong. A second omission from this chapter is an assessment of the skill in executing surgical procedures, and of the many other aspects of care before, during, and after surgery. It seems that information about these matters is often sought only indirectly by an examination of outcomes such as complications and deaths, outcomes to be studied in detail later in this book.

Chart 4–1

The first chart in the series on the epidemiology of surgical procedures shows the considerable increase that has occurred in the United States in the incidence of all surgical procedures taken as a group. According to McCarthy and Finkel (1980a) this is a relatively recent phenomenon. From around 1930 "until the early 1970s the rate of surgery in the United States was fairly stable" (at something between 50 and 70 procedures per 1,000 persons), whereas between 1971 and 1977 the population increased by about five percent and the number of operations by 34 percent (ibid., pp. 884, 892).

The rates for the small selection of surgical operations shown in the chart illustrate the finding that not all procedures have shared in this trend. Some have increased (in relative or absolute terms) more than others, while still others have actually decreased.

Not shown in the chart are differences in the experience of different population subgroups. For example, the increase has been relatively greater among females than among males, and among persons 65 or older as compared to those in any other age group (ibid., p. 886).

To some extent these changes may have been appropriate—the consequence of useful developments in science and technology, and of the improvements in access to care due to better coverage by government programs and voluntary health insurance. It is believed, however, that at least some of the increase in surgery represents an increased propensity to operate without sufficient justification. This may be because there are too many surgeons, because reimbursement by third parties is too readily available, and because some surgical procedures are as yet of unproven value. The harm that unnecessary surgery may cause the patient, and in particular the financial drain that it represents, have produced an insistent demand for some kind of control on surgery.

The data in this chart are from the Hospital Discharge Survey of the National Center for Health Statistics. The methods of that survey should be carefully examined before making comparisons with data from other sources. The data in this case pertain to a sample of nonfederal, short-stay hospitals and include a maximum of three procedures per discharge. The definition of what constitutes a surgical procedure or operation is particularly critical, as are the conventions for coding diseases and procedures. For example, coding conventions introduced in 1979 have greatly increased the number of surgical procedures reported (National Center for Health Statistics 1982, p. 8).

Chart 4-1

Rates per 1,000 Persons per Year, for All Surgical Operations and for a Selection of Specified Procedures. Nonfederal, Short-stay Hospitals, U.S.A., 1965 and 1977.

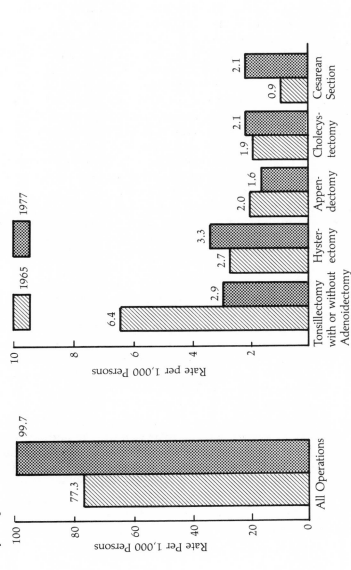

Source: National Center for Health Statistics 1978, Table K, p. 10; and National Center for Health Statistics 1979, Table 21, p. 49.

Chart 4–2

The next seven charts report some findings on geographic variability among small areas in the United States. It is fitting to begin with the work of Paul Lembcke, a distinguished pioneer in studies of regional organization, hospital performance, and quality assessment.

This chart shows the 23 service areas of the Council of Rochester Regional Hospitals distributed according to two variables: the appendectomy rate and the mortality rate from appendicitis in each area. Inspection of the scatter diagram suggests that these two variables are unrelated. Lembcke reports, however, that if one accepts the experience of the Rochester Service Area (with its teaching hospitals) as the standard, one finds that the six service areas that have significantly higher appendectomy rates also have a significantly higher mortality rate from appendicitis, when the mortality data from all six areas are pooled.

Several features of this study should be noted because they are important elements in methodology and have a bearing on the inferences to be drawn from the findings. Only "primary" appendectomies (those for suspected appendicitis) are included, so as not to cloud the picture by counting appendectomies performed incidentally in the course of another abdominal operation. The appendectomy rates are adjusted for age and sex so as to correct for differences in the incidence of the disease attributable to these factors. The service areas used are nonoverlapping geographic units that are delineated so as to make them as self-contained as possible with regard to their use of hospital services. In this instance, 75 to 95 percent of the hospitalizations of the residents of the several areas were within their own areas. As a result, hospital data could be related to their corresponding population base, and the hospitals in an area could be considered to be responsible for the care provided in that area, unless the area was large and served by many hospitals.

The most reasonable interpretation of these data is that the incidence and severity of appendicitis are similar (within age and sex groups) in all areas, and that the higher appendectomy rates represent unnecessary surgery, and possibly a lower level of surgical skill, since they seem to be associated with higher rather than lower death rates from "appendicitis." This is, however, a hypothesis that needs to be confirmed by more direct evidence. A great deal of what comes later in this book is an exposition of that kind of evidence.

Chart 4–2

Hospital Service Areas Distributed by the Appendectomy Rate and by the Death Rate from Appendicitis in Each Area. Rochester Hospital Regional Council, Western New York State; Appendectomies in 1948, and Average of Deaths from Appendicitis, 1944–1948.

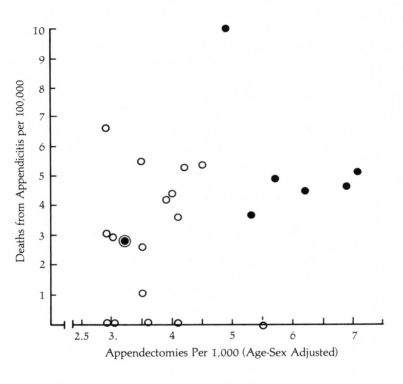

● Rochester Service Area: Considered To Serve as "Standard"

● Service Areas with Appendectomy Rates Significantly Higher (*p* < 0.001) than the Rate for the Rochester Area

Source: Lembcke 1952, Table 1, p. 279.

Chart 4–3

This chart, drawn from the same study used for the preceding chart, reveals what Lembcke called "a curious difference" between categories of service areas in the effect of urban or rural location.

The Rochester area was used by Lembcke as a standard partly because it contained a medical school and its affiliated hospitals. In this service area both the appendectomy rates and the death rates from appendicitis were on the low side (as shown also in the preceding chart) and there was no difference to speak of between rural and urban locations. By contrast, when the four service areas with the highest appendectomy rates were examined, there were rather large differences between the urban and rural localities within these areas, particularly with regard to the incidence of appendectomies. And once again the higher incidence of appendectomies was associated with a higher rate of mortality from appendicitis.

Lembcke says that the differences between the urban and rural rates are not due to different age distributions. Rather, in his words, "a reasonable inference is that in areas served by hospitals where operations are not controlled strictly, the simple fact of greater accessibility to hospital and medical care is a deciding factor" (Lembcke 1952, p. 281). He could have added that greater access to surgery, together with fewer controls on that surgery, would also explain the higher mortality rates.

That proximity to a hospital could, in some ways, be inimical to health, is indeed a sobering thought.

Chart 4-3

Rates for Primary Appendectomies and Death Rates from Appendicitis in Specified Hospital Service Areas, by Urban or Rural Residence. Rochester Hospital
Regional Council, Western New York State, Specified Years.

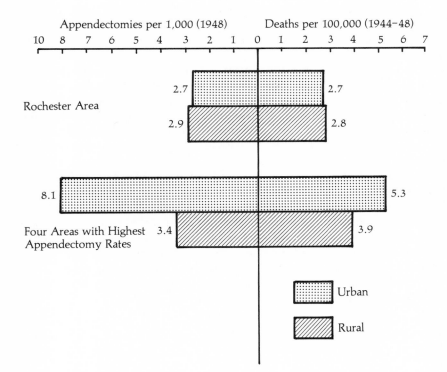

Source: Lembcke 1952, text p. 281.

Chart 4–4

This chart and the next illustrate some findings of a study that obviously follows in the footsteps of Lembcke. In fact, I suspect that the boundaries of the ten regions of Kansas, which are the units of analysis, owe at least something to the work of Lembcke (see Poland and Lembcke 1962). Each region is a reasonably good "service area," since over 80 percent of patients hospitalized in any given region come from within the region, and there is "little variation among regions in terms of 'non-regional' patients" (Lewis 1969, p. 881). Metropolitan Kansas was excluded from the regional comparisons partly because it attracts patients from all over the state.

This investigation does differ from Lembcke's in that the population studied is restricted to those enrolled in a reasonably generous Blue Cross plan with uniform benefits. This is an advantage because it standardizes, at least to some extent, the effect of economic factors that may influence clients to seek care, and physicians to provide it. A weakness is the investigator's inability to correct for variations in age and sex because the data were not available.

The chart shows that the mean rates (which include Metropolitan Kansas) vary by type of procedure. More germane to our immediate interests is the wide variation in rates for any given operation among persons with similar insurance coverage who reside in different regions. While all the operations show significant variability in their regional incidence, the variability is greater for some than for others; the reasons seem unrelated to the seriousness or expected necessity of the operation.

In the next chart we see some results of the investigator's effort to find out what accounts for these differences.

Chart 4-4

Range, Mean, and 95 Percent Confidence Limits of the Rates Per 10,000 Persons for Specified Surgical Operations, Indicating Variation Among Ten Health Planning Regions. Blue Cross Subscribers, Kansas, 1956.

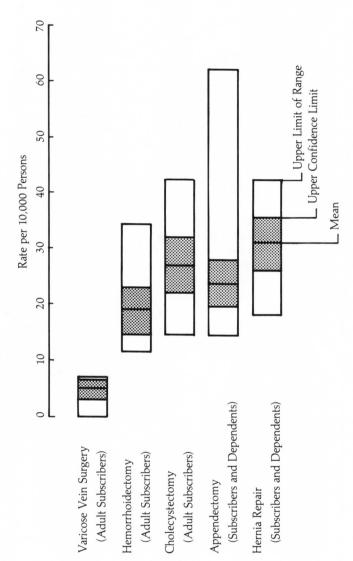

Source: Lewis 1969, Table 3 and text, p. 882.

Chart 4–5

This chart shows some results of the effort to explain the interregional differences in surgical rates depicted in the preceding chart. Lewis chose, as possible explanatory variables, four characteristics of each region. These were hospital beds per 1,000 persons, surgeons plus general practitioners per 100,000 persons, board-certified surgeons per 100,000 persons, and the percent of persons who have Blue Cross insurance. The last of these variables proved to be unrelated to variations in surgical rates. Hemorrhoidectomies and varicose vein operations were not related to any of the remaining three variables, even though these operations are considered to be highly discretionary. The incidence of each of the other three operations (as well as that of tonsillectomies, which was not shown in the preceding chart because of a large difference in scale) was related to one or more of the three variables. Depending on the operation, from 49 to 70 percent of the interregional difference was explained.

The chart shows the findings for the incidence of appendectomies, which was related to all three variables, and for which 70 percent of the interregional variation was explained. The chart is, of course, a very crude visual representation of the relationships that are more precisely measured by multiple regression. In particular, comparisons by rank lose much information that using the rates themselves would provide. Nevertheless, one can still see patterns that suggest at least weak correlations between the ranks of the ten regions according to the incidence of appendicitis, and their ranks according to the prevalence of each of (1) surgeons and general practitioners, (2) board-certified surgeons, and (3) hospital beds. Even by visual inspection it is clear that the best correlation is obtained when the effect of the three independent variables is combined by the very crude method of computing a mean rank.

This investigation suggests that the greater availability of surgeons and hospital beds increases surgical rates in a population that has good health insurance coverage. It does not tell us what level of surgical use is appropriate. It will be recalled that Lembcke used the relevant death rates to reach the inference that some of the higher appendectomy rates were probably unnecessary and harmful. Lewis does not have that information.

Chart 4-5

Ten Health Planning Regions Distributed According to Their Ranks with Respect to the Incidence of Appendectomies and Their Ranks with Respect to Each of Three Specified Independent Variables, and All Three Variables Weighted Equally. Blue Cross Subscribers, Kansas, 1965.

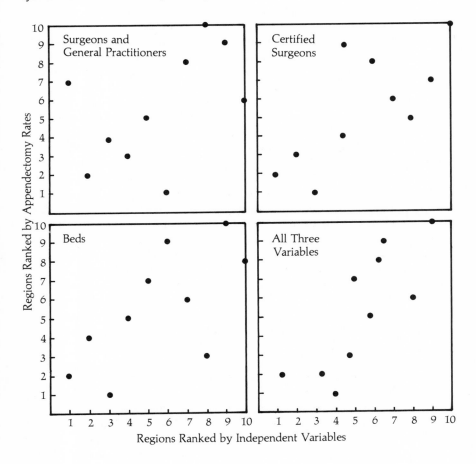

Source: Lewis 1969. Based on Tables 1 and 3, pp. 881 and 882.

Chart 4–6

This chart shows the extent of variation in the age-adjusted rates for appendectomies among 13 hospital service areas in Vermont. The variation is considerable and significant (when tested by chi square) though not as large as the variation reported for the ten regions of Kansas by Lewis in his somewhat earlier study. This is also illustrated in the chart, so that the reader can compare the two. This comparison can only be a rough one, however, since the degree of variability observed is influenced by the sizes of the populations of the several service areas, the sharpness of separation into service areas, the length of time during which data were collected, and by other features of method. For example, in this instance, the data from Vermont are adjusted for age, though not for sex, whereas the Kansas data are not adjusted for either age or sex.

In Vermont, as in Kansas, there was a great deal of variability also in the incidence of surgical procedures other than appendectomies (Gittelsohn and Wennberg 1977, Table 7.8, p. 100; Wennberg and Gittelsohn 1973, Table 3, p. 1105). The findings in Vermont are also similar to those in Kansas in showing a positive correlation between the prevalence of surgeons and the incidence of surgery ($r = 0.6$). An additional finding in the more recent Vermont study is that the complexity of the surgical operation was a factor in this relationship. The most complex procedures are positively related to the prevalence of general surgeons, but negatively related to the prevalence of general practitioners who do surgery. The least complex procedures are positively related to the prevalence of both kinds of physicians. The prevalence of physicians who do not perform surgery is negatively related to the incidence of surgery, but it is positively related to the performance of diagnostic procedures such as laboratory tests, x-rays, and electrocardiograms (Wennberg and Gittelsohn 1973, Table 4, p. 1105).

The delineation of service areas in Vermont followed closely the method used earlier by Lembcke. Service areas were constructed by assigning townships to the hospital which was the predominant source of care, and a very high correspondence was achieved by the simple device of excluding from the study those townships that were divided in their sources of care. In addition, the prevalence of hospital beds and physicians in each service area was adjusted to reflect the proportion of hospitalizations that occur outside that area.

Chart 4-6

Appendectomy Rates by Hospital Service Areas. Vermont 1969–1971, and Kansas, 1965.

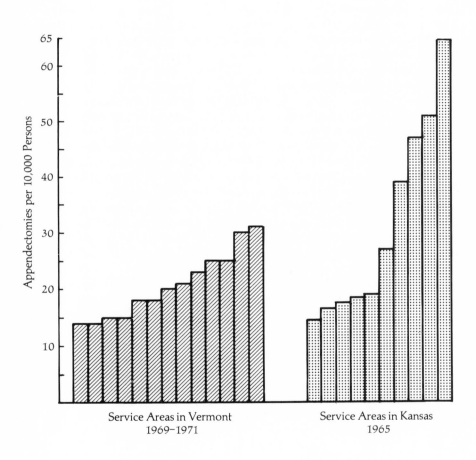

Source: Gittelsohn and Wennberg 1977, Table 7.8, p. 100; and Lewis 1969, Table 3, p. 882.

Chart 4–7

This second chart derived from the Vermont study represents the geographic variability in the probability of having a tonsillectomy.

An interesting methodological refinement in the Vermont study was the recognition that surgical removal of an organ generally precludes a second operation for the same purpose. The incidence of a surgical procedure in successive age groups was, accordingly, corrected for the reduction in the number of persons subject to that procedure. Because tonsillectomies occur very frequently, it is particularly important to exclude from the computation of the rate for any age group those persons who have had a tonsillectomy at an earlier age. This chart allows for that by showing the cumulative probability of having had a tonsillectomy by any given age. For example, by age 24 only nine percent (0.09) of persons in service area 13 will have had their tonsils removed, whereas at the other extreme, in service area 7, 63 percent (0.63) of 24-year olds will have had their tonsils removed. This does not mean, of course, that any cohort of actual births will experience the probabilities depicted in the chart as the cohort ages. The curves shown in the chart are only representations of the forces that have resulted in a tonsillectomy correctly and in the recent past. A cohort of births in each service area would follow its corresponding curve only if these forces were to remain constant. (In the chart the data for areas 10 and 11 are shown only partially to avoid cluttering the chart even more.)

The remarkable geographic variability in the occurrence of tonsillectomies, which was the largest of any surgical procedure observed in this study, calls for an explanation. In the words of the investigators:

> The estimated probability of about 60% for Area Seven is to be contrasted with values of 11%, 19%, 20%, and 27% in four directly adjacent communities, which, for the most part, are served by different groups of physicians operating in different hospitals. The 5 communities are similar in population density, topography, and per capita income; and it is unlikely that the differential tonsillectomy rates can be related to variations in the incidence of tonsillitis, recurrent sore throat, or otitis media. Rather, the major source of variation appears to be in differing attitudes by physicians as to indications for the procedure. (Gittelsohn and Wennberg 1977, p. 95)

Chart 4–7

The Probabilities that Tonsils and Adenoids Are Removed by Specified Ages in Each of 13 Hospital Service Areas. Vermont, 1969–1971.

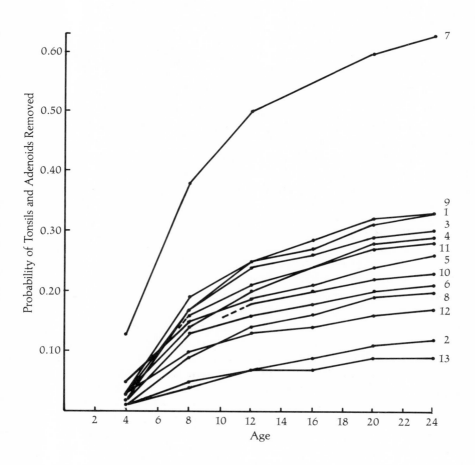

Source: Gittelsohn and Wennberg 1977, Table 7.2, page 96.

Chart 4–8

This chart, which shows the variations in appendectomy rates among hospital service communities in Michigan, demonstrates that the tradition we first encountered in the work of Lembcke in the Rochester region is alive and, one hopes, well. The purpose of this more recent enterprise is to collect information concerning communities that are served by individual hospitals or groupings of hospitals and, by conveying that information to the hospitals concerned, to create an awareness of each hospital's performance and of its responsibility for more effective planning. The information includes data on use of service, cost, and a variety of events that reflect on health status.

One can compute the number of persons served by a hospital if it can be assumed, without too much error, that of all *hospitalizations* that originate in a large area around the hospital, the proportion occurring at that hospital equals the proportion of that area's *residents* which is served by that hospital. The area in which the population served by a hospital resides is sometimes called the catchment area, and this often overlaps with the catchment areas of other nearby hospitals. To delineate geographic service areas that are mutually exclusive, the various areas of overlap must be divided among the hospitals that share them so as to minimize the crossing of boundaries to receive hospital care (Donabedian 1973, pp. 473–85). Such nonoverlapping areas are relatively easy to draw in rural areas, as illustrated in earlier charts. But the high density of both people and hospitals (as well as the functional differentiation of hospitals) in many parts of Michigan preclude the precise matching of a hospital, its service population, and a geographic area of residence. In this study, the solution was (1) to cluster hospitals that have highly overlapping service areas, and (2) to draw more relevant catchment areas so as to exclude those subparts (in this case zip code areas) in which less than a specified percent of hospitalizations occur at a certain hospital or cluster of hospitals. The resulting catchment areas are the service communities which contain the more immediate service populations of each hospital or cluster. The hospital performance indices are computed for only these populations. To compute the appendectomy rates used in this chart, the cutoff point was set at a very high level (50 percent of hospitalizations) in order to reduce variability due to errors in matching appendectomies to the population to which they pertain.

Chart 4–8

Frequency Distribution of "Hospital Service Communities" by Appendectomy Rate. Forty-nine Hospital Service Communities, Lower Peninsula of Michigan, 1978.

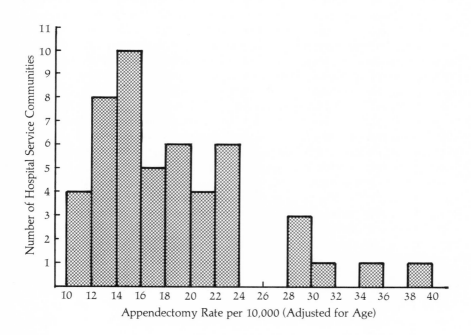

Source: Griffith et al. 1981, with additional data provided by Peter Wilson.

Chart 4–9

This chart begins a series of international comparisons which supplement the findings of geographic comparisons within the United States and lead to rather similar speculations. In this instance, women in the United States are shown to have a rate of surgery that is, overall, twice as high as that for women in England and Wales during the periods specified. The United States also has twice as many surgeons, including trainees, per unit population. (Not shown in the chart is the finding that when only fully trained surgeons are counted, the surgeon–population ratio for the United States is 4.5 times that for England and Wales.)

The juxtaposition of relative surgical rates and relative supply of surgeons represents the inference, drawn by the investigator, that the two phenomena may be causally related. Bunker recognizes, of course, that there are many other factors that influence surgical rates, and he provides a masterly exposition of the subject. For example, people in England and Wales should have greater access to surgery because they are all participants in a national health service. But relative shortages in personnel and resources have led to long waiting times for the more discretionary operations, even though surgical services are said to be run more efficiently in Britain. Besides, surgeons in Britain function only as hospital-based consultants who, because they are paid what corresponds to a salary, have no financial incentive to operate. Finally, though the chart eliminates the effect of sex differences by showing only the data for women, there remain many demographic, socioeconomic, and geographic factors that influence morbidity and the behavioral response to it.

All these factors, and perhaps others as well, influence the relative frequencies of the selected specific surgical operations that are also shown in the chart. Differences in "surgical philosophy" no doubt account for the relatively larger incidence of simple mastectomy, and adenoidectomy without tonsillectomy, in England and Wales.

The reader should note that in this chart (as well as in some others that follow) a method has been used that creates a visual equivalence between a ratio and its reciprocal, so that the lengths of the bars on the left of the vertical line can be directly compared to those on the right. The reader should also be aware of a lack of complete comparability in the data from the two countries. Bunker notes the differences and concludes that they do not affect the comparisons materially (p. 136).

Chart 4–9

The Prevalence of Surgeons and the Incidence of Specified Surgical Procedures for Women in the United States Expressed as Ratios of the Corresponding Rates for England and Wales. Surgeons 1967; Surgical Operations for the United States in 1965, and for England and Wales in 1966.

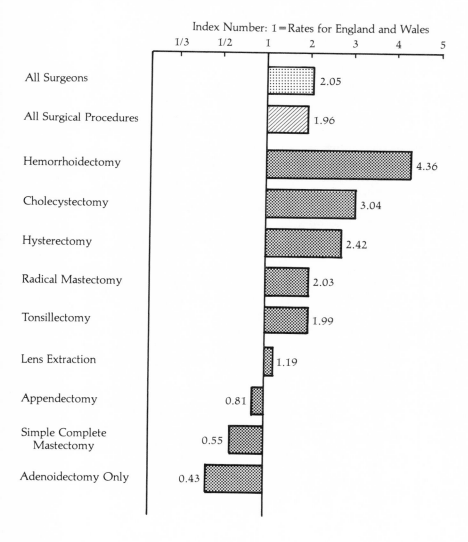

Index Number: 1 = Rates for England and Wales

All Surgeons	2.05
All Surgical Procedures	1.96
Hemorrhoidectomy	4.36
Cholecystectomy	3.04
Hysterectomy	2.42
Radical Mastectomy	2.03
Tonsillectomy	1.99
Lens Extraction	1.19
Appendectomy	0.81
Simple Complete Mastectomy	0.55
Adenoidectomy Only	0.43

Source: Bunker 1970, p. 136, and Table 2, p. 137.

Chart 4–10

In this chart we see a comparison of surgical rates and health care resources that is very similar in method and intent to that shown in the preceding chart. Vayda points out, however, that comparisons between Canada and England and Wales, which are shown in this chart, are more precise because the data on surgery are collected and recorded in a more comparable manner in the two countries. Furthermore, the rates used to construct this chart are standardized for differences in the age compositions of the two populations. Still another distinctive feature is the introduction of information on mortality rates from the diseases that correspond, at least roughly, to the surgical operations shown in the chart. The reader will recall that this kind of comparison between surgical rates and mortality rates was used by Lembcke (Charts 4–2 and 4–3) to help explain the unusually high appendectomy rates that he observed in some of the service areas in the Rochester region.

The findings in this chart are that Canada has relatively higher surgical rates than England and Wales, but that the corresponding mortality rates are either similar or higher in Canada. Higher morbidity rates in Canada could explain these findings. But they are more likely to result from a greater propensity to operate, which is encouraged and made possible by a greater prevalence of surgeons and acute hospital beds in Canada, a finding which the chart also shows. The incentives of the fee-for-service method of payment in Canada could be another contributing factor. If, however, the morbidity rates and other relevant population characteristics are comparable in the two countries, any excess in age-adjusted female mortality rates is to be attributed, at least in part, to the higher surgical rates and to other deficiencies in the quality of surgical care. The differences in the relative frequencies of the different types of mastectomy "probably reflect differences in preferred modes of treatment" (Vayda 1973, p. 1227).

The reader will note how critical a determination of the comparability of population characteristics, including the incidence and severity of disease, is to the interpretation of this chart and many of the earlier charts in this chapter.

Chart 4–10

Rates for the Incidence of Selected Surgical Operations in Females and for the Roughly Corresponding Causes of Death, as Well as for the Prevalence of Surgeons and Acute Care Hospital Beds in Canada, Expressed as a Ratio of the Corresponding Rates in England and Wales, 1968.

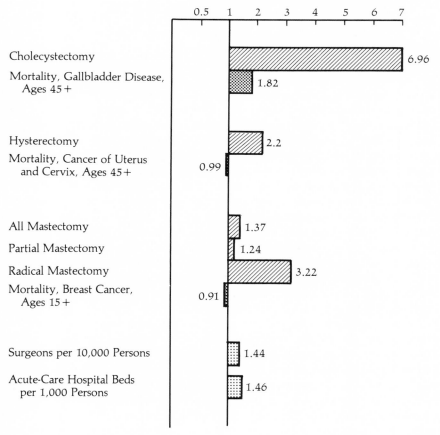

Index Number: 1 = Rates for England and Wales

Source: Vayda 1973, Tables 2 and 3, pp. 1226 and 1227. I have adjusted the death rates for England and Wales to the age distribution for Canada, based on data in Table 3, p. 1227.

Chart 4–11

This chart shows that wide variations in the incidence of surgery among small geographic units is not peculiar to the United States. A comparison of counties in the Canadian province of Ontario reveals that the ratio of the highest to the lowest rates ranges from 4.8 to 8.2. This ratio is used here as a rough representation of the variance in rates among counties, permitting a convenient graphic representation of the percent of variance explained by intercounty differences in the prevalence (1) of "active-treatment" beds, and (2) of specialists and generalists, who can be considered jointly because the contribution of the prevalence of generalists to the observed variation in surgery is small.

This study extends the earlier work of Lewis. As the chart shows, the prevalence of "active-treatment" beds is a very important explanatory variable in four of the five procedures. In the remaining one (appendectomy) the prevalence of physicians is much more important; one does not know why. Though we also do not know which comes first—the demand that eventuates in surgery or the availability of surgeons and hospital beds—we find, once again, an association between the two. But the variable that is most powerful in explaining the incidence of any given surgical procedure in a county is the incidence of the other four procedures. As much as 84 percent of the variation in surgical rates was explained by this. A classification of procedures by "complexity" and by degree of "discretion" did not lead to any clear conclusions. In the chart, the procedures are shown in order of decreasing discretion. Obviously, colectomy does not fit the pattern of a correspondingly decreasing variability in surgical rates. Possibly this is because colectomy was rated the most complex of all the operations, so that surgeons who are able to perform it are very unevenly distributed.

This study corrects for differences in age and sex, and uses a rigorous statistical technique. But it does have the disadvantage of using counties rather than service areas as units of analysis. For example, the flow of patients into counties with teaching centers may explain, in part, why residents of these counties were found to have low surgical rates, even though the prevalence of physicians and hospital beds was high. But intercounty travel does not explain why the rates in counties with teaching centers are also among the lowest when compared to other counties. One may conclude that surgery is done more discriminatingly in the shadow of a teaching institution.

Chart 4-11

Ratios of the Highest to the Lowest Rates of Specified Surgical Operations (Standardized for Age and Sex) among 49 Counties, and Percent of the Variance in Surgical Rates Explained through Multiple Regression by Specified Variables. Ontario, Canada, 1974.

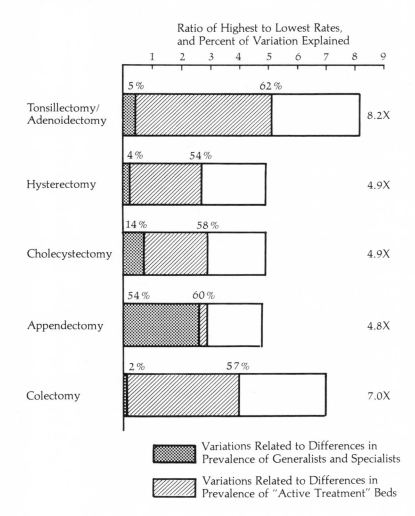

Ratio of Highest to Lowest Rates,
and Percent of Variation Explained

Tonsillectomy/ Adenoidectomy	5% 62% 8.2X
Hysterectomy	4% 54% 4.9X
Cholecystectomy	14% 58% 4.9X
Appendectomy	54% 60% 4.8X
Colectomy	2% 57% 7.0X

Variations Related to Differences in Prevalence of Generalists and Specialists

Variations Related to Differences in Prevalence of "Active Treatment" Beds

Source: Stockwell and Vayda 1979, Tables 2 and 3, p. 392.

Chart 4–12

With this chart we make a transition from the study of geographic differences in surgical rates to an examination of the relationship between surgical rates and the characteristics of the individual patients. For example, this chart shows that surgical rates are higher for whites, urban residents, and members of families headed by a person of intermediate education. The differences related to race and residence are statistically significant. So is the difference between families headed by a person with less than eight years of education and those headed by a person with nine to fourteen years of education. These disparities are observed *after* the rates have been adjusted for differences in the age and sex composition of the population groups being compared. But when an adjustment for differences in income is added, there remain no significant relationships between surgical rates and race, residence, or education of the head of the family. Thus income emerges as an important differentiator of the use of surgical services among persons whose need for surgery has been made more comparable through adjustments for differences in age and sex.

It is not easy to interpret these findings: low surgical rates could mean either insufficient surgery relative to need, or an ability to avoid surgery that is useless or that can be replaced by medical treatment. The investigators lean toward the latter explanation for the lower rates among the best educated. We are tempted to accept the former explanation for the low surgical rates among nonwhites who live outside metropolitan areas, a subgroup that the investigators show to have low rates even after age, sex, and education have been accounted for. It is not totally unreasonable to suggest that some disadvantaged groups are subject, at the same time, to more of the surgery that is unnecessary and less of the surgery that is needed. Only direct assessment of surgical care can settle the issue.

The data used in this study come from the Health Interview Survey of the National Center for Health Statistics. The sample includes only persons who are alive and not in an institution. The information is subject to error and bias due to deficiencies in reporting. Data based on hospital records can be obtained from the Center's Hospital Discharge Survey.

Chart 4–12

Rates of Surgical Procedures (Standardized for Age and Sex) by Race, Residence, and Education of the Head of the Family. U.S.A., 1970.

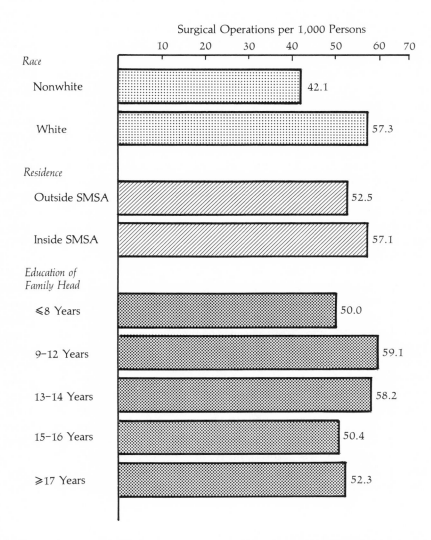

Source: Bombardier et al. 1977, Table 1, p. 700. Data are from the U.S. Health Interview Survey.

Chart 4–13

We see in this chart, which is based on data from Hannover, West Germany, that demographic and socioeconomic differences in surgical rates are not restricted to the United States. The left-hand side of the chart shows a higher incidence of appendectomies in females compared to males and in white collar workers compared to blue collar workers. On the right-hand side there is an important piece of new information: the percent of appendices which, when examined by the pathologist, show the presence of inflammation. When the corresponding bars on the two sides of the chart are compared, it appears that there is an inverse relationship between the incidence of appendectomy and the percent of inflamed tissue for each of the two comparisons, by sex and by occupation. The elucidation of the significance of the ratio of normal to abnormal tissue in appendectomies will be a major theme (and learning device) in this book. For now, we can proceed by drawing the most obvious inference, which is that there is a higher proportion of "unnecessary" appendectomies among females and among white collar workers. The sex-related differences may be due, in part, to the greater difficulty of making the diagnosis in adolescent and young adult females. The occupational differences are more difficult to explain. Under the health care system in West Germany, all workers have equal access to care, and surgeons have no financial incentive to operate. But appendectomy is very fashionable in West Germany, where the appendectomy rate in 1966 was almost four times that in the United States. Perhaps the white collar worker is more apprehensive, and the surgeon more responsive to his expectations and fears. In the words of the authors, "It may be now that during the game called the 'diagnostic process' the primary doctor and the patient will settle upon the diagnosis of appendicitis and that the surgeon will not dare to refuse appendectomy unless he is able to exclude appendicitis for sure" (pp. 326–27).

In this study the data are not adjusted for age, but I did adjust the rates for the occupational groups for differences in sex. The data on tissue findings are very incomplete, since only about 15 percent of appendices removed are examined pathologically. It is not known whether the findings are also biased by age, sex, or occupation. Fortunately, all tissue is examined at one "pathologic institute," so that source of variability has been removed.

Chart 4-13

Appendectomy Rates by Sex and Occupation, and Percent of Appendices that Showed Acute Appendicitis on Pathological Examination. Hannover, Federal Republic of Germany, 1966–1967.

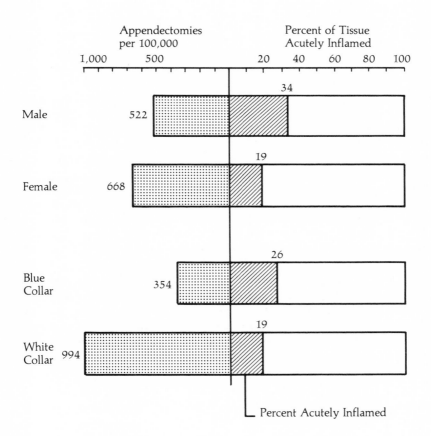

Source and Note: Lichtner and Pflanz 1971, Tables 3, 4, and 7, pp. 317, 318, and 322. I adjusted the rates in order to remove the effect of different proportions of men and women in the two occupational groups.

Chart 4–14

In this chart we continue our examination of the effects of the personal attributes of clients on surgical rates by introducing a new indicator of quality and then by expanding that concept. The indicator of quality is the training and status of the surgeon, and by using that indicator we raise questions not only about the justification of surgery but also about the quality of surgical technique and management.

The panel on the left-hand side of the chart shows that in one urban hospital black patients admitted for cholecystectomy or hernia repair were much more likely to be operated upon by resident staff than were white patients. It also shows that this situation has not changed much over a period of 20 years in the recent past. In the panel on the right-hand side, the secular trend is depicted as a percentage change relative to the values for 1952. Between 1952 and 1962 the experience of blacks remained relatively unchanged, whereas whites experienced some increase in the proportion of surgery done by the resident staff. After 1962 there was a decline in the ratio for both blacks and whites, possibly due to the introduction of Medicare and Medicaid.

The authors believe that ability to pay is not the only factor in the differential allocation of patients, since irrespective of whether the patient has private health insurance, or seeks care in the emergency service of the hospital, blacks are more likely to be assigned to the resident staff than are apparently comparable whites. The authors also argue that the surgical care given by residents is expected, on the average, to be of lower quality than that given by the average attending surgeon. Unfortunately, this allegation, though a reasonable one, is not supported by an examination of either the process or the outcomes of care. Some subsequent charts will provide conflicting information on this matter. But no realistic observer can doubt that our medical care system is markedly differentiated along socioeconomic lines.

Chart 4-14

Percentages and Relative Percentages of Patients of Specified Race Who have Inguinal Hernia Repairs and Cholecystectomies Performed by Resident Staff. The Johns Hopkins Hospital, Baltimore, Maryland, 1952–1972.

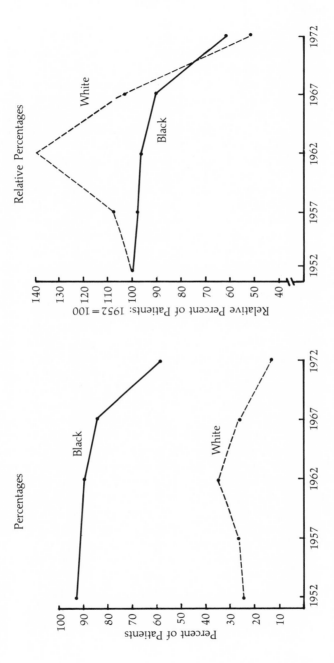

Source: Egbert and Rothman 1977, Table 1, p. 90. I computed the relative percentages.

Chart 4–15

The behavior of physicians as informed consumers of health services has been suggested by some as one means of identifying good quality. For example, Maloney et al. (1960) have suggested that the characteristics of physicians chosen by other physicians for their own care, and that of their families, can be taken to stand for care of better quality, even though, as Bynder (1968) has argued, physicians may not always be free to seek the best care available. The study from which this chart is derived has the somewhat broader purpose of studying surgical care among several occupational groups. This particular chart, however, addresses the standards of surgical care enjoyed by the wives of physicians in comparison to the generality of women in the United States. There is also a comparison with women in the Oxford area of England.

Each of the three curves in the chart shows the percent of women who have had a hysterectomy by the time they attain any given age. Though they start a little later, the probability of having a hysterectomy increases so rapidly among the wives of physicians that by age 65 over half of them will have had the operation. This compares with 33 percent for all women in the United States, and 17 percent for women in the Oxford area. In another analysis, the investigators show that cumulative appendectomy rates for males in the United States and in the Oxford area are very similar at successive ages, but that those for male physicians in Santa Clara County (California) are considerably higher, and that the difference begins to show at age ten.

The investigators wonder whether the higher surgical rates for physicians and their wives are the norms which will eventually prevail for everyone else. If, as many believe, a considerable proportion of hysterectomies and appendectomies in the United States are "unnecessary," can we expect an even greater incidence of unnecessary surgery? On the contrary, are there advantages to at least some of the operations that physicians and their wives now enjoy and that others can now only aspire to? In other words, what is the appropriate propensity to operate?

In a note on method, the investigators warn that these comparisons "must be regarded with some caution, since the national and Oxford figures represent cross-sectional data obtained on a population at a given point in time, whereas the data on physicians and their wives represent life-history information on each subject . . ." (p. 1053).

Chart 4-15

The Percent of Women Who Can Be Expected To Have Had a Hysterectomy by the Time They Attain Specified Ages. Wives of Physicians, Santa Clara County, California, 1968; All Women, U.S.A., 1968; and All Women, the Oxford Area of England, 1962–1965.

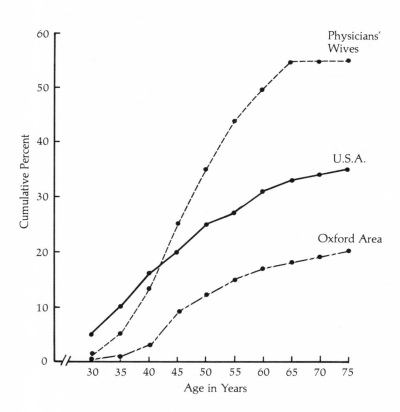

Source: Bunker and Brown 1974, Figure 2, p. 1053. Reprinted, by permission of the *New England Journal of Medicine* (290:1051–55, 1974).

Chart 4–16

The characteristics of providers are also an important influence on surgical rates. We have already seen that the availability of surgeons tends to increase surgical rates, possibly beyond the level of optimal usefulness. One also finds that a relatively small proportion of surgeons accounts for a large proportion of surgical procedures.

This chart is in the form of a Lorenz curve, produced by first arranging physicians who performed one or more tonsillectomies by the number of such operations that they performed during 1969–1971, and then plotting the cumulative percent of physicians against the cumulative percent of the total of tonsillectomies performed by these physicians. Had all the physicians performed equal numbers of operations, the plot would have been the diagonal shown in the chart. A curvilinear plot indicates inequality in the contribution of several surgeons to the total number of tonsillectomies. The more curvilinear the plot, the larger the inequality, the area enclosed between the curve and the diagonal being a measure of inequality.

The phenomenon depicted in this chart has already been described and discussed under the headings of "service concentration" and "error concentration," for example in connection with Charts 3–1 and 3–4. Gittelsohn and Wennberg comment as follows on their own findings:

> More than 80% of the procedures were carried out by two dozen practitioners and more than half of all cases were accounted for by 10 physicians. . . . For the most part, T&A's are not referred, with nearly 90% of the cases performed by local physicians in the hospital serving the residence community. The tonsillectomy rates in the smaller communities of the state thus primarily reflect the decision processes and efforts of a small number of physicians practicing in the local hospital. Such localization is the key to understanding the wide variance in tonsillectomy rates in the 13 hospital service areas. (pp. 98–99)

Eleven of the 13 service areas are served by one hospital and the rest by two each. These hospitals could also be held accountable for the appropriateness of the surgical rates in their respective areas. Gittelsohn and Wennberg point out that "there are major differences in procedure rates, types of procedures performed, and diagnostic labeling between areas served by teaching and community hospitals. Towns, primarily feeding patients into teaching hospitals, experience low overall rates, while there is a wide variance in rates between the community hospital areas" (pp. 99–100).

Chart 4–16

Number and Percent of Physicians Who Perform Specified Percentages of All Tonsillectomies and Adenoidectomies. Persons 25 and Younger, and Physicians Who Perform One or More Such Operations, Vermont, 1969–1971.

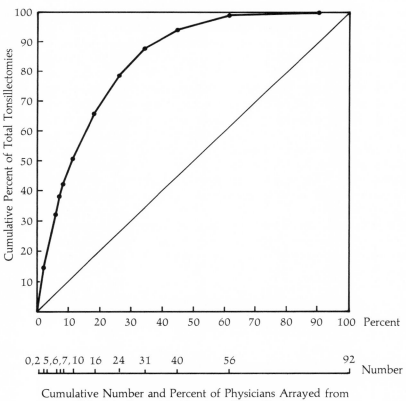

Cumulative Number and Percent of Physicians Arrayed from
Highest to Lowest in Number of Tonsillectomies
and Adenoidectomies Performed

Source: Gittelsohn and Wennberg 1977, Table 7.2, p. 96.

Chart 4–17

The remarkable concentration of the performance of tonsillectomies in the hands of relatively few surgeons (as shown in the previous chart) can be regarded as an example of a more general phenomenon, which is illustrated in this chart. The chart shows the percent distribution of physicians who performed one or more operations during 1970, by the annual number of operations that they performed. This is shown graphically in two ways: as a histogram and as a cumulative distribution. For example, one can tell from the curve of cumulative distribution that 65.3 percent of those who operated during 1970 did fewer than 100 operations a year, or about two a week. Similarly, from the histogram one can tell that 39.8 percent did less than 25 operations, and that 10.8 percent did between 25 and 49 operations.

The observation that many surgeons do very little surgery, whereas others do a great deal, has led to a variety of inferences. One is that those who do a lot may tend to operate unnecessarily. Another is that those who do little may not do enough to remain competent, especially when they attempt the more complex, less common operations. Still another inference is that we have an excess of surgeons, which would explain why many of them are not fully occupied. Although physicians are supposed to be able to generate a demand for their own services, perhaps surgeons, who more often have to depend on referrals, are less able to do so. Alternatively, though it is suspected that a great deal of unnecessary surgery takes place, some surgeons may be underoccupied because they resist the temptation, while others succumb to it *because* they are underoccupied!

The definition of what constitutes a surgical operation is critical to these findings, as is an adjustment for the complexity of the procedures—an adjustment that the investigators make in another part of their analysis. Physicians who do surgery also do other work that may not be well represented by the number of operations performed. Surgeons acquire patients as they mature. While the data shown in the chart exclude interns and residents, they do reflect the differences among surgeons at different stages of their careers. Finally, the illustrative areas selected for this study may not be fully representative of the United States as a whole. The reader is referred to the original publication for a consideration of these and other issues.

Chart 4-17

Percent Distribution and Cumulative Percent Distribution of Physicians by Number of Annual, In-Hospital Surgical Operations. Physicians Who Performed One or More Such Operations, Four Selected Areas within Three Geographic Regions, U.S.A., 1970.

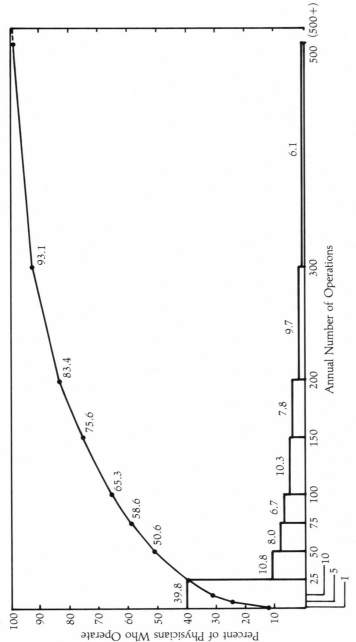

Source: Nickerson et al. 1976, Table 3, p. 923.

Chart 4–18

The postulates that there is a relationship between the prevalence of surgeons and surgical rates that is not entirely justifiable, and that the workloads of some surgeons may be too large while those of others are too small, are related to still another postulate. This asserts that surgeons are influenced in their decisions to operate by the financial rewards of doing so. Thus surgeons who are underemployed strive to generate a demand for their services, and some surgeons attempt to do more than they should.

This chart pertains to the question of financial incentives. It is derived from a study of the surgical services received by members of the United Steelworkers Union in seven regions of the United States. These workers were covered by a contract providing uniform benefits in all regions. There was free choice of physician, and physicians were paid according to a fee-for-service schedule. Physicians, however, tended to charge patients fees beyond the scheduled fee paid by the insurance plan. The chart shows that the frequency with which such additional fees were charged was inversely related to the frequency with which surgery was performed. In regions where extra charges were infrequent, surgical operations were much more frequent; where extra charges were frequent, surgical operations were much less frequent.

What one sees, of course, is the traditional relationship between price and demand. In this instance it can be assumed, though there is no direct evidence to support it, that members of the union in all regions were reasonably similar and that their health status was generally comparable. If so, the differences observed do not reflect differences in need but the impact of different pricing practices. It is difficult to say whether these represent differences in costs to the physician, in the content or quality of care, or in the expectations of physicians for income. One plausible explanation is that physicians have considerable control over their prices and may elect to achieve a satisfactory income either through performing more procedures at lower price or fewer procedures at higher price. (For more see Donabedian 1976, Chapter 2, and especially pp. 64–71.)

The seven geographic areas shown in the chart are, reading from left to right: Minnesota (various areas); Michigan (various areas); Detroit, Michigan; Pennsylvania (Bethlehem and Allentown); Western Pennsylvania; Ohio (Cleveland, Youngstown, etc.); and Illinois (Chicago and nearby).

Chart 4–18

Geographic Areas by Rates for Nonobstetrical Surgery and by Frequency of Additional Charges by Surgeons. Members of the United Steelworkers Union Covered by Blue Shield Contracts, U.S.A., July 1, 1957—June 30, 1958.

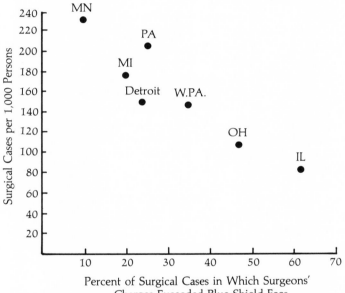

Source: United Steelworkers of America, 1960, p. 75.

Chart 4–19

After what may have been a surfeit of epidemiological data on the incidence of surgery, we will end with a piece of dessert which, however, provides much food for thought. Accordingly, the next chart shows the epidemiological and experimental findings of a study designed by Raymond Franzen and conducted under the auspices of the American Child Health Association, with financial support from the Metropolitan Life Insurance Company and with the full cooperation of the departments of Education and Health of New York City. The study is an old one, but as we shall see repeatedly in this book, age only adds luster to studies of classic elegance and continuing relevance.

In this case, an examination of a sample of 1,000 eleven-year-old children in 11 New York City schools showed that 611 had already had a tonsillectomy, as illustrated in the first bar of the chart. Two physicians (out of a pool of 20 school medical examiners) were sent later to each school to examine, using their usual procedures, all 389 children who had not already had a tonsillectomy. As a result, there were two independent judgments as to whether each of these children needed a tonsillectomy. The second bar in the chart shows that as a result of one examination an additional 174 children were found to require tonsillectomy. This is 45 percent of those children who still had their tonsils. The result of the examination by the second physician was to add another 99 students who were thought to require tonsillectomy, as shown in the third bar of the chart. This is 46 percent of the children whom the first physician had not already judged to require a tonsillectomy. After these two examinations only 116 students remained who were judged by both examiners to be capable of retaining their tonsils. But, when this hardy remnant was examined by still another physician from an entirely different group of examiners, an additional 51 children (or 44 percent of the remnant) were found to require a tonsillectomy. After three examinations by three different physicians only 65 children remained free of any tonsillar taint. Thus, the 45 percent law of tonsillectomy inexorably took successive bites out of a population of children until almost no tonsils remained to be extirpated!

Chart 4–19

Number and Percent of 11-Year Old Children Who Were either Found To Have Had a Tonsillectomy or for Whom Tonsillectomy Was Recommended at Specified School Medical Examinations. Eleven Schools in New York City, 1933.

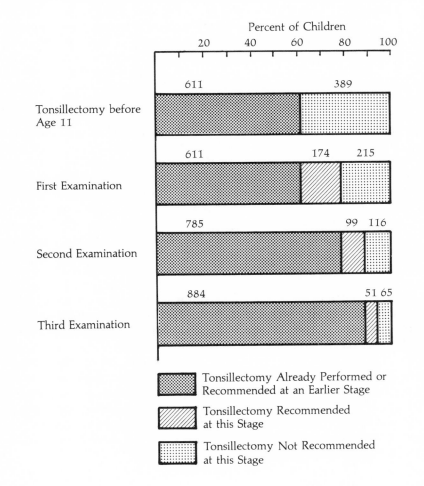

Source and Note: American Child Health Association 1934, Figure 10, p. 84. The numbers of children are shown over each of the bars.

Chart 4–20

This first chart in the series of retrospective studies of the justification of surgery serves as a convenient bridge to this section because it is so similar to some of the material shown in the preceding one. Here, 19 hospitals in Southwest Michigan are arranged in descending order according to the proportion of all primary appendectomies in each hospital that yielded tissue which the pathologist judged to show "no disease." The chart also shows the range of variation in normal tissue removal found among the surgeons in each hospital. It is obvious that the several surgeons in each hospital differ widely in this regard, and that the average performance of the surgical staff as a whole differs widely among hospitals.

A more rigorous analysis would have corrected for demographic and socioeconomic differences among the patients of each surgeon and hospital, and would have indicated how much of the remaining variability might easily have arisen by chance. One suspects, however, that these refinements would have been inadequate to explain why one surgeon removed normal tissue in over 70 percent of the appendectomies he performed, whereas at the other extreme there were surgeons in several hospitals who removed no normal tissue at all. If 70 percent is too high a proportion, one wonders if zero percent is too low. How is one to tell?

It is also unlikely that the judgments of the pathologists are always accurate, or that they are equally accurate or inaccurate across hospitals.

These data come from the archives of the Commission on Professional and Hospital Activities in Ann Arbor. The Commission sells a service which permits a hospital to send in coded abstracts of its medical charts and to get back tabulations that show many aspects of the performance of the hospital and of its physicians. Comparisons among departments and physicians are easily made. The commission can also provide information about the performance of a given hospital as compared to others that are similar to it. These data are useful for epidemiological studies, for administrative management, and for quality assessment and assurance. Studies that have used these data will be encountered repeatedly in this book.

Chart 4–20

Percent of Primary Appendectomies in which "No Disease" Was Reported After Pathological Examination of the Removed Tissues. Surgeons in each of 19 Selected Hospitals, Southwest Michigan, 1956–1957.

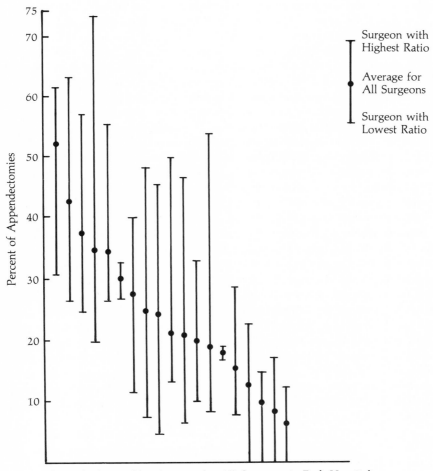

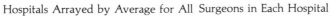

Hospitals Arrayed by Average for All Surgeons in Each Hospital

Source: Weeks, undated.

Chart 4–21

For this chart, the hospitals in Baltimore were classified into two categories: those that were affiliated with a medical school ("university hospitals") and those that were not ("community hospitals"). Then, in each category of hospitals, patients were classified according to the source of payment for their care. The chart shows, for each of the eight resulting classes of patients, the percent of appendectomies for which the pathologist reported the removed tissue to be either not diseased or doubtfully diseased.

In looking at the lightly shaded bars in the chart, one finds that the proportion of appendectomies in university hospitals that yield essentially normal tissue does not vary appreciably according to the source of payment. For reasons that we could speculate about, the university hospitals are insensitive to this variable. But one also notices that even in a university hospital over 30 percent of primary appendectomies yield essentially normal tissue. Is all of this correctable "error"? Is some of it correctable error and the remainder a justifiable, even necessary, margin needed to make sure that few cases with diseased appendices are missed? We do not as yet know. While we search for an answer (as we shall) we could decide to accept the removal of normal tissue in 30 percent of appendectomies as an "empirically derived" standard by which the performance of other hospitals can be judged. By this criterion, the surgeons in the community hospitals, taken as a group, remove normal tissue too often. Even more remarkable is the association in a community hospital between the likelihood of performing an appendectomy that yields normal tissue and the source of payment for the operation. This likelihood is lowest for patients on welfare who, most probably, are cared for by the house staff. It is higher for patients who pay for their own care, still higher for patients who have health insurance other than Blue Cross, and highest for persons who have Blue Cross insurance. This progression suggests that in cases that are not clear-cut, there may be a financial incentive for the surgeon to recommend, and for the patient to accept, an appendectomy when the patient has adequate health insurance coverage.

Unfortunately, there is no way to tell how comparable the patients in the several categories are. And we can only speculate about what biases, if any, have been introduced by the pathologists in the several institutions. Finally, the data come in a manner that does not permit statistical testing.

Chart 4-21

Percent of Apendectomies Classified by Pathological Examination as "Unnecessary" or "Doubtful" in Two University and Three Community Hospitals, by Type of Hospital and by Source of Payment for Care, Baltimore, Maryland, 1957 and 1958.

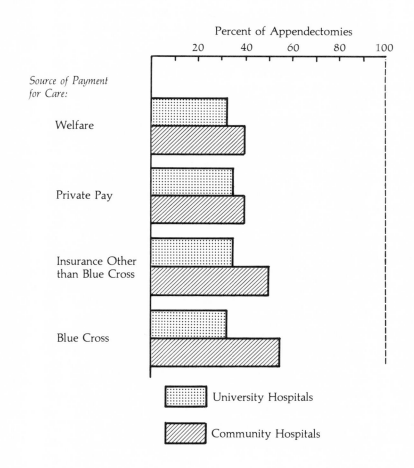

Source: Sparling 1962, Figure 3, p. 67. Used by permission, American Hospital Association.

Chart 4–22

The study from which this chart is derived is an early example of the concern for unjustified hysterectomies. It also begins to extend the basis for assessing whether surgery is justified or not. Though the absence of pathological findings continues to be the key factor, this investigator also took into account the presence of signs and symptoms that may have justified the operation. "It was difficult to establish hard and fast criteria for justification for hysterectomy," but the investigator made a "critical evaluation of each hysterectomy" and classified each case accordingly (p. 364).

One sees that 39 percent of all hysterectomies in all the 36 hospitals studied were open to criticism, whereas 61 percent were probably justified. The chart also illustrates the remarkable variability in hospital performance by showing the findings in the four hospitals at each end of the distribution. In the four hospitals with the worst performance, only 24 percent of hysterectomies seemed to be justified. Not shown in the chart is the investigator's judgment that even among the operations that were justified, some could be criticized because the uterus was removed abdominally when a vaginal operation would have been preferable.

The completeness of the operation is also an important issue. If the cervix (neck) of the uterus is not removed with the rest of the organ, the patient remains exposed to the risk of subsequent cancer in this part. In this group of cases, gynecologists performed 31 percent of hysterectomies, general surgeons performed 36 percent, and general practitioners performed 33 percent. The percent of subtotal hysterectomy was 35 percent when performed by gynecologists, 50 percent when performed by general surgeons, and 72 percent when performed by general practitioners. In an earlier study of unnecessary hysterectomies that was the prototype of this one, Miller (1946) concedes that, in the hands of an experienced surgeon, total hysterectomy is a better choice because the added risk of removing the entire organ is less than the risk of later cancer in the cervix, when that part is left in place. "While this advantage seems real and sufficient enough to many of us," he goes on to say, "I question whether it justifies the potential added risk to the patient entailed by forcing total hysterectomy upon the occasional operator" (p. 807). It is important to remember that the best quality in the abstract may not be the best in any particular situation.

Chart 4-22

Percent Distribution of Hysterectomies by Judgments Concerning the Justifiability of the Operation. A Selection of 35 Nongovernmental Hospitals, California, 1948.

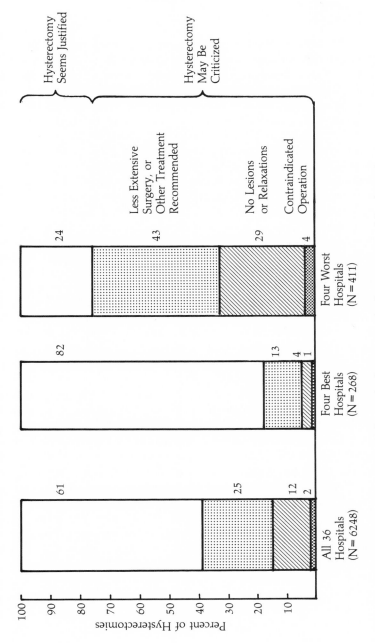

Source: Doyle 1953, Table 4, p. 364. I computed the weighted percentages for the two groups of four hospitals.

Chart 4–23

The work represented by this chart is a major landmark in the development of quality assessment and has earned for Lembcke a secure place among the leading pioneers in that enterprise. It is presented at this point because it illustrates the justification of surgery by a still larger set of considerations beyond the pathological findings in the tissues removed at operation. The central significance of the work, however, rests on those features that Lembcke hoped would make it a "scientific method" for quality assessment: one that would produce valid, reproducible judgments. The procedures used to achieve this goal included (1) a very precise specification of discrete diagnostic categories, (2) a specification of the aspects of care to be judged (for example, justification of surgery, completeness of the operation, necessity for hospitalization, and so on), (3) an explicit, detailed specification of criteria in advance of making any judgments about each of these aspects of care, and (4) where necessary, checks on the validity and reliability of basic diagnostic information, such as that contained in pathological or radiological reports. But Lembcke recognized that, in spite of all these refinements, the method might misjudge some cases because the criteria could not be hoped to allow for all possible contingencies. Therefore, he introduced a factor of "tolerance." This was done by specifying that the percent of cases that should comply with the criteria need not be greater than a given percentage, which generally represented the observed level of compliance in a good teaching hospital.

The findings shown in this chart document the very high ratio of criticized gynecological operations in this one hospital. We can also see that the audit, conducted by an examiner from outside the hospital, had a remarkable effect in reducing operations that were criticized without, however, influencing the frequency of those that were justified. Lembcke says that these results were obtained "without drastic disciplinary measures." During the second and third quarters of the study, surgeons who were not doing well were spoken to. Later, the criteria were distributed to everyone. The excellent response suggests that the surgeons knew what needed to be done but had perhaps grown careless in their work. Unfortunately, the problem is not always this simple, nor the results of quality monitoring so favorable.

Chart 4–23

Number of Justified and Criticized Operations on the Uterus, Ovary, and Fallopian Tubes that Resulted in Sterilization or Castration. One Hospital, U.S.A., circa 1954.

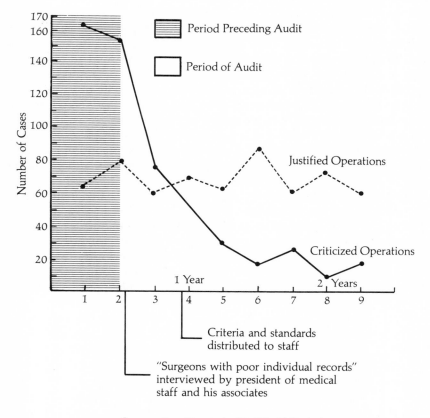

Consecutive Quarterly (13-Week) Periods

Chart 4–24

McCarthy, Finkel, and Ruchlin report that, on the average, 18.7 percent of all recommendations for elective surgery are not confirmed by a consultant's "second opinion." This is based on a study of 6,799 consultations in several mandatory programs in the greater New York City area during an eight-year period, 1972–1980.

This chart shows the large variation according to diagnosis that the overall average conceals. Here we encounter some surgical operations, such as hysterectomies, which we have already learned to look upon with suspicion. Our attention is also drawn to some new categories that we need to be alert to: for example, certain orthopedic operations and prostatectomy. What is interesting is that some other procedures are found not to merit all their notoriety. Among these are varicose vein surgery and tonsillectomy. But the number of these operations is so large that even a modest proportion of unjustified excess can add up to a large amount of waste. This reminds us that the procedures that demand relatively greater attention are those that have a higher proportion of nonconfirmation, are frequent, are costly, and are associated with a high ratio of expected risk to expected benefit.

In this chart I have taken the precaution of showing the line that indicates 100 percent, so as to create an accurate visual image of the ratio of nonconfirmed cases. This also gives me the opportunity to warn the reader that a graph may present a distorted image of the facts—often unintentionally, but sometimes in order to manipulate or mislead.

Chart 4-24

Percent of Recommendations for Surgery of Specified Categories that Were Not Confirmed by Surgical Consultants. Selected Mandatory Second Opinion Programs, Greater New York City Area, 1972–1980.

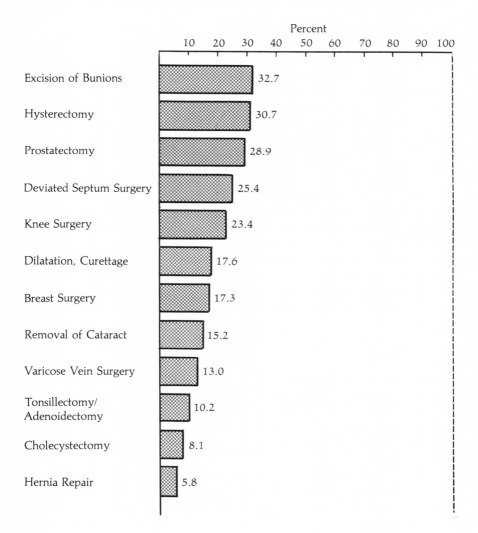

Percent

| | 10 | 20 | 30 | 40 | 50 | 60 | 70 | 80 | 90 | 100 |

Excision of Bunions — 32.7

Hysterectomy — 30.7

Prostatectomy — 28.9

Deviated Septum Surgery — 25.4

Knee Surgery — 23.4

Dilatation, Curettage — 17.6

Breast Surgery — 17.3

Removal of Cataract — 15.2

Varicose Vein Surgery — 13.0

Tonsillectomy/ Adenoidectomy — 10.2

Cholecystectomy — 8.1

Hernia Repair — 5.8

Source: McCarthy, Finkel, and Ruchlin 1981, Table 3-3, p. 39.

Chart 4–25

The variation in the nonconfirmation ratio by type of procedure which was illustrated in the preceding chart is mirrored in the variation by specialty shown in this one.

On the right-hand side of the chart we see the variability in the non-confirmation ratio according to the specialty of the consultant who offers the second opinion. Since cases are referred to consultants in keeping with some prior agreement on the legitimate domains of the several specialties, the results reflect the relative susceptibility to differences of opinion about the justifiability of surgery in these domains of practice. It is also likely that the several consultants differ in the stringency of their criteria and standards, and that this attribute is to some degree correlated with specialty.

On the left-hand side of the chart one sees the ratios of nonconfir-mation by the specialty of the surgeon who made the initial recommen-dation. The discrepancy between some of the corresponding bars on the two sides of the chart suggests that a difference of opinion about the justifiability of surgery is more frequent when a procedure is recom-mended or done by someone outside the specialty considered to have jurisdiction over that procedure. This is quite apparent in the domain of orthopedics. The observed discrepancy probably occurs because the reviewing consultant is an orthopedist, whereas many of the operations are proposed by practitioners who are not orthopedists. In a recent pa-per, Finkel, McCarthy, and Miller (1982) report findings that support this conjecture by showing that in one second opinion program 72 percent of recommendations for foot surgery were made by podiatrists. When the consultant who reviewed the initial recommendation for surgery was a podiatrist, 95 percent of these recommendations were confirmed; but only 50 percent were confirmed when the reviewing consultant was a board-certified orthopedic surgeon. As a result of this experience, and the additional observation that the podiatrist consultants were more likely to order additional tests, including X-ray examinations, those respon-sible for the second opinion program decided not to use podiatrists as consultants.

More generally speaking, however, McCarthy, Finkel, and Ruchlin report that the nonconfirmation ratio for all surgical procedures was not significantly higher when the initial recommendation was made by an internist, as compared to a surgeon, or when it was made by a surgeon who was not board-certified, as compared to one who was.

Chart 4–25

Percent of Recommendations for Surgery that Were Not Confirmed by Surgical Consultants, by the Specialty of the Surgeon Making the Initial Recommendation, and by the Specialty of the Consultant Surgeon. Selected Mandatory Second Opinion Programs, Greater New York City Area, 1972 – 1980.

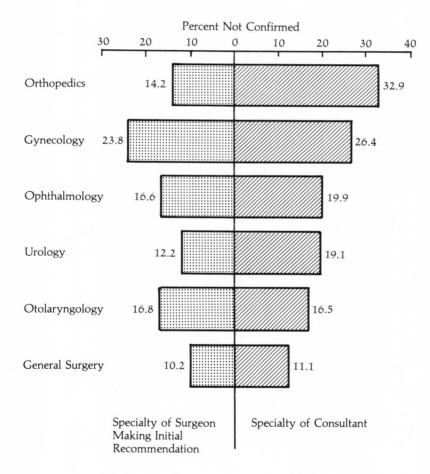

Source: McCarthy, Finkel, and Ruchlin 1981, Tables 3-4 and 3-5, pp. 40–41.

Chart 4–26

This chart offers an example of the reasons given for not confirming an initial recommendation for surgery.

From February 1972 through April 1979, the researchers at Cornell University Medical College had information about 1,055 patients who sought a second opinion concerning the appropriateness of elective gynecological surgery, either voluntarily or because of a mandatory second opinion program. The board-certified gynecologists who served as consultants refused to confirm the need for surgery in 38.3 percent of voluntary and 24.7 percent of mandatory referrals. The chart summarizes the consultants' reasons for refusing to confirm in almost 93 percent of the nonconfirmed cases known to have occurred during this period. The explanations are inferences made by the research staff based on the consultants' notes. I have further classified the categories reported by McCarthy and Finkel into two groups, one suggesting questions concerning the original diagnosis and the other questioning the treatment recommended.

If the judgment of the consultant is accepted as valid, one would conclude that surgery is clearly unnecessary whenever the consultant says that there is no apparent pathology to justify it. Fourteen percent of cases fall in this category. For the rest, the situation is not so clear-cut. It is this ambiguity that permits differences of opinion as well as "honest" mistakes. This is also the main reason for urging collegiate consultation. The purpose of quality monitoring is not to discover and stop fraud (though it can do that) but to redirect the practice of honest practitioners into more strictly appropriate channels.

The chart shows another important finding. Often the consultant neither approves nor disapproves surgery, but recommends additional investigation and observation, leaving open the possibility of surgery being needed later on. As another possibility, the consultant may recommend that either the original procedure or an alternative one be done on an outpatient basis, reducing the cost to the insurer and, perhaps, to the patient as well.

Chart 4–26

Percent of Patients for Whom a Recommendation To Have Gynecological Surgery Was Not Confirmed by Gynecologist Consultants, Distributed According to the Inferred Reasons for Nonconfirmation. Greater New York City Area, February 1972–April 1979.

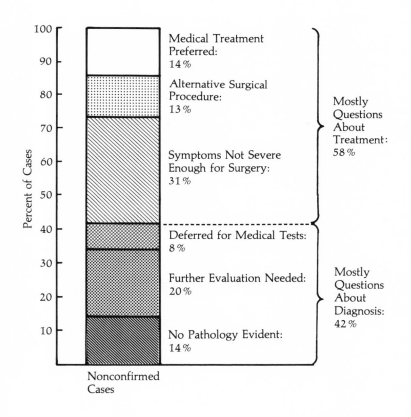

Source: McCarthy and Finkel 1980b, Table 5, p. 408, with my diagnostic and therapeutic groupings.

Chart 4–27

The proponents of second opinion programs must show that these can reduce the incidence of surgery and do so selectively, only through a reduction of "unnecessary" surgery, so that the patients are not harmed. More realistically, they must show that the programs do more good than harm, and that the net monetary benefit is greater than the monetary cost. Some of these issues are addressed in this chart and in the next two.

In the first bar of this chart we see that in 18.7 percent of cases the consultants do not confirm the initial recommendation to have surgery. In the second bar we see a picture of what has happened to confirmed and nonconfirmed cases during the six months following the consultants' judgment. We note first that the second surgical opinion seems to have made a difference. Patients whose need for an operation was confirmed had surgery in 85.9 percent of cases ($69.8 \div 81.3 \times 100$); those whose need was not confirmed had an operation in only 32.6 percent of cases ($6.1 \div 18.7 \times 100$). The noncompliance represented by the latter has its counterpart in the confirmed group. Of these, 14.1 percent failed to have surgery even though it was recommended once by their own doctor and again by the consultant.

Because there is no control group of patients, we are not certain of the net effect of the second surgical opinion. The observed incidence of surgery in this group was 75.9 percent, which is only 10 percent lower than the 85.9 percent among those whose need for surgery was endorsed by the second opinion. Since this confirming opinion is likely to have encouraged some reluctant patients to accept surgery, we can surmise that the program's effect must be something smaller than a ten percent reduction for these patients. And since these are candidates for "elective" surgery, and only some of these at that, the effect of second opinion programs on all surgical interventions must be even smaller than the foregoing estimates. But in addition to reducing the incidence of "elective" surgery, the program has produced a more favorable mix of operations, by encouraging surgery recommended by the consultant and discouraging surgery that the consultant does not confirm. There may also be a "sentinel effect," which is a subject we shall return to.

The findings of follow-up beyond the first six months are not revealing because most of the effect occurs soon after the second opinion; also, the later course of events is clouded by the difficulties of remaining in touch with the original group of patients.

Chart 4–27

Percent Distribution of Persons Who Had an Initial Recommendation for Surgery, by the Nature of the Second Opinion of the Consultant; and the Percent Distribution of Persons at Subsequent Follow-up, by the Consultants' Opinion, and by Whether or Not Surgery Was Done. Selected Mandatory Second Opinion Programs, Greater New York City Area, 1972–1980.

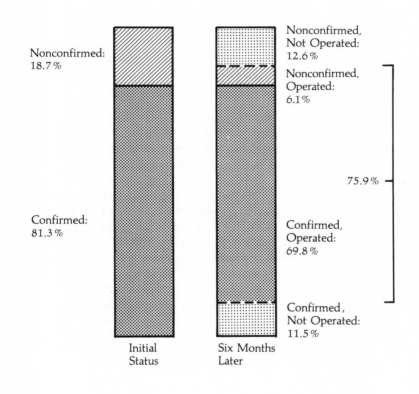

Nonconfirmed: 18.7%

Confirmed: 81.3%

Initial Status

Nonconfirmed, Not Operated: 12.6%

Nonconfirmed, Operated: 6.1%

75.9%

Confirmed, Operated: 69.8%

Confirmed, Not Operated: 11.5%

Six Months Later

Source: McCarthy, Finkel, and Ruchlin 1981, Tables 3-2 and 4-2, pp. 38 and 50, with minor computations.

Chart 4–28

This chart shows that noncompliance with the recommendations of the consultant who provides the second surgical opinion varies markedly by the type of procedure in question.

The right-hand side of the chart shows the percent of persons who went ahead and had the operation even though the consultant surgeon had disagreed with the earlier recommendation of the patient's own doctor. Noncompliance occurred in about a third of all cases, varying between 8.3 percent for knee surgery and a remarkably high 52.6 percent for hysterectomies. When questioned about noncompliance, 80 percent of patients said they decided to ignore the consultant's opinion because their symptoms either persisted or worsened. An additional 12 percent simply decided to follow the initial advice of their own doctors. In the majority of cases the operation was done within 90 days of the second, disapproving, opinion.

The left-hand side of the chart shows another kind of noncompliance: the decision not to have the operation even though two doctors (the patient's own as well as the consultant) recommended surgery. This happened in 14.2 percent of all cases, and it varied in frequency from none (for knee surgery) to 26.7 percent (for surgery of the foot, excluding bunionectomy).

When questioned about this behavior, eight percent of patients said the symptoms had disappeared, 51 percent said either that the condition was tolerable or that they thought surgery could be postponed, 12 percent feared surgery or thought it was too risky, and 14 percent mistakenly thought that the consultant had said the operation was not needed. Another 15 percent had consulted still another (third) doctor and were, ostensibly, following his advice not to have the operation.

The reasons for having or not having an operation obviously come into play to different degrees for different procedures. But the absence of a discernible correlation between the two sides of the chart precludes a simple explanation of the nature and degree of noncompliance.

Chart 4-28

Percent of Cases, Classified by Type of Procedure, Who Had Not Complied with the Recommendations of the Consulting Surgeons within Six Months. Selected Second Opinion Programs, Greater New York City Area, 1972–1980.

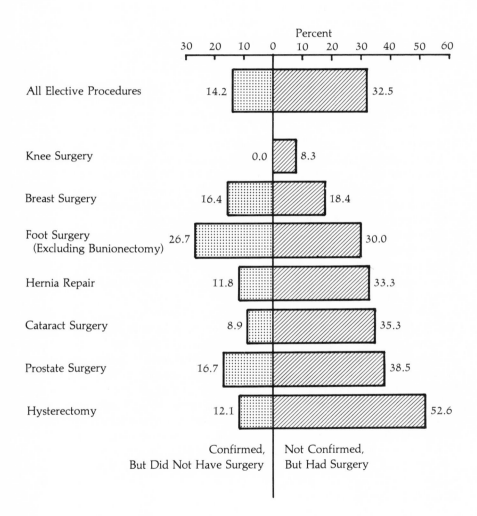

Source: McCarthy, Finkel, and Ruchlin 1981, Tables 4-3 and 4-4, pp. 52 and 53.

Chart 4–29

We are also indebted to McCarthy, Finkel, and Ruchlin for one of the few studies of the monetary costs and benefits of quality monitoring activities. The study is restricted to the experience of one mandatory second opinion program. It includes all persons 15 years old or older who had an initial recommendation to have surgery between January 1, 1977 and December 31, 1978, and it takes account of the subsequent experience of this cohort during 1979. There were 2,284 patients in all, the consultants having confirmed the need for surgery in 1,918, and declined to confirm it in 366. The analysis includes 342 of the nonconfirmed cases.

The second bar of the chart shows the best estimates of the actual costs incurred by the 342 patients whose need for surgery was not confirmed. The costs are made up of two categories: resource use and productivity loss. The former are expenditures for medical care, including those for surgery done contrary to the consultants' judgments, while the latter includes the monetary value of work loss, of restricted activity, and of travel.

The first bar of the chart is an estimate of what the costs incurred by the 342 nonconfirmed cases would have been in the absence of a second opinion program. To obtain the estimate, it was assumed that the nonconfirmed patients would have behaved as did the cases for whom the need for surgery was confirmed. The data were derived, therefore, from the actual experience of 342 patients randomly sampled from the confirmed group.

The difference between the costs incurred by the two groups, each made up of 342 patients, is the benefit attributable to the second opinion program. The cost of the program is made up of three elements: expenditures directly attributed to the consultation, the cost of time and travel needed to obtain the consultation, and the administrative cost of the second opinion program. The savings are the difference between the benefits and the costs. The cost–benefit ratio is $(1,135,950 - 601,159) \div (203,300) = 2.63$. This means that for every dollar spent, the program yields \$2.63. When the savings of \$331,491 are divided by the 2,284 patients in the cohort, one finds a saving of \$145.14 for each patient who obtains a second opinion. My own calculations suggest that this represents a net reduction of about five percent in the expected cost of elective surgery in this population.

Chart 4–29

Estimates of the Observed Costs of Elective Surgery with a Mandatory Second Surgical Opinion Program, and of the Expected Costs without Such a Program, and of the Costs and Savings Attributed to the Program. Welfare Fund of the Building Service Local 32B-J, New York City, January 1, 1977– December 31, 1979.

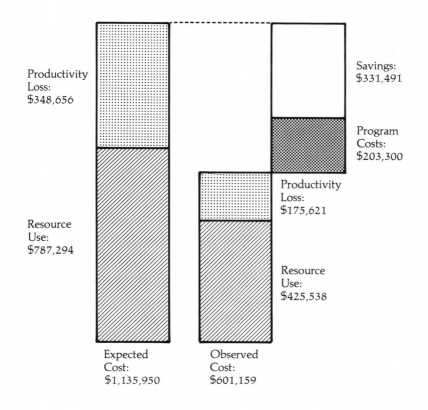

Source: McCarthy, Finkel, and Ruchlin 1981, Tables 6-2, 6-12 and 6-23, pp. 117, 134 and 147.

Chart 4–30

For an estimate of the magnitude of the "sentinel effect" we go to a study by Martin et al. (1980, 1982) of the effects of a mandatory second surgical opinion program for Medicaid beneficiaries in Massachusetts that included eight elective procedures. The chart shows only the data for hysterectomies, and in only one geographic area. The first two bars of the chart show the incidence of hysterectomy in the study area and a comparison area before the introduction of the program in the former. By comparing the second pair of bars with the first pair, we can see a 23 percent reduction in the incidence of surgery in the study area after the institution of the program there, whereas the comparison area (the "non-equivalent control") shows only a six percent reduction. Because this latter change was not statistically significant, while the change in the study area was, the entire difference in incidence rates in the study area (17.10–13.10) was considered to be caused by the program, even though this could be an overestimate.

The more direct effect of the program, that of dissuading patients from having an operation that the consultant has not approved, is very difficult to estimate because patients both comply and fail to comply with the approvals as well as the disapprovals of the consultant. To allow for the likelihood that some of the nonconfirmed cases would not have had an operation even in the absence of the program, the investigators used the noncompliance ratio for confirmed cases to compute a "minimum estimate" of the direct effect of the program. Accordingly, 37 percent of the total reduction in the incidence of hysterectomy is attributed to a direct effect on patients.

The final bar of the chart shows a subdivision of the total *expected* incidence of hysterectomies in the study area into (1) the 76.6 percent that actually took place, (2) the 8.7 percent reduction attributed to the direct effect, and (3) the 14.6 percent reduction attributed to the "sentinel effect," which occurs because some future recommendations for surgery are discouraged. These findings are illustrative rather than representative, since, as Martin et al. show, there are large differences by type of operation and population, and estimates are markedly affected by the assumptions and methods of the analysis. Furthermore, the underemployed surgeon may make up for doing less of some operations by doing more of others that are not so closely monitored. Is there a "compensatory effect" as well as a "sentinel effect"?

Chart 4–30

Hysterectomy Rates Before and After the Introduction of a Mandatory Second Surgical Opinion Program. Medicaid Beneficiaries, Bay State Area and a "Nonequivalent Control" Area, Massachusetts, May 1, 1975–December 30, 1978, and May 1, 1975–February 28, 1978, Respectively.

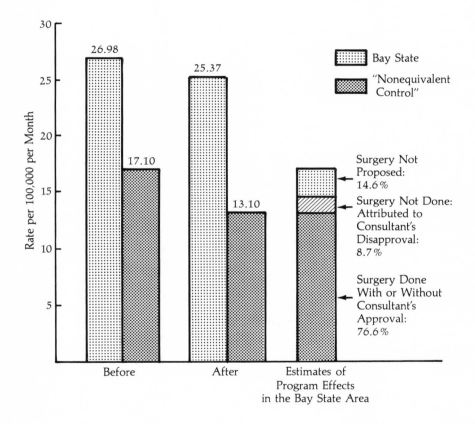

Source: Martin et al. 1980, pp. 104 –105 and Tables 27 and 36, pp. 119 and 138.

Chart 4–31

The work of Martin et al. (1980) also provides some interesting information on how patients responded to the first consultant's decision that surgery was not needed, and on the replicability of this negative opinion. In this program, patients who wanted an operation even though the consultant had advised against it were required to have another consultation, after which they could decide as they pleased. The first bar of the chart shows that in 14 percent of cases the first consultant advised against surgery. The second bar shows that 44 percent of patients who were so advised chose to challenge this negative opinion by seeking a second consultation. In the third bar we find a rather disquieting reminder of "the 45 percent law of tonsillectomy," as illustrated earlier in Chart 4–19. While the second consultant agreed with the first one in 35 percent of the cases that he saw, he disagreed in 65 percent of the cases and confirmed the need for surgery. The final bar of the chart shows the total effect of these several events. Of all the patients who were referred for consultation, 86 percent received the approval of the first consultant, an additional four percent were approved only by a second consultant, two percent were disapproved by two consultants, and eight percent did not challenge the disapproval of the first consultant.

Martin et al. also tell us about the subsequent behavior of patients during three to twelve months or more (Table 21, p. 98). If one lists the opinions of the initial medical advisor and those of the first and second consultants, in that order, the percent of persons in each category who are known to have surgery is as follows:

Yes	Yes	Not challenged:	88.5% have surgery
Yes	No	Not challenged:	14.0% have surgery
Yes	No	Yes:	80.0% have surgery
Yes	No	No:	44.4% have surgery

The presence of several kinds of compliance and noncompliance in all categories makes it difficult to decide precisely what effects are attributable to the program. We also see that some of those who challenge the first consultant's opinion are very determined to have surgery, perhaps because they trust their own physicians most.

The findings are heavily influenced by the nature of the population studied; by the fact that some patients chose not to have any consultations, while others were excused from the requirement to do so; and by the selected nature of the surgical procedures included in the program.

Chart 4-31

Percent Distribution of Persons in Each of Relevant Subgroups, by the Nature of the Consultants' Opinions and by the Nature of Their Own Reactions to These Opinions. A Mandatory Second Surgical Opinion Program for Eight Surgical Procedures in Medicaid Beneficiaries, Bay State and Central Massachusetts Regions, Massachusetts, May 1, 1977– April 30, 1978, and October 1, 1977–September 30, 1978, Respectively.

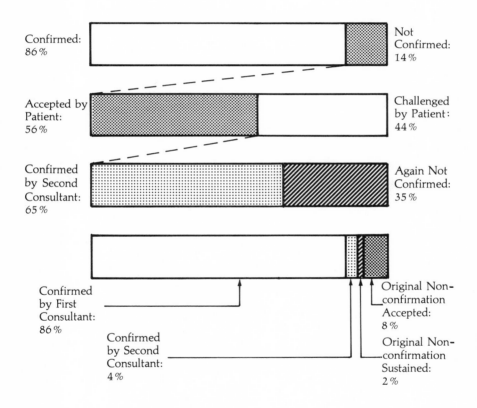

Source: Martin et al. 1980, Exhibit XIII, p. 78.

Observation of the
Process of Care

FIVE

In order to assess the process of care one must know how the practitioner conducts himself: what he does and what he fails to do, as judged by the standards of what needs to be done in each case. Ordinarily, one obtains information about the care from the records kept by physicians and other health care practitioners. But, even at their best, these records tend to be incomplete. Sometimes they are so rudimentary as to be next to useless as a basis for quality assessment. Then observation of practice, whether directly or through videorecording, is used either to replace or to supplement the medical record. The management of the interpersonal process is an aspect of care that is particularly difficult to know except through what we are told about it, or through some form of direct observation, the less obtrusive the better.

To illustrate the observation of practice as a method of quality assessment I shall draw mainly on the landmark study of general practice in North Carolina by Peterson et al. 1956. I shall supplement this with information from a study of general practice (as reported by Clute 1963) in the Canadian provinces of Ontario and Nova Scotia which was carefully patterned on the earlier work in North Carolina.

Of course, many years have passed since these studies were done, so that no one can claim that what we shall see represents general practice today. Our emphasis will be on the method used and on the relationships that it reveals. There is every reason to believe, however, that we have here a true picture of general practice at the time and in the places studied. I also suspect that many of the problems revealed by these studies are with us, at least to some extent, even now.

Considerable attention was given in both studies to drawing representative samples of the relevant practitioners; in both, the ratio of participation was remarkably high—90 percent in North Carolina, 86 percent in Ontario, and 88 percent in Nova Scotia. Each practitioner was visited by a physician who spent about three days with him, so as to observe the care given in the office, during home visits, and, in the Canadian study, during visits to the hospital as well. Two internists undertook this task in North Carolina; in Ontario the observers were an internist and a pediatrician with additional training in internal medicine, and in Nova Scotia the observer was a highly qualified general practitioner with additional training in public health. In all studies, the observer was guided in his judgments of the quality of care by a carefully designed schedule that specified the information to be obtained under the headings of clinical history, physical examination, laboratory procedures, therapy, preventive care, and clinical records. The schedule also gave guidance on what would constitute quality at each of several levels, and expressed these levels in numerical scores that, when added, gave an overall numerical measure of performance. This method of specifying the criteria is described and discussed in some detail in Volume II of this work (Donabedian 1982, pp. 24–26, 245–46, and 278–79).

It is regrettable that there was no formal attention to assessing the interpersonal relationship between clients and practitioners, even though the method of assessment was particularly well suited for this purpose. Clute does, however, include in his elegantly written narrative examples of humane and considerate conduct, as well as of some that was insensitive and inept.

It is reasonable to ask whether the mere fact of being observed changes a practitioner's behavior, whether the judgments on what is observed are reliable, and whether specialists are the best judges of the work of general practitioners. There are no completely satisfactory answers. The investigators assure us that, perhaps after a short initial period of adjustment, the practitioners under observation fell into their usual routines. They also emphasize that the observers were careful not to expect a standard of care that was not realistic for everyday practice. The work of the observers was subjected to repeated checking to assure accuracy, uniformity, and comparability. Some visits were repeated to see whether two observers obtained similar results, and whether this was also true when the same observer visited the same practitioner twice. On all these grounds, we are assured that the results are trustworthy.

Chart 5–1

This chart shows the overall findings of the studies of general practice described in the introduction to this section. Though the same method was used to assess the quality of care in the three locations shown, the findings may not be fully comparable. In both North Carolina and Canada, a quantitative score was computed, expressed as the percent of the possible total points. But in the Canadian studies, laboratory procedures were weighted much less. The scoring for the two Canadian studies was identical, but all of the observations in Nova Scotia were made by a single general practitioner and may have been somewhat biased, even though considerable attention was paid to assuring comparability. In the North Carolina study, the observing physician was also asked to assign a qualitative score, expressed in the Roman numerals I through V, prior to the computation of the numerical score. The correlation between the qualitative and quantitative scores was so high that many of the findings of the North Carolina study are reported only in terms of the former. The numbers shown on the chart in parentheses are either the range of quantitative scores that correspond to each category, or the mean score, when this is the only datum reported.

Peterson et al. say that there is some overlap between adjacent categories of their qualitative scale. The Canadian investigators recognize this by allowing for a category that "could not be labelled unequivocally as satisfactory or as unsatisfactory." Nevertheless, the distinctions between physicians were usually clear and consistent. Good physicians tended to do well in all aspects of care, whereas poor physicians were correspondingly poor in most aspects, or all.

Clute described "satisfactory" care as either outstanding or having deficiencies that "were not likely to have serious consequences" to the patient. By contrast, there were "grave misgivings" that unsatisfactory care would expose the patient to "serious risk" (pp. 313–14). Peterson et al. describe the physician who was above average as knowing clinical medicine, challenged by his practice, interested in the patient, and willing to accept responsibility. At the other end of the scale were physicians who most often "lacked fundamental clinical medical knowledge and skill," though some seemed to have the knowledge but were no longer challenged by their work or interested in their patients (pp. 47–48). On pages 18–20, Peterson et al. eloquently describe the two contrasting modes of practice.

Chart 5-1

Percent Distribution of General Practitioners by the Observed Quality of Their Practice. North Carolina, and the Canadian Provinces of Ontario and Nova Scotia, during Specified Time Periods.

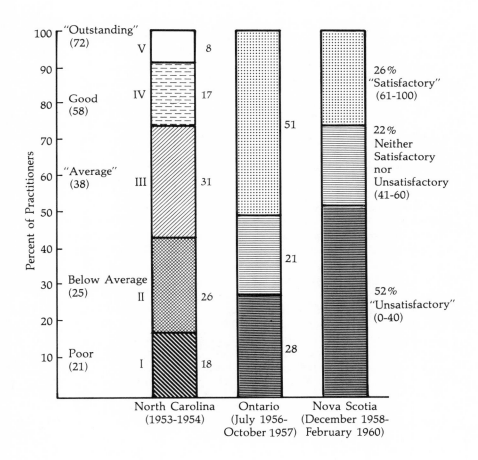

North Carolina (1953-1954)   Ontario (July 1956-October 1957)   Nova Scotia (December 1958-February 1960)

Sources and Note: Peterson et al. 1956, pp. 18–20, and Clute 1963, pp. 313–314. Numbers in parentheses are mean quantitative scores.

Chart 5–2

The observers who visited the general practitioners in the studies reported by Peterson et al. and by Clute were guided by a schedule that
listed the components of management which needed to be assessed.
Each component was characterized by two or three descriptions, and
each description was assigned a score. This chart shows a selection of
components accompanied by descriptions that characterize a level of
quality to which a score of zero was assigned and that therefore represent
unacceptable performance. Because there was a great deal of consistency
in the performance of each practitioner, each description is taken to
represent the practitioner's performance as a whole.

Peterson et al. describe the performance of the best physicians as

> outstanding in nearly all respects. In obtaining clinical histories, these phy-
> sicians carefully organized their questioning to develop the symptomatol-
> ogy surrounding the presenting complaint. Thoroughness, attention to
> detail, and the logical sequence of questions . . . indicated ample medical
> knowledge. In performing the physical examination they were thorough
> and showed that they were using the information obtained from the history
> purposefully in their search for physical stigmata of disease. In the choice
> of laboratory procedures these physicians again demonstrated the train of
> thought on which they built their evidence for diagnosis. The ease with
> which this train of thought and plan of investigation could be grasped by
> the observer was characteristic of these very good practices.

By contrast, the poorest physicians

> demonstrated an entirely different concept of the methods of patient
> care. . . . In history taking, questions were few, usually disconnected and
> lacking in incisiveness. These gave little evidence that the physician was
> thinking in terms of probable diagnoses. They were not planned or de-
> signed to explore the function of specific organs or physiological units. The
> physical examination was usually sketchy and it was frequently difficult
> to understand, in view of the patient's history, why one area was chosen
> for examination and another ignored. The laboratory tests performed by
> these physicians were few, often poorly performed and showed the same
> lack of direction. Under these conditions the indications for specific treat-
> ment were usually lacking or unclear. . . . Throughout the handling of each
> patient this lack of direction and purposefulness made it difficult for the
> observer to follow the physician's reasoning (pp. 18–19).

Chart 5-2

Percent of General Practitioners Whose Performance Could Be Described in Specified Ways that Denote Unacceptable Performance. North Carolina, 1953–1954, Ontario 1956–1957, and Nova Scotia 1958–1960.

	North Carolina	Ontario	Nova Scotia
PHYSICAL EXAMINATION			
Disrobing: Examinations performed with patient dressed or almost completely dressed.	45	16	33
Percussion of Lungs: Not done, or chest thumped perfunctorily.	77	70	62
Examination of Heart: Auscultation of base or other single area of the heart.	65	33	36
Examination of Abdomen: No examination or examination with the patient sitting or standing.	16	14	19
Rectal Examination: Not usually done. (Not examined when indicated.)	83	59	56
Ophthalmoscopy: Never done. (Not done when indicated.)	66	70	90
DIAGNOSTIC PROCEDURES			
Urinalysis: Not done or rarely done. (Or omission of protein or sugar.)	11	19	64
Hemoglobin: No determination or determination by Tallquist method only.	26	19	43
X-rays: No radiographic work performed and patients not referred . . . ; or improper careless use including . . . procedures beyond doctor's skill and training.	18	10	17
THERAPY			
Use of Antibiotics (and Sulphonamides): Given indiscriminately to all patients or to most patients with upper respiratory infections. (Lack of knowledge of general principles . . . , indiscriminate use, inadequate use, . . . dosage, . . . duration. . . .)	67	27	45
Anemia: "Shot-gun" preparation used always.	85	—	—
OTHER ASPECTS OF PERFORMANCE			
Sterile Technique: Breaks in technique, inadequate sterilization of skin or instruments . . . , use of unsterilized syringes, needles, or stylets.	43	10	46
Clinical Records: Only information concerning medications, fees, or isolated data such as blood pressure recorded.	36	35	62

Sources: Peterson et al. 1956, pp. 27–46, and Clute 1963, tables and text, pp. 290–304.

Chart 5–3

The purpose of the studies described by the preceding two charts was not simply to document the quality of general practice, but to use this information to discover which factors were associated with good practice or with bad, so that improvements could be proposed. Quite understandably, there was particular interest in the possible correlation between the practitioners' education and training and the quality of care they provided.

Peterson et al. report that the performance of the practitioners who were graduated from medical schools that emphasized clinical training was no different from that of practitioners who had graduated from schools that emphasized scientific endeavor and research. The practitioners' scores on the Medical College Aptitude Test were also irrelevant to current performance. Some other aspects of student performance, postgraduate training, and continuing education were, however, found to be pertinent.

This chart shows the associations between quality of care given and academic standing in medical school, as these associations are modified by age. The first three triplets of bars classify the practitioners simultaneously by age group and by rank in their class, the latter being shown in academic thirds. There is a significant positive correlation in the youngest group of physicians, but none thereafter. One possible conclusion is that the effects of different degrees of undergraduate learning become weaker with time and finally disappear.

The relationship to age (irrespective of academic standing) is shown in the fourth triplet of bars. The physicians who are older than 45 practice at a significantly lower level of quality.

The final triplet of bars also shows the relationship between age and the quality of performance, but now quality has been measured by the numerical ("quantitative") score which Peterson et al. constructed and used. In drawing this part of the chart I chose a scale that would permit a rough visual comparison of the relationship between age and quality as revealed by the two methods of scoring that quality, the qualitative one and the quantitative or numerical one. The purpose is to show the similarity of the results with either method of scoring. As I have already said, the results of the two methods of scoring were highly correlated.

Chart 5-6 has more information about the relationship between age and the quality of performance in general practice.

Chart 5-3

Mean Qualitative Scores of the Observed Quality of Practice of General Practitioners in Specified Categories of Academic Rank and Age, and Mean Quantitive Scores of Quality by Age Group. North Carolina, 1953–1954.

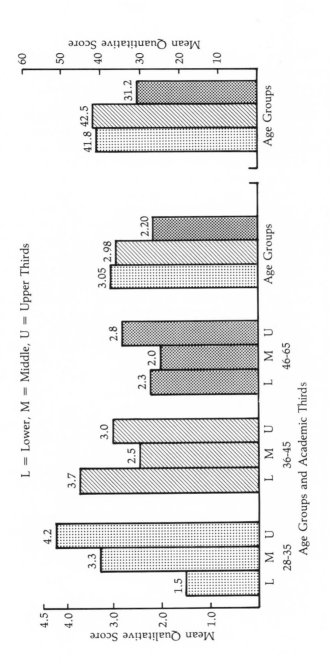
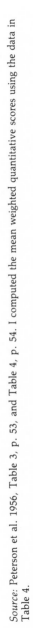

L = Lower, M = Middle, U = Upper Thirds

Source: Peterson et al. 1956, Table 3, p. 53, and Table 4, p. 54. I computed the mean weighted quantitative scores using the data in Table 4.

Chart 5–4

The postgraduate training of the physician is, of course, another factor that might be expected to influence the quality of his general practice later on. In the left-hand panel of this chart we see the relationship between the number of months of internship and residency that the practitioner had and the qualitative score awarded to his current performance. There appears to be an association which does not, however, achieve statistical significance because there are only eight physicians in the category of "0–10 months," and only five in the category of "over 30 months." Further analysis led to the conclusion that only the length of training in internal medicine made a definite contribution to the quality of general practice, as shown in the right-hand panel of the chart. Also as shown, a minimum of about three months of such training was needed for a subsequent association to be seen, and the gains were small beyond a period of about five to eight months of training in internal medicine. Two additional important findings are not shown in this chart. First, it was not important that the training took place in a teaching hospital or one approved to educate house staff. Second, the salutary association of performance with training was found only in the physicians who were younger than 46. As was shown in the preceding chart to be true of class rank, the effects of postgraduate training appear to erode under the buffetings of time.

The findings in the Canadian provinces of Ontario and Nova Scotia were rather different. In Ontario there was a correlation between the total duration of training and the quality of general practice, but only if at least some of that training had been in a teaching hospital. It was not possible to determine whether training in internal medicine had an effect different from that of other forms of training. In Nova Scotia there was no association between performance and the length, type, or location of training. Clute concludes that the "findings are too indefinite either to confirm or to contradict Peterson's conclusions that 'the better medical student tends to become a better physician' and that 'the more training a physician has received in internal medicine the more likely he is to become a good physician' " (Clute 1963, p. 326).

Chart 5–4

"Qualitative" Scores of the Observed Performance of General Practitioners, by Months of Postgraduate Training in All Specialties, and by Months of Postgraduate Training in Internal Medicine. North Carolina, 1953–1954.

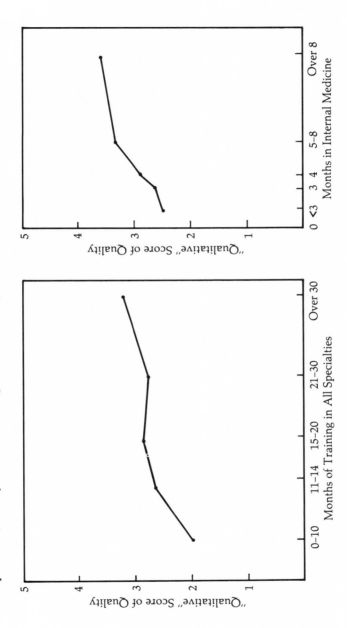

Source: Peterson et al. 1956, Tables 6 and 10, pp. 61 and 65. I used the data in Table 6 to compute the mean qualitative scores (or ranks) weighted by the number of practitioners in each category.

Chart 5–5

Since both class rank in medical school and length of training in internal medicine influence the performance of the younger general practitioners, it would be interesting to take a look at the joint effects of these two variables. In this chart, the physicians who were 28 to 35 years old at the time of the survey are categorized by whether they stood in the lowest or highest thirds of their classes in medical school, and by whether or not they had at least four months of postgraduate training in internal medicine. Each of the two variables appears to have an effect, and the two seem to reinforce each other, but the effect of class rank is clearly the more powerful of the two. In fact, the quality-enhancing effect of longer training in internal medicine is not statistically significant for practitioners of either low or high standing in medical school. By contrast, the quality-enhancing effect of high class rank is large and statistically significant both for physicians with short training and for those with long training in internal medicine.

Though standing in medical school and postgraduate training in internal medicine may be important, they do not explain many differences in performance, especially since, as we have seen, their effects dwindle with time until they seem to have no influence on general practitioners who are more than 45 years old. Some other factor seems to be more constantly at work. Peterson et al. believe that this is the individual practitioner's "interest in medicine." In their words, "there were physicians who had been good medical students and had received good training, who were not exceptional physicians. There were others whose performance as students was unusually poor, whose internships were of indifferent quality, who nevertheless became superior physicians" (p. 73).

Peterson et al. say that they have a good cross section of the graduates of a rather wide selection of medical schools. They are inclined to believe, therefore, that their findings are valid for general practitioners in general, though not necessarily for physicians who choose other careers. One must keep in mind, nevertheless, the possibility that the relationships between quality and the several variables studied in this survey have been distorted by the contingencies that lead some physicians, sometimes circuitously, to end up in rural general practice.

Chart 5–5

"Qualitative" Score of the Observed Performance of General Practitioners Who Were 28 to 35 Years Old, Categorized by Specified Combinations of Class Rank in Medical School and Length of Postgraduate Training in Internal Medicine. North Carolina, 1953–1954.

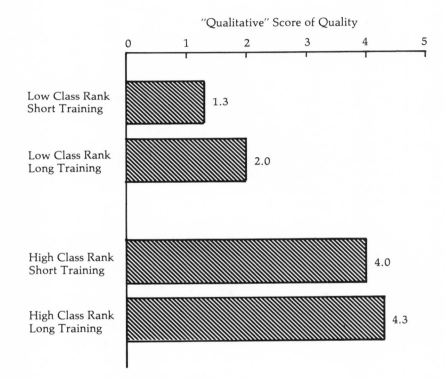

Source: Peterson et al. 1956, Table 14, p. 69.

Chart 5–6

This chart consolidates the findings concerning the association between age and the quality of general practice. The quantitative score used is the percent of all applicable points that the physicians' typical performance has earned. As I have already pointed out, comparisons among the three studies are hazardous and are made more so by the exclusion of all physicians older than 60 from the Canadian surveys.

It is tempting to interpret this chart to mean that the average performance of general practitioners begins to deteriorate toward the end of middle age. Though in describing some of the preceding charts I may have seemed to favor this interpretation, I must now point out that it may not be justified. This is because these are studies of physicians who have already attained a variety of ages. These are, in other words, "cross-sectional" surveys, rather than "longitudinal" studies in which groups of individuals are observed as they age. One cannot be certain, therefore, that the characteristics associated with age have developed as a result of, or together with, the process of aging, rather than being there from the beginning, even when the physicians in question were young.

The investigators are fully aware of this problem, but they tend to attribute the findings to aging. Clute points out that "the physicians' scores did not depend on their knowledge of recent advances—except to a slight degree—but were determined by their use of, or their failure to use, the long established, basic procedures of clinical medicine" (p. 320). According to Peterson et al. there may actually be some initial improvement in quality, perhaps due to learning through practice, particularly by the less well-trained physicians. Further analysis shows that if there is any such improvement, it involves the clinical records, therapy, and the use of the laboratory. In other aspects of practice there is a linear downward trend, and in *all* aspects the most aged physicians perform the worst. There were physicians, however, in both Canada and North Carolina who gave excellent care despite their advanced age. According to Peterson et al., "the identification of the individual who will become a good doctor despite indifferent training or the doctor whose interest in practice will not lag after a few years will probably be as productive of better quality of practice as any other measure" (p. 73).

Chart 5–6

Mean "Quantitative" Scores of the Observed Quality of Care, by the General Practitioners' Age Group. North Carolina, 1953–1954; Ontario, 1956–1957; and Nova Scotia, 1958–1960.

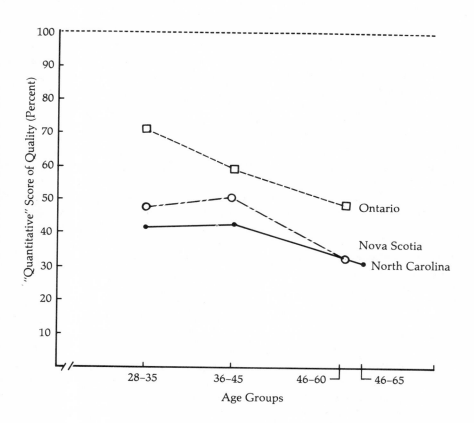

Source and Note: Peterson et al. 1956, Table 4, p. 54, and Clute 1963, Table 82, p. 319. I have used the data reported by Peterson et al. to compute mean scores adjusted by number of physicians and by weights of the components of clinical performance.

Chart 5–7

Peterson et al. found that opportunities for continuing education contributed to better practice, at least to some extent. Physicians who bought and read more journals ranked higher in quality; so did physicians who devoted more time to postgraduate study, except that there was a concentration of superior physicians in the group that spent 40–59 hours on such study, rather than 60 hours or more. The former was the one group whose performance was significantly better than that of the others. Physicians who went away for formal courses also performed significantly better than those whose educational activities were limited to meetings of the local medical society or hospital staff. Taking care of patients in the hospital, and being otherwise "active" in the hospital's affairs, were not associated with better performance.

Many other features of practice were examined by Peterson et al. and by Clute in search for causes or predictors of good practice. As shown in this chart, Peterson et al. found that owning certain items of diagnostic equipment (a microscope, a centrifuge, a calorimeter, an electrocardiograph, and a basal metabolism machine) was correlated with the quality of care. In both North Carolina and Canada, physicians who saw their patients by appointment gave better care than those who did not. In North Carolina there was no correlation between how many hours a practitioner worked and the quality of his work, but in the Canadian studies it appeared that, on the whole, the busier doctors gave somewhat better care.

Group practice, which was loosely defined as working with one or more other physicians, was not associated with quality in the Canadian studies. In North Carolina, physicians in "group practice" gave distinctly better care, but they were also younger, had better academic records, had more training, had more diagnostic equipment, and purchased more journals. This shows how difficult it is to isolate the contributions that each of several associated attributes may make to the quality of care. We also do not know whether certain attributes of practice made the physicians better, or whether good physicians sought out certain forms and conditions of work. Finally, we are reminded repeatedly that superior care was sometimes observed under adverse conditions, and poor care under conditions that should have been favorable. While this may be chastening to the planner, we can also rejoice that man is not completely the captive of his circumstances.

Chart 5–7

Mean "Qualitative" Scores of the Observed Quality of the Performance of General Practitioners, by Yearly Hours of Postgraduate Study, by Number of Journals Purchased, and by Possession of None or More of Five Items of Laboratory Equipment. North Carolina, 1953-1954.

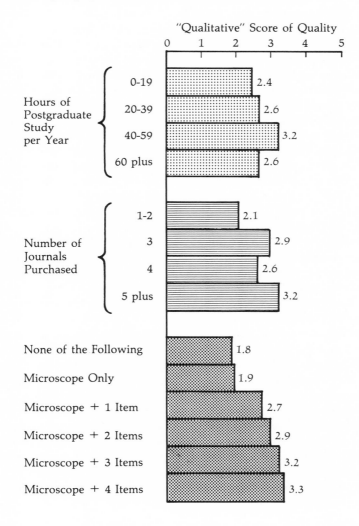

Source: Peterson et al. 1956, Tables 19, 25, and 31, pp. 81, 88, and 107. I used the data in Table 25 to compute mean scores (ranks) weighted by the number of practitioners in each category.

Chart 5–8

I have drawn on a preliminary study of nursing care to show that direct observation is a useful tool in the assessment of hospital care as well. Although hospital records are more ample; observation is still necessary if one wants to assess the interpersonal exchange in the management of patients. This study also alerts us to the possible presence of differences in quality even beyond the barriers of initial access to care.

Out of 80 hospitals in the Detroit area, 19 agreed to participate. In these hospitals, 229 randomly sampled patients were each observed for a two-hour period by one of a visiting team of qualified nurses who had already found out a great deal about each patient's needs. All interactions between patients and nurses, or other personnel under the supervision of nurses, were rated using the Quality Patient Care Scale (Wandelt and Ager 1970). This instrument contains 68 items, divided among six "areas" of nursing care, and is notable for its attention to the psychosocial needs of patients. Thus while a great deal of structure was imposed on the observations, it was still up to the observers to indicate how well each of the 68 items was performed by awarding it a score from 1 to 5—and in this they may have differed from one another, though they had been trained to be consistent.

The ratings are uniformly much below the highest possible score of 5. They also suggest that younger males receive better care than older ones, whereas this relationship to age is reversed for females. Nonwhites receive worse care than whites, and patients with cancer are not as well handled as those with other medical or surgical diagnoses. Not shown is the finding that patients who had a "poor" prognosis were not treated as well as those in other prognostic categories. We do not know what the combined effect of all these adverse circumstances might be, but one suspects that an old, black male with advanced cancer would not fare well in this environment.

The differences observed are small and not uniformly significant; they reflect care given by professionals and nonprofessionals, and they pertain to only this one set of hospitals. Most importantly, we cannot say that nurses make unwarranted distinctions among patients, because the differences in care could have resulted from the way in which patients are distributed among hospitals. This does not mean, however, that we need not look carefully to see if health care personnel are impartial in the care they give.

Chart 5–8

Scores of the Quality of Nursing Care, by Specified Characteristics of Patients in 19 Hospitals. Wayne, Oakland, and Macomb Counties, Michigan circa 1972.

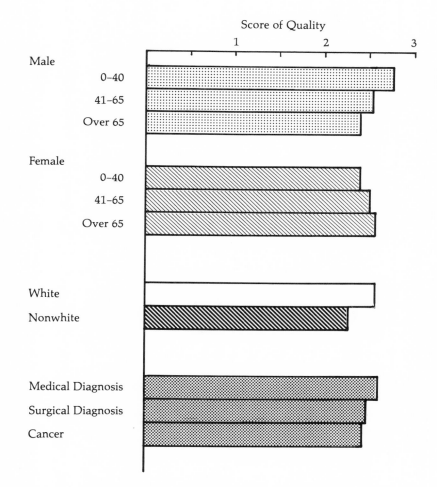

Source: Janzen 1974, Tables 3, 4, and 5. I used the data in Table 3 to compute the mean scores, giving equal weight to each of the six components of care.

Audits of the
Records of Care

SIX

Direct observation, the method that we have just studied, is not often used in a formal assessment of the process of care. More frequent, by far, is the use of the medical record, particularly of hospital care, where it is a reasonably adequate account of the process of technical care and some of its immediate consequences. Some records of ambulatory care may also be good enough to use, for example those from the outpatient department of a hospital or a group practice. But in all these places, because of frequent deficiencies in the record, the assessment is restricted to a subset of technical matters, and there are doubts about the validity of the judgments concerning even these. As a result, critics of quality assessment often argue that the *record,* rather than the care itself, is being assessed. I shall have more to say about this in a subsequent chapter. Now, I shall pay more attention to the kinds of criteria used and to the findings.

Assessments of the records of care can be handily classified as using "implicit" criteria, "explicit" criteria, or some of each. As I described in Chapter 2 of the second volume of these *Explorations,* there is a gradation in explicitness and specification (Donabedian 1982, pp. 19–29). At one extreme, the judgment of quality is based on a mental process that remains completely unspecified. One relies entirely on the "implicit" norms, criteria, and standards of the assessor. A step toward structuring the process of assessment is to guide it by selecting in advance the information to be used or the aspects of care to be judged. Abstracting the record is an example of the former, and drawing the attention of the assessor to specific elements of medical management is an example of the latter. Another step toward greater explicitness is to ask the assessor to explain and justify the judgments he has made. This is, in effect, a "postspecification" of the criteria and standards. More often, explicit criteria are "prespecified" by panels of competent practitioners. When this specification is complete, the assessment of quality is reduced to determining whether those elements of care detailed in the criteria are noted in the record.

Preformulated explicit criteria and standards are meant to ensure that the best professional opinion is used uniformly and consistently in judging the quality of care. They are generally formulated by panels of physicians who draw on their own knowledge and experience, as well as on the pertinent literature, to specify any one or more of the following: the circumstances that justify admission to the hospital; the findings that justify the diagnosis; the diagnostic and therapeutic procedures that are necessary for, or consistent with, the diagnosis; the state of the patient that signifies readiness to be discharged; the length of stay that is generally sufficient to achieve that state; and the outcomes of care to be attained, expressed as satisfaction with care and as changes in health status, knowledge, and behavior.

To specify any of these, it is necessary also to specify the "referent" of the criteria, which is the thing to which the criteria are meant to pertain. The referent is most often a diagnosis, but it can also be something else—usually a condition (such as headache) or a procedure (such as blood transfusion). Because the validity of the explicit criteria depends, among other things, on the precise match of the cases being assessed to the referent, only rather restricted subsets of cases can be assessed in this way. Even then, the criteria often do not anticipate all the variations in the cases being judged. One way of handling this problem is to introduce "contingencies" or "branching," which means that certain subsets of criteria are conditional on certain characteristics of the cases being assessed, whereas when other characteristics are present, other criteria apply. When this procedure is fully developed one obtains "algorithmic criteria" or "criteria maps" which take the form of a logic flow chart with multiple branching.

The studies described in this chapter will be classified in a progression according to the criteria used, the categories being implicit criteria without guidance, implicit criteria with guidance, explicit criteria, and a mix of implicit and explicit criteria used together. Within each of these subsections the studies will be arranged according to the site of care, the major categories being hospital and ambulatory care, respectively. Other characteristics of the criteria, including whether they are "linear" or "branched," will be described as the occasion arises. Examples of "algorithmic" criteria will be given in Chapter 13, where different types of criteria are described.

Chart 6–1

In order to illustrate the use of implicit criteria without guidance I have chosen the second of two studies, by Morehead and her associates, of the quality of hospital care received by members of the Teamsters Union and their families. The findings are based on a random sample of hospital claims paid during May 1962 to hospitals in New York City. The method used was to submit photostatic copies of the complete hospital record of each hospitalization to highly qualified physicians who were asked to assess the necessity for admission and the quality of care. The necessity for admission was to be judged "solely on the basis of the patient's medical needs." The instructions regarding the judgment of quality were as follows: "We are asking you to judge the quality of medical care in line with your clinical judgment and experience. You will use as a yardstick in relation to the quality of care rendered, whether you would have treated this particular patient in this particular fashion during this specific hospital admission" (p. 13). But, having made their judgments based on their own implicit criteria, the assessors were asked to reveal some of their reasons by specifying why any case was given less than the highest rank.

Initially, hospital care was described as excellent, good, fair, or poor, but later these classes were combined in pairs to form two categories: "optimal," and "less then optimal." For a large subset of admissions (those in medicine, surgery, and pediatrics) there were two such judgments, one by each of two separate assessors. In 78 percent of these cases the two assessors began by agreeing on whether the care given was to be called optimal or less than optimal. After the judges were asked to reassess the cases on which they disagreed, there was agreement on 92 percent of cases.

This chart shows that after normal deliveries and tonsillectomies were excluded, care was judged to be less than optimal in 43 percent of cases; in 15 percent of cases there were questions about the need for admission to the hospital. Both of these percentages varied markedly by medical or surgical specialty. These findings do not represent the hospital care received by others in New York City, nor do they necessarily represent the overall performance of doctors who include Teamster families in their practices.

Chart 6-1

Percent of Hospitalized Cases Judged To Have Received "Optional" Care, and Percent of Cases Whose Admission Was Judged To Have Been Necessary, by Medical or Surgical Specialty. Members of the Teamsters Union and Their Families for Whom Hospital Claims Were Paid to New York City Hospitals in May, 1962.

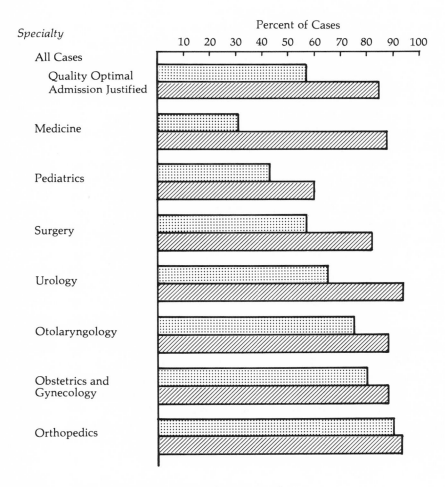

Source: Morehead et al. 1964, Tables 3 and 8, pp. 47 and 52.

Chart 6–2

Morehead and her coworkers not only developed and tested an important method for assessing the quality of hospital care, but they made an additional significant contribution by examining the effects of several factors on the quality of care and on the need to be admitted to the hospital. As expected, the qualifications of the physicians who undertook the care of the patient, and of the surgeon who actually did the operation, were found to be important.

In this chart, and in some of those that follow, physicians and surgeons are put into three classes. In Class I are those who are either board certified or are fellows of a College of specialists. In addition, these doctors almost invariably have an appointment at a voluntary or municipal hospital. In Class II are the doctors who are not recognized as specialists by the criteria already described, but whose skill is presumably attested to by their having obtained staff appointments at a voluntary or municipal hospital. Class III includes the physicians who are neither considered to be specialists, nor have the privilege of an appointment at a voluntary or municipal hospital; they may, however, be on the staff of a proprietary hospital. Class IV is made up of the house staff in voluntary and municipal hospitals. The chart introduces still another classification by distinguishing cases that are surgical from those that are not.

The chart shows that Class I physicians perform better than Class II physicians, and these, in turn, do better than those in Class III. It also looks as if the performance of the doctors in Class I is more homogeneous, in that the quality of care is equally high for surgical and medical conditions. In Classes II and III, surgical care appears to be better than nonsurgical care, and the disparity between the two types of care seems to become greater as the qualifications of the physicians are lower. These differences between surgical and medical conditions suggest that the care of the latter is undertaken by physicians who are more varied in their abilities, and under conditions that are less uniformly controlling. The house staff of voluntary and municipal hospitals performed remarkably well according to this study, particularly in surgical care. This is a tribute to their training and the quality of the supervision of their work. It may also reflect the tendency of house staff to keep more complete records.

(For differences in the appropriateness of hospital use by type of physician and other variables see Chart 3–21.)

Chart 6–2

Percent of Hospitalized Cases Judged To Have Received "Optimal" Care by Type of Care, and by Qualifications of the Physician Responsible for Care. Members of the Teamsters Union and Their Families for Whom Hospital Claims Were Paid to New York City Hospitals, May 1962.

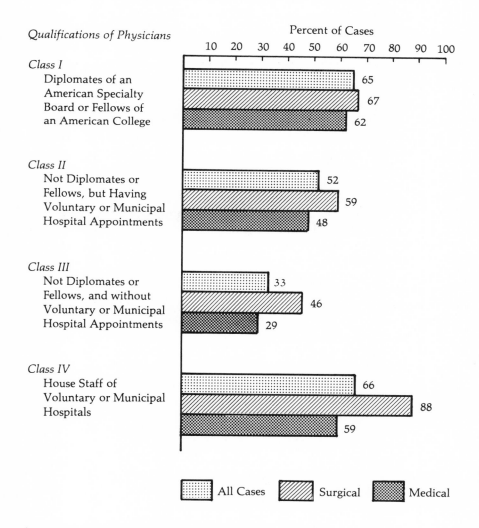

Source: Morehead et al. 1964. Computed from data in Table III, p. 92.

Chart 6–3

We saw in the preceding chart that the qualifications of physicians influence the quality of the hospital care they give. In this chart we take a look at the effects of some hospital characteristics.

Morehead et al. classified the hospitals in New York City according to whether they were (1) affiliated with a medical school, (2) approved by the American Medical Association to train interns and residents, (3) accredited by the Joint Commission on Accreditation of Hospitals, and (4) a nonprofit, voluntary (community) hospital, a municipal hospital, or a proprietary hospital presumably run for profit. The chart shows that hospitals affiliated with medical schools (which are all also accredited and approved to train house staff) provide the best care by far. A comparison with the other categories of hospitals in the chart shows that the medical school affiliation, with all it entails, is the key variable. In its absence, average performance is at a much lower level, even though other desirable attributes may be present. For example, approval for training residents and interns has no perceptible effect, and care in voluntary (and municipal) hospitals is only a little better than that in proprietary hospitals. All hospitals that are affiliated with medical schools, or are not affiliated but are approved for training house staff, must be accredited. The effect of accreditation can, therefore, be observed only in the lowest two categories in the chart. What we see is a curious effect. Accreditation appears to be associated with somewhat better care in voluntary hospitals but not in proprietary institutions. It is tempting to suggest that a hospital may appear to comply with the requirements of accreditation without making a serious enough effort to improve the quality of care.

In interpreting these findings we should remember that they show mainly the quality of technical care, and that this care is being judged by experts with intimate ties to the leading teaching institutions in the area. It is not known how successfully the identity of the hospitals could be concealed when a photostat of the entire record was available for review. Finally, these findings reflect the many characteristics of a specific population, in a particular place, at a particular time. Proprietary hospitals are particularly idiosyncratic, and the requirements for accreditation have changed a great deal. All this should lead us to be cautious, at least for now. But subsequent studies will help confirm some of the more important findings of this one.

Chart 6–3

Percent of Hospitalized Cases Judged To Have Received "Optimal" Care, by Type and by Accreditation Status of Hospitals. Members of the Teamsters Union and Their Families for Whom Hospital Claims Were Paid to New York City Hospitals, May 1962.

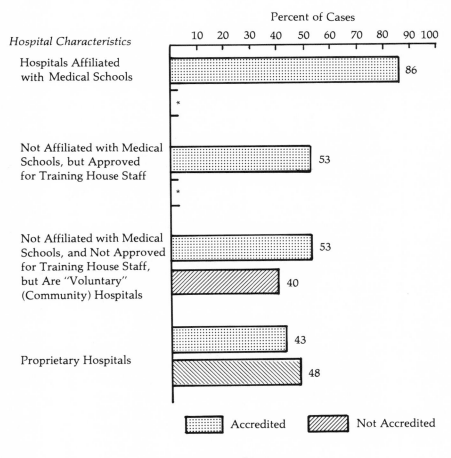

*No cases in this category.

Source and Note: Morehead, personal communication, to supplement information in Morehead et al. 1964. The asterisks mean that there are no unaccredited hospitals in these categories.

Chart 6–4

The characteristics of the physicians who provide care are, obviously, not unrelated to the attributes of the hospitals in which they work. It would be interesting, therefore, to see how these two sets of characteristics influence the quality of care, separately and jointly.

We already know that, in comparison to other hospitals, the quality of care was found to be much higher in hospitals that were affiliated with medical schools. We now see that, in these hospitals, having formal recognition as a specialist (through either board certification or fellowship in a College of specialists) does not contribute any further to the quality of care. If anything, physicians who do not have such qualification perform even better than those who do. The medical school and the hospital appear to assure the competence of their staff, perhaps through careful initial selection and incentives for continued excellence.

Irrespective of their qualifications, the performance of physicians in voluntary and municipal hospitals without medical school affiliation is at a markedly lower level. While formal qualifications as a specialist are not sufficient to ensure the highest levels of quality, they do, however, seem to confer a small advantage over other physicians in this category of hospitals.

The performance of physicians in proprietary hospitals is much more variable, through being more closely related to physician attributes. On the average, qualified specialists perform even better here than their counterparts do in voluntary or municipal hospitals. Physicians who are not specialists, but who do have staff appointments at voluntary or municipal hospitals, do no better here. But in proprietary hospitals there is a third category of physicians: generalists who cannot take care of patients in any other kind of hospital. In only 29 percent of cases was the care these physicians gave judged to be "optimal." Not shown in the chart is the additional finding that 44 percent of admissions by these physicians were judged to be questionable.

We may conclude that in the best hospitals the institution itself controls the quality of care. But when the hospital does not do so, the patient must depend entirely on the qualifications of his physician. This is, of course, a preliminary interpretation subject to confirmation. Moreover, there is nothing here to suggest that the *same* physicians vary their performances depending on the hospital in which they work.

Chart 6–4

Percent of Hospitalized Cases Judged To Have Received "Optimal" Care, by
Type of Hospital and by Qualifications of the Physician Responsible for
Care. Members of the Teamsters Union and Their Families for Whom
Hospital Claims Were Paid to New York City Hospitals, May 1962.

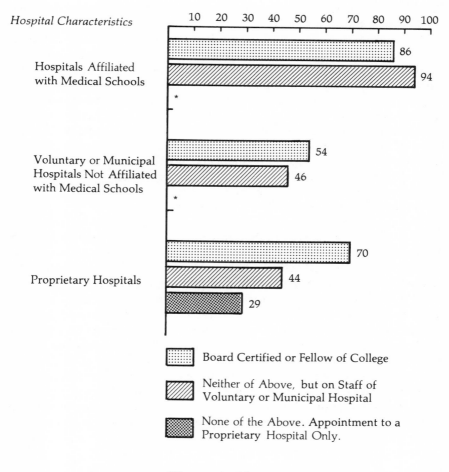

*No cases in this category.

Source and Note: Morehead et al. 1964, Table 7, p. 51. The asterisks mean the absence of this
category of physicians.

Chart 6–5

There is a category of studies falling in between those that use fully implicit criteria and those that use fully explicit criteria. In this intermediate position are the methods that specify, with varying detail, the procedures for assessing the care, but which also allow the assessor considerable room to judge what is good and what is not. The studies described in a preceding section on the observation of practice were of this kind. In this section I will describe two additional applications, this time to assessing the clinical record.

In the first of the two studies, random samples of 40 cases with each of selected (presumably representative) diagnoses were drawn from each of three departments in each of four hospitals (of which only three are shown in the chart.) Three pairs of physicians, two for each specialty, separately reviewed the complete medical record of each case pertaining to that specialty. The record review was guided by a highly detailed schedule that specified the information to be abstracted from the record, provided guidance about what the standards of care should be, and specified how the assessors' judgments of "good," "fair," or "poor" about the many components of care were to be combined into a corresponding overall judgment for the entire management of each case. The method is described in greater detail in Donabedian 1982, pp. 26–29.

The chart shows several findings. It gives an overall impression of the quality of hospital care, even though we cannot be sure that the selected diagnoses represent all care in these departments. Hospitals A and B are affiliated with medical schools; hospital C is a community hospital. The presence or absence of affiliation, and perhaps the nature of the affiliation, appear to be related to the quality of care, as noted also by Morehead et al. in the study we have just reviewed. In this chart we get the additional impression that there is a consistency in the relative level of performance for each hospital in all three departments, with one exception. That exception draws attention to the replicability of judgments, which is also shown in this chart. It appears that if the procedure is carefully specified, two judges can agree on the ranking of the hospitals, though one judge may be consistently more lenient than the other. The one exception (Judge One, for surgery) appeared to have been careless.

Chart 6–5

Percent of Patients Who Received "Superior" or "Good" Care in Three
Departments in Each of Three Hospitals, as Judged by Each Member of a Pair
of Judges, There Being a Different Pair for Each Department. Boston, 1953.

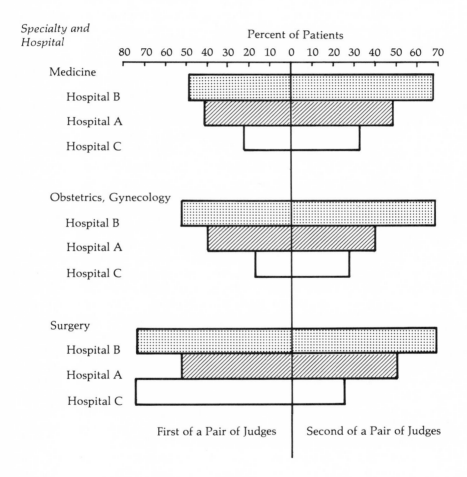

Source: Rosenfeld 1957, Table 1, p. 859.

Chart 6–6

Our second example of a method that uses guided implicit judgments about the clinical record comes from the field of nursing. The process of judgment is structured by a schedule that lists the seven "nursing functions," which are the aspects of nursing care shown in the chart. Under each of these functions there are items, ranging in number between four and sixteen. The items are, in effect, questions about more detailed aspects of nursing care, which the assessor must answer as "yes," "no," "uncertain," or "does not apply." These are the judgments which require nursing expertise, drawing upon the internalized, implicit criteria and standards of the assessor. Once they are made, the rest proceeds in a routinized manner. Each of the answers is assigned a numerical score, and the scores are added to obtain subtotals for each nursing function and a grand total for all functions. The numerical scores of the grand total and subtotals are interpreted as "excellent," "good," "incomplete," "poor," and "unsafe," with the numerical boundaries between categories being placed at 80, 60, 40, and 20 percent of each subtotal or total, respectively.

The method is an excellent example of guided or structured implicit assessment. It also shows how the definition of quality and the procedures for judging it are adapted to the responsibilities and ideology of a profession other than medicine. Particularly notable is the mix of those nursing functions that are dependent on prior decisions by the physician and those that are not. Among the latter is the function of direction and teaching, an aspect of quality that has received much more attention in assessing nursing care than in assessing the performance of physicians. Also notable is the separate attention to reporting and recording.

The procedure also illustrates some important features in constructing scales for measuring quality. All inapplicable items of performance are, of course, excluded from these scales. The remaining scores are obtained by simple addition, which means that possible interactions among items and among functions are ignored. In this particular procedure, items (and, consequently, functions) have been assigned different weights. In this way one obtains a weighted numerical measure of performance which is useful for comparisons, but which has less meaning by itself. That is why the descriptive equivalents ("excellent," "good," etc.) are so important. The method is described fully in Phaneuf 1976. The weighting of the criteria is discussed at length in Donabedian 1982, pp. 223–91.

Chart 6–6

Percent Distribution of Cases Judged To Have Received Nursing Care of Specified Quality in Specified Aspects of Care. Recipients of Care from 20 Community Nursing Agencies. Greater New York City Area, circa 1967.

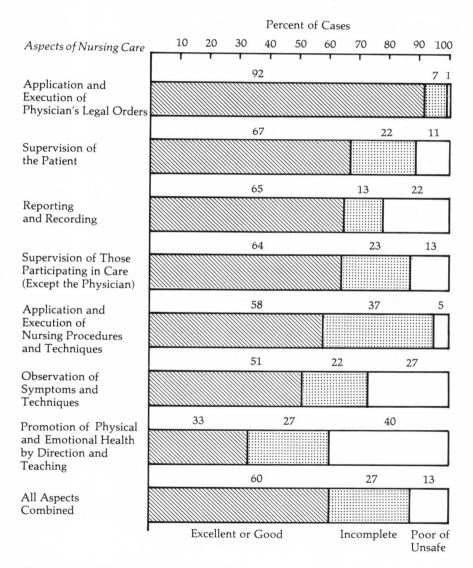

Source: Phaneuf 1968, Figures 1–5, pp. 57–59.

Chart 6–7

This chart comes from a study on which I will draw extensively, because its detailed findings have not been published in accessible form, because I think it is a worthy companion to the work of Peterson et al. in North Carolina, and because it represents the intermediate stage in an important line of development in the assessment of ambulatory care in more formally organized settings. The story begins in 1949 with the work of Makover (1951) at the Health Insurance Plan of Greater New York (HIP) and continues, as will be shown later, with the more recent studies of Morehead et al. in neighborhood health centers.

This study included 407 family physicians. It was believed that the clinical skills of each physician could best be judged by care for "major" diseases such as diabetes, hypertension, coronary artery disease, peptic ulcer, anemia, and kidney disease, supplemented by a selection of other chronic illnesses. Almost 90 percent of the assessments were made by one of two board-certified internists who reviewed medical records and then discussed the findings with each physician. The reviewers relied primarily on their own implicit criteria and standards. They were, however, guided by a schedule that listed the aspects of care to be assessed, described what constituted "good," "fair," and "poor" performance, and assigned numerical weights to each of these descriptors. In these ways the approach was very similar to that used by Peterson et al., except that the information was not obtained by direct observation.

The chart shows the percent of physicians in each category of length-of-training who were awarded scores of 76 or more out of 100. We see that longer periods of training are associated with a higher proportion of physicians who have higher scores, but that approved training is more efficacious in this respect. Some additional findings not shown in the chart are that (1) training in internal medicine was more effective than "rotating training," (2) certification in internal medicine was almost a guarantee of receiving the highest scores (p. 24), and (3) taking postgraduate courses had little relationship to performance (p. 48). These findings seem to agree partly with the observation of Peterson et al. and partly with those of Clute, for example as shown and discussed in Chart 5–4. While the agreements add credibility to the findings, we should remember that HIP physicians may not be typical.

Chart 6-7

Percent of Family Physicians Whose Performance in Caring for Selected Cases of Major Illness Was Judged To Be in the Highest of Three Classes, by Length of Postgraduate Training in Approved and Unapproved Programs. Groups Affiliated with the Health Insurance Plan of Greater New York, circa 1954.

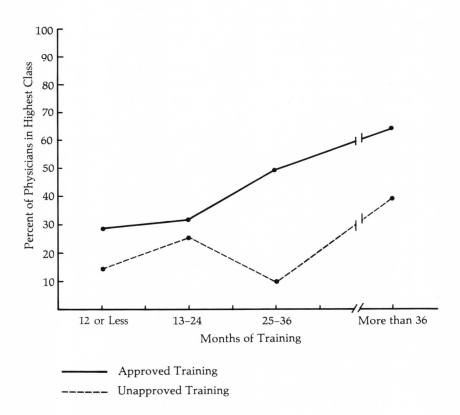

Source: Morehead 1958, Table 4, p. 60.

Chart 6–8

It is important to know whether, in addition to postgraduate training (the effects of which are shown in the preceding chart), the earlier medical education of physicians has an effect on subsequent performance. Because students of the more highly regarded medical schools, and those who do better in school, are more likely to receive additional training in approved programs and to have longer periods of training, it is necessary to disentangle the possible effects of these associations. Accordingly, Morehead classified 379 family physicians by whether or not they had attended a medical school in the United States or Canada. A subset of 102 physicians who had graduated from five medical schools in New York City could be ranked as having been either in the upper third of their classes or in the lower two-thirds. Within each of these categories the findings are shown separately for those physicians who had two years or less of approved postgraduate training and for those who had more.

For each category of family physicians the chart shows the percent of physicians who scored 76 percent or higher (Class I) and the percent who scored 60 percent or lower (Class III). Performance is better for physicians who graduated from medical schools in the United States or Canada, and for those who ranked higher in the kind of medical school represented in New York City. Though this is true irrespective of length of training, longer training seems to have a particularly strong effect on graduates of United States and Canadian schools, and on those who performed well in school. The three variables studied can, therefore, be considered to have mutually reinforcing effects.

The effect of training in unapproved programs (not shown in the chart) could be studied only partially. Physicians who had only two years or less of unapproved training performed equally well or badly irrespective of the type of medical school they had attended. Among graduates of other than United States or Canadian schools, those who had more than two years of unapproved training performed somewhat better than those who had less (Table 10, p. 63). The effect of longer durations of unapproved training on graduates of U.S. and Canadian schools could not be studied because there were very few physicians in this category.

The general applicability of these findings is, of course, limited by the peculiarities of the assessment method and of the population studied. I have also taken a liberty in showing the data represented by the bar with an interrupted outline, even though Morehead omitted this information because it is based on the performance of only eight physicians.

Chart 6–8

Percent of Family Physicians Whose Performance in Caring for Selected Cases of Major Illness Was Judged To Be in the Highest and Lowest of Three Classes Respectively, by Type of Medical School and Class Standing, and within Each of These Categories by Length of Postgraduate Training in Approved Programs. Groups in the Health Insurance Plan of Greater New York, circa 1954.

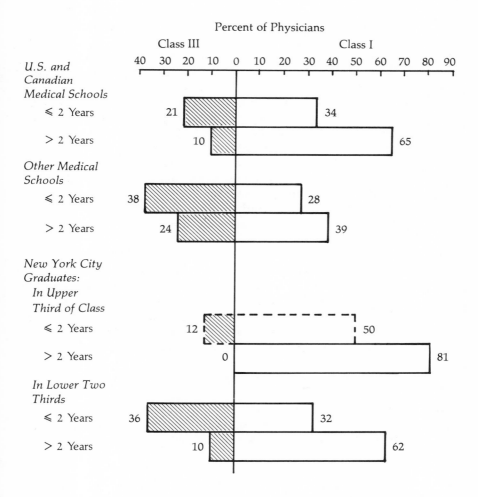

Source: Morehead 1958, Tables 9 and 12, pp. 62 and 64.

Chart 6–9

The third chart in the series drawn from the study of family practice in the Health Insurance Plan of Greater New York shows the proportion of each age group of family physicians who scored 76 percent or higher (Class I) and the proportion who scored 60 percent or less (Class III). In general, greater age is associated with lower levels of performance. This does not, of course, necessarily mean that age causes a deterioration in performance. In this instance, for example, many more of the younger physicians had received longer periods of training in approved programs. But age continued to be associated with some deterioration in performance among physicians who had received two or less years of approved training, as well as among those who had received more (Table 8, p. 62). Morehead concludes that training is more important than age as a determinant of performance by these physicians (p. 48).

A reasonable interpretation of these findings (and of the rather similar findings of Peterson et al. in North Carolina, as shown in Chart 5–3) is that the longer years of family practice associated with older age do not compensate fully either for initial deficiencies in technical training or for the tendency to fall behind the advances in medical science. This is, at least, the judgment of more fully qualified internists who review the care provided by less fully trained generalists.

Though the findings of this study are not always the same as those reported by Peterson et al. (1956) and by Clute (1963), the many similarities suggest that general practice in several settings is subject to the influence of similar forces, and that the effects of these forces can be detected irrespective of whether performance is assessed by direct observation or by a review of records supplemented by interviews with the physicians. Even the interviews may not be necessary. Longer experience with the method led Morehead to conclude that the interviews "did not seem to elucidate further understanding of the clinical handling of the case—a very sensitive area when compared to that of record keeping" (Morehead 1967, p. 1646).

To permit the reader to compare the effects of several factors on performance I have shown the data on performance in a uniform way, and drawn to the same scale, in several charts in this section. In this chart the bars showing the several age groups are varied in width in order to roughly represent the widths of the corresponding age intervals.

Chart 6-9

Percent of Family Physicians Whose Performance in Caring for Selected Cases of Major Illness Was Judged To Be in the Highest and Lowest of Three Classes Respectively, by Age of the Physician. Groups Affiliated with the Health Insurance Plan of Greater New York, circa 1954.

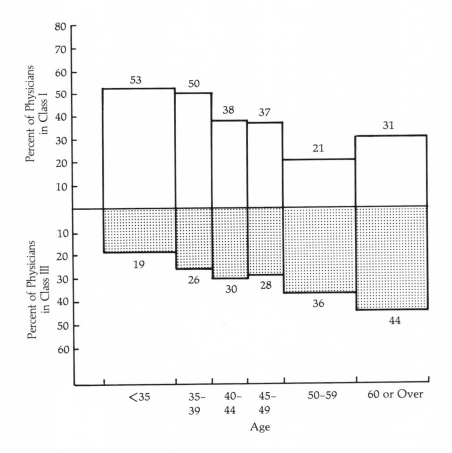

Source: Morehead 1958, Table 7, p. 61.

Chart 6–10

The preceding three charts have illustrated the importance of education and training to the performance of family physicians and prompted us to think about the further importance of continuous learning to maintaining clinical skills. Hospital appointments (the subject of this chart) are awarded in recognition of prior accomplishments but also provide an opportunity for professional renewal and growth. The consequences should be seen in the physicians' performance in both hospital and office care. There is ample evidence to support this view in many charts in several sections of this book.

The findings illustrated in this chart, as well as some others not included, show how important hospital affiliation is to performance outside the hospital, even when the latter is conducted in a group practice. Family physicians who have never held a hospital appointment do worse than those who have, and those who have relinquished a previous appointment seem to do somewhat worse than those who hold a current one. A longer affiliation with the hospital also seems to be associated with better performance, at least up to a point. How active the physician is in hospital work is also important, as shown by the associations between the monthly number of hospital visits and the proportion of physicians in the highest and lowest performance groups. The rank of the appointment is also a factor: the higher the rank the more likely are the physicians to perform well.

Other findings not shown in the chart suggested that, on the whole, an appointment in internal medicine is more likely to be associated with better performance in family practice than an appointment in another department, and that physicians who are appointed only to the outpatient service of a hospital do not do as well as those who have a more inclusive appointment.

None of these relationships represents the effects of hospital affiliation exclusively, because physicians who do not have hospital appointments, or do not hold the better posts, are more likely to have come from unapproved schools, and not to have had approved training, or to have had less of it. Physicians who have never held a hospital appointment are much more likely to be in the older age groups. Multivariate analysis is needed to estimate precisely the separate contributions of these interrelated factors.

As in previous charts, Class I physicians scored 76 percent or better, and Class III physicians scored 60 percent or less.

Chart 6–10

Percent of Family Physicians Whose Performance in Caring for Selected Cases of Major Illness Was Judged To Be in the Highest and Lowest of Three Classes Respectively, by Specified Characteristics of the Physicians' Hospital Appointments. Health Insurance Plan of Greater New York, circa 1954.

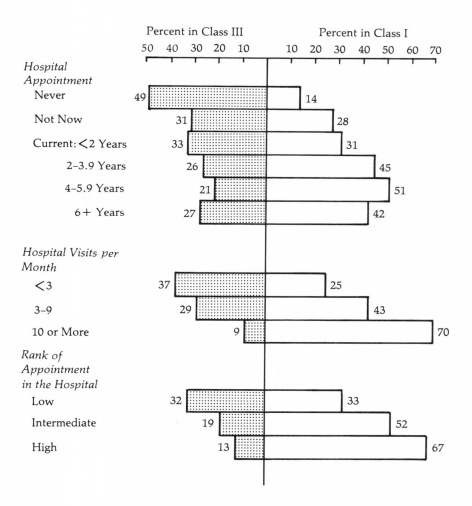

Source: Morehead 1958, Tables 18, 19, 20, and 47, pp. 67, 68, and 84.

Chart 6–11

The preceding four charts have shown that better education, more post-graduate training, and the continuing learning associated with hospital affiliation very likely contribute to higher performance by family physicians in caring for ambulatory patients. It is reasonable to expect that the extent of involvement in group practice and the degree of commitment to it would also be relevant.

At the time this study was done, physicians affiliated with this plan (HIP) could choose to continue to practice in their own offices, devoting various proportions of their time to patients enrolled in HIP while also caring for their own private patients. Alternatively, physicians could choose to see their HIP patients at facilities operated by the several groups affiliated with the plan, and do so either full time or part time.

The chart shows that the quality of care practiced on HIP premises is better than that practiced in the physicians' own offices. In either setting, physicians who devote more of their time to HIP clients perform better. The performance of physicians who work at HIP facilities for a large proportion of their time is particularly good. Data not shown in the chart indicate that these effects can be observed irrespective of the amount of postgraduate training received by physicians.

These findings do not necessarily mean that the same physicians perform differently in the two settings, since partially overlapping sets of physicians, devoting various proportions of their time to HIP patients, are involved in the comparison between sites. It is reasonable to propose, nevertheless, that even the same physicians might perform better when they are likely to be observed by colleagues, and when they have readier access to consultation, diagnostic services, and other assistance.

The lowermost panel of the chart suggests that the longer the affiliation with the plan, the more likely is the physician to perform better. Further analysis showed the relationship to be stronger for physicians with two years or less of approved training, but to be absent for physicians who gave 50 percent or more of their time to HIP. Affiliation with a group practice may either help improve performance or slow its deterioration. In time the less able physicians may also be more likely to leave, with or without prompting by their colleagues. This may be partly why those who become partners in the group are more likely to perform better than those who are still only on contract.

Chart 6–11

Percent of Family Physicians Whose Performance in Caring for Selected Cases of Major Illness Was Judged To Be in the Highest and Lowest of Three Classes Respectively, by Specified Attributes of the Degree of Commitment to Group Practice. Health Insurance Plan of Greater New York, circa 1954.

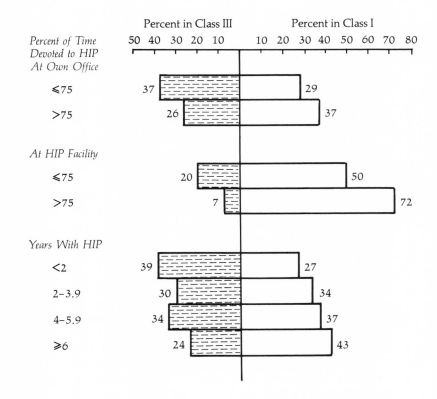

Source: Morehead 1958, Tables 24 and 27, pp. 71 and 73, with some additional computations.

Chart 6–12

In this chart we see associations between performance and several attributes of private office practice which supplement the relationships to the seemingly more fundamental attributes of education, training, hospital affiliation, and closeness of association with group practice shown in several preceding charts.

The top panel shows that family physicians who do not have help in their offices do not perform as well as those who have a full-time office assistant or are helped by their wives. The middle panel shows a striking positive relationship between the proportion of patients seen by appointment and the physicians' performance, an association also found by Peterson et al. in North Carolina (Chart 5–7, text).

The lowermost panel of the chart shows that the larger the size of the medical record (and the closer to the format endorsed by HIP) the more likely is the physician to fall in the highest class of performance by earning a score of 76 percent or more. But this variable was not associated with the probability of scoring 60 percent or less (Class III).

Morehead does not analyze further the association of performance to the size of the medical record, but she does show that the associations with having an office assistant and an appointment system continued to be present when the data were subclassified, first by whether the physicians had less or more than two years of approved postgraduate training, and then by whether they devoted more or less than 50 percent of their time to the group practice. We can conclude that training and attachment to the group do not completely explain the observed relationships to performance, even though these variables could still play a part, along with other variables whose effects were not tested.

One can only speculate about how the relationships observed in this chart are brought about. For example, we do not know to what extent an appointment system brings about better care, and to what extent the better family physicians insist on seeing their patients by appointment. The effect of record size is particularly intriguing, since the judgment about the quality of care depended so much on what was entered in the record.

Morehead summarizes her findings by concluding that the relationships of performance to physician training, time devoted to group practice, and features of practice such as its location and how much of it is in the hospital are so large and consistent that they are not likely to have arisen by chance (p. 45).

Chart 6–12

Percent of Family Physicians Whose Performance in Caring for Selected Cases of Major Illness Was Judged To Be in the Highest and Lowest of Three Classes Respectively, by Specified Features of the Physicians' Private Office Practice. Health Insurance Plan of Greater New York, circa 1954.

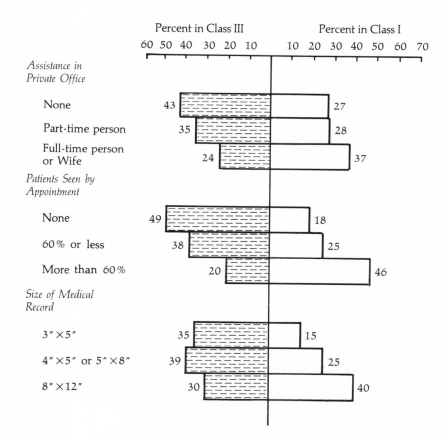

Source: Morehead 1958, Tables 33, 37 and 39, pp. 77, 79, and 80, with additional computations.

Chart 6–13

We have already encountered the use of explicit criteria to assess hospital care as reflected in the medical record. The work of Lembcke on the justification of gynecological surgery (Chart 4–23) represents the debut of explicit criteria as a key tool for assessing quality. Subsequently, a group of investigators at The University of Michigan rediscovered this method and used it to assess the appropriateness of hospital admissions and lengths of stay (Charts 3–7 to 3–12). Since then, Payne, a member of the original Michigan group, has played a leading role in further developing the method and using it to assess the quality of hospital and ambulatory care.

To obtain the data shown in this chart, 16 diagnostic categories were selected because they were illustrative of a wide range of hospital care, were important, and lent themselves to assessment using explicit criteria. Expert panels specified the criteria for each of the 16 major categories and some additional subclasses. They then assigned a weight ranging from 0.5 to 3.0 that was supposed to represent the "importance" of each criterion item "recommended" for the diagnostic management of each case. A representative sample of discharges with the selected diagnoses was drawn from all 22 nonfederal, short-term hospitals in Hawaii. Well-trained abstractors searched the medical record for the presence of the items of performance that the criteria specified. Where possible, pertinent information was also obtained from the records of office care. Having this information, it was easy to construct the Physician Performance Index, which was the percent of the weighted total of pertinent criterion items that were present in the medical record. The appropriateness of admission and length of stay could also be determined.

In this chart we find that two factors, the size of the hospital and whether the physician has the appropriate ("modal") specialty to take care of the case, influence the quality of care and, to some extent, the appropriateness of hospital stay. Care is better in larger hospitals and in the hands of specialists. In noting the importance of specialization, these findings are consistent with those of Morehead et al. as shown in Charts 6–2 and 6–4.

Chart 6–13

Physician Performance Index and Percent of Cases that Are Appropriately Admitted and Have an Appropriate Length of Stay, According to Specialty Status of Physician and to Size of Hospital. Hospital Discharges in Any One of 16 Diagnostic Categories, Nonfederal Short-term Hospitals, Hawaii, 1968.

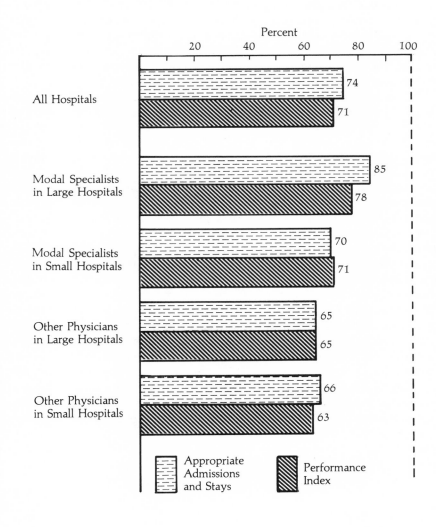

Source: Payne et al. 1976, Table 3, p. 14.

Chart 6–14

In this chart, which is the second in the series drawn from, or based upon, the work of Payne et al. in Hawaii, we see the relation between practice setting and hospital care. There is a gradient, in both quality and appropriateness of hospital stay, in which physicians who work in a large multispecialty group practice which is part of the Kaiser-Permanente system rank first, physicians in other multispecialty group practices rank second, and physicians who are in solo practice rank last. This finding is rather easily explained by differences in specialization. The percent of hospitalized cases treated by modal specialists in the three practice settings was 93, 71, and 34 percent, respectively.

Besides reflecting the performance of physicians and hospitals, the findings are influenced by the sample of diagnoses selected and by the nature of the criteria used. The content of the criteria is, of course, important. In this study, as in almost all studies of physician performance, the emphasis is on technical care. In this case, the criteria are restricted even more than usual by the exclusion of therapy from the assessment of many diagnoses. The form of the criteria and the procedures for scaling are also important. The criteria for this study were essentially "linear," a format that is often referred to rather slightingly as a "laundry list." It is generally believed that such criteria are rather difficult to match with their referents. It is feared that in the attempt to make the criteria comprehensive, procedures are included that are not necessary in every case. This may encourage waste, especially if the several criterion items are not weighted, so that their relative importance cannot be appreciated. In this case the criteria were weighted, but the range in weights is rather small, and the simple addition of scores to arrive at the performance index assumes that there are no interactions among the criterion items. Besides, one cannot tell what values of the index correspond to descriptions such as "excellent," "good," "acceptable," or "unacceptable." Frequency distributions could have helped, but these have not been reported.

These comments are meant to identify methodological problems that require attention. They are not meant to detract from the importance of the study as a major advance in quality assessment. The study is also notable for attempting to assess an entire episode of care that includes, but is not confined to, hospitalization, and for describing the care received by everyone in a large, self-contained community.

Chart 6–14

Physician Performance Index and Percent of Cases that Are Appropriately Admitted and Have an Appropriate Length of Stay, According to Type of Practice. Hospital Discharges in Any One of 16 Diagnostic Categories, Nonfederal Short-term Hospitals, Hawaii, 1968.

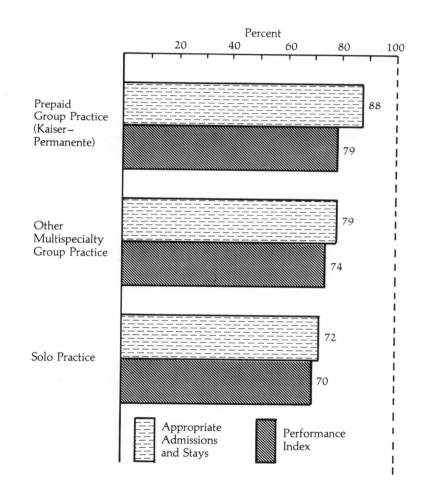

Source: Payne et al. 1976, Table 3, p. 14.

Chart 6–15

We have a more detailed picture of what Payne et al. found about the quality of care in Hawaii from the results of additional analyses made by Rhee. Because physician performance varied according to diagnosis, Rhee constructed a standard z score for each case, and used it to compute average scores of physician performance. This procedure holds the mean performance by all physicians for each diagnosis to be zero and the standard deviation to be 1. As a result, we have a picture of relative position, rather than of absolute performance.

In this chart, which is the first of several based on the work of Rhee and his associates, we see the effects of specialization. Three levels of specialization are recognized: board certified physicians with a certified or claimed subspecialty, board certified physicians without a subspecialty, and board eligible physicians irrespective of subspecialty. All other physicians are considered to be general practitioners, even when they reported that they limited their work to a specialty. Recognized specialists do not always confine their work to the area (or "domain") in which they are specialized. To study the possible effects of this practice, Payne et al. asked their consultants to assign each diagnostic category used in their study to the one or more specialties considered to be most appropriate to it. A specialist who cared for a case within his domain was considered to act as a "modal" specialist, whereas one who stepped outside the legitimate bounds of his specialty became "nonmodal" every time he did so.

The chart shows that the performance of recognized specialists is superior to that of generalists, but only when the former remain within their domains of specialization. Though the performance of specialists when they practice within their domains improves with increasing specialization, this relationship is not statistically significant. The decisive difference is brought about by having sufficient training to become board eligible. Actual certification, through passing the required examinations, conferred no additional benefit in this study. The performance of specialists, taken as a group, deteriorates significantly when they practice outside their domains. The chart also suggests that the more highly specialized a physician is, the larger is the adverse consequence of practicing outside his domain, but this was not a statistically significant finding.

Important though these findings are, only one percent of the variance in performance among physicians was explained by the degree of their specialization.

Chart 6-15

Standardized Physician Performance Scores, by Specialty Status and Domain of Practice. Hospital Discharges in Any of 15 Diagnostic Categories, Nonfederal Short-term Hospitals, Hawaii, 1968.

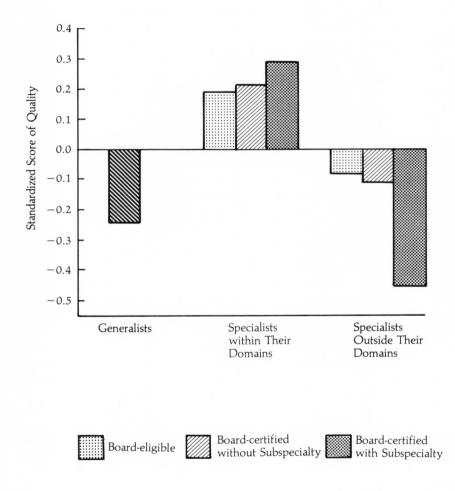

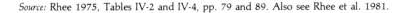

Source: Rhee 1975, Tables IV-2 and IV-4, pp. 79 and 89. Also see Rhee et al. 1981.

Chart 6–16

Using the data and methods described in the immediately preceding charts, Rhee examined the effect of undergraduate education on the technical quality of the care provided by physicians during episodes of illness that included care in the hospital. To do this, hospital discharges were categorized not only by the specialty status of the physician, and by whether the specialized physician was or was not practicing within his "domain" in caring for each particular case, as was done in the preceding chart, but also by the type of medical school from which the physician was graduated. U.S. medical schools were classified into quartiles using the average of two ratios: the proportion of graduates in teaching or research, and the proportion who had attained board certification. Foreign medical schools were classified using a method devised by Knobel (1973) based on selected indicators of wealth, education, health status, and health care resources that characterized their respective countries.

The chart shows a very regular gradient for specialists, as long as they practice within their "domains": performance relative to the average declines as the implied ranking of the medical school goes down. General practice, and the practice of specialists outside their "domains," does not show a similarly consistent relationship. For these forms of practice, the performance of physicians who graduated from the U.S. schools assigned to the fourth quartile of the classification appears to be better than that of many other U.S. graduates, but not much better than that of foreign graduates. Because many of the differences observed were found not to be statistically significant, the safest conclusion to be drawn from the findings is that physicians who graduated from the most highly placed U.S. medical schools do perform better, but that the differences among all the others are of doubtful importance.

To remove the disturbing influence of a correlation between medical credentials and organizational affiliations, the data shown in the chart were adjusted for type of hospital and form of ambulatory practice, as well as for years in practice. When these adjustments were made, and the effect of specialty status was also controlled, the type of medical school explained only two percent of the variance in physician performance. One should also remember that the findings pertain only to the sample studied. They may not apply to all the graduates of the medical schools represented in the study, and certainly not to those that were not included.

Chart 6–16

Standardized Physician Performance Scores, by Specialty Status, Domain of
Practice, and Type of Medical School from which Physicians Were Graduated.
Hospital Discharges in Any One of 15 Diagnostic Categories, Nonfederal
Short-term Hospitals, Hawaii, 1968.

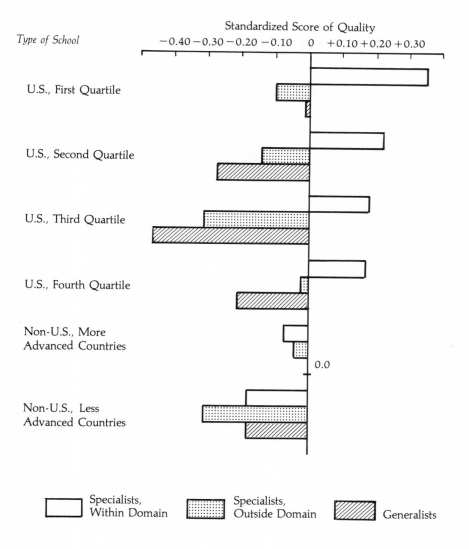

Standardized Score of Quality

Type of School   −0.40 −0.30 −0.20 −0.10   0   +0.10 +0.20 +0.30

U.S., First Quartile

U.S., Second Quartile

U.S., Third Quartile

U.S., Fourth Quartile

Non-U.S., More
Advanced Countries

0.0

Non-U.S., Less
Advanced Countries

Specialists,   Specialists,
Within Domain   Outside Domain   Generalists

Source: Rhee 1977, Table 2, p. 573.

Chart 6–17

From Rhee's more detailed analysis of the data collected by Payne et al. in Hawaii we also get information about the possible effect of the duration of practice, which is, of course, associated with age.

The reader will recall that by constructing a measure of the variation in physician performance for each diagnostic category Rhee was able to obtain a standardized mean score for all diagnoses. The left side of the chart shows these scores of performance for physicians in three categories of duration of practice. On the right hand side, the scores are adjusted for associated differences in the category of medical school from which the physicians graduated and their specialty status (as shown in the preceding charts), as well as for the organization of office practice and type of hospital (as will be described for succeeding charts). I have varied the widths of the three bars in each of the two panels in order to convey a rough impression of the relative duration of each segment.

The findings remind us a little of the earlier reports of Peterson et al. concerning general practice in North Carolina (Charts 5–3 and 5–6). Judging by the unadjusted means, the quality of episodes of care that include a hospital stay begins by being relatively low, improves significantly during the physicians' middle years, and is somewhat lower thereafter. Adjustment for the factors mentioned above reduces these differences by only a little; the pattern remains highly unlikely to have occurred by chance.

Although these data do not come from a study that follows physicians as they age, it is tempting to see in them the resultant of two opposing tendencies: one of learning through experience and continuing education, and the other of partial obsolescence through failure to keep up with new knowledge. In extreme old age other forms of deterioration may also set in. The findings in the chart are clouded, however, not only by the "cross-sectional" nature of the study, but also by the method of judging quality through searching medical records for the presence of prespecified activities (mainly of a diagnostic nature) that are considered to represent good care. Could it be that more experienced physicians can do as well with less investigation, or that they record less of what they actually do?

Chart 6–17

Standardized Physician Performance Scores by Years in Practice. Hospital Discharges in Any of 15 Diagnostic Categories, Nonfederal Short-term Hospitals, Hawaii, 1968.

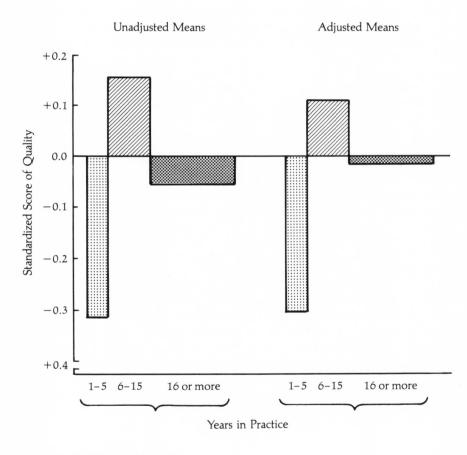

Source: Rhee 1976, Table 7, p. 743.

Chart 6–18

Rhee's more detailed analysis of the data amassed by Payne et al. provides additional information about the relationship between performance and organizational factors shown earlier in Charts 6–13 and 6–14.

This chart shows some of the effects of the organization of office practice as modified by specialty status, restriction to specialty "domain," and other variables that may influence practice. Rhee classified office practice into seven categories which he thought represented progressively higher degrees of formal organization. This chart shows the findings only for solo practice at one extreme of the scale and large multispecialty group practice (irrespective of prepayment) at the other end.

The first pair of bars demonstrates that physicians who practice in large multispecialty groups provide significantly better care for episodes that include hospital stay than do physicians in solo practice. The second pair of bars confirms the earlier report by Payne et al. that the difference mentioned above is due to the greater proportion of specialists in the larger group practices. Within their clinically appropriate "domains" specialists in the larger multispecialty groups are seen to perform only a little better than their counterparts in solo practice. As shown in the third pair of bars, even this small difference is wiped out when further adjustments are made for differences in category of medical school, type of hospital, and years in practice. The final pair of bars shows that performance suffers when specialists care for patients who fall outside their fields of particular competence, irrespective of whether this happens in solo practice or in a large multispecialty group practice.

Not shown in the chart is the important observation that, at least in Hawaii, physicians in small and medium-sized group practices perform no better than their counterparts in solo practice, and in some kinds of groups (notably in medium-sized multispecialty groups with at least some prepayment) they do considerably worse. In the larger multispecialty groups (those with at least the equivalent of 16 full-time physicians) prepayment is not, itself, related to performance. It is obviously necessary to go far beyond the surface characteristics of group practice to understand which features of organization safeguard and promote quality, and which do not.

Chart 6–18

Standardized Physician Performance Scores, by Specialty Status, Domain of Practice, and the Manner in Which Office Practice Is Organized. Hospital Discharges in Any of 15 Diagnostic Categories, Nonfederal Short-term Hospitals, Hawaii, 1968.

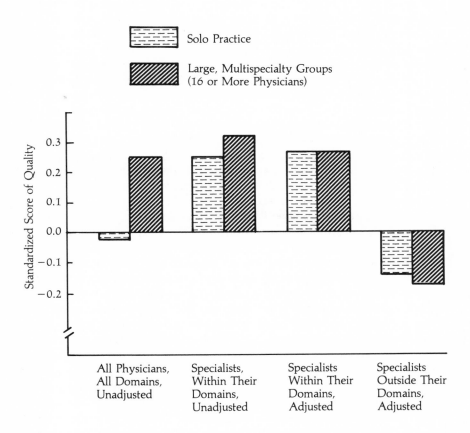

Source: Rhee 1975, Tables V-5 and V-6, pp. 115 and 120. Also see Rhee 1976, Table 8, p. 744.

Chart 6–19

The study of organizational factors that influence the qualtiy of care leads inevitably to the attributes of the hospitals in which physicians practice. The earlier work of Morehead et al. (Charts 6–2, 6–3, 6–4) has already alerted us to the importance of this factor, and in particular to that of a hospital's affiliation with a medical school. The findings in Hawaii, whether reported by Payne et al. (Chart 6–13) or by Rhee (as in this chart and the next), add to the evidence.

Rhee classified the nonfederal, short-term hospitals in Hawaii mainly according to size, location, and teaching function. The five teaching hospitals trained interns and residents, but none had more than "limited affiliation with a medical school" (p. 171). The hospital owned by the Kaiser Foundation is recognized separately as the only one formally associated with a large, prepaid multispecialty group practice.

The progression of categories shown in the chart implies a rough scale of increasing tightness in formal organization and control. Whether or not this is the case, the chart does show that larger size and the presence either of house staff or of prepayment contribute significantly to technical quality, at least quality as judged by prespecified explicit criteria and as documented in the medical record.

Of all the variables whose effects were studied by Rhee, hospital attributes were, in fact, the most important. They explained 16 percent of the observed variation in physician performance. When adjustments were made to account for associations between hospital attributes on the one hand, and specialty status, duration of practice, and organization of office practice on the other, the effect of hospital attributes was, as is shown in the chart, somewhat reduced. But even then, hospital attributes accounted for 12 percent of the observed variation in physician performance. Compare this to the contribution (after adjustment for the effect of the other variables) of two percent by the category of medical school from which the physician was graduated (Chart 6–16), one percent by specialty status (Chart 6–15), two percent by duration of practice (Chart 6–17), and one percent by the organization of office practice (Chart 6–18). The decisive preeminence of hospital characteristics is evident. But perhaps the more important finding is that all of these factors combined account for only 18 percent of the variance in physician performance. There is much about the quality of care that we do not, as yet, understand.

Chart 6-19

Standardized Physician Performance Scores by Type of Hospital. Hospital Discharges in Any of 15 Diagnostic Categories, Nonfederal Short-term Hospitals, Hawaii, 1968.

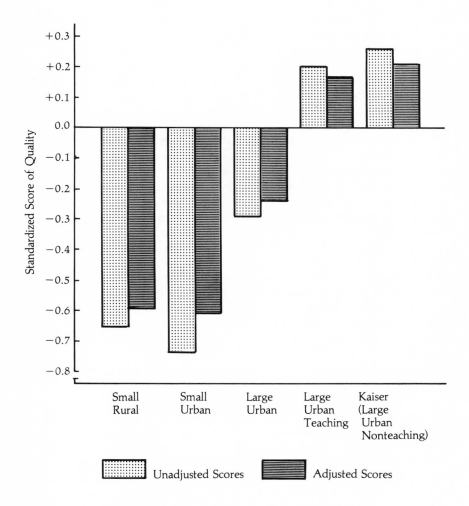

Source: Rhee 1975, Table VI-5, p. 150. Also see Rhee 1976, Table 9, p. 745.

Chart 6–20

In this chart we see the joint and separate effects of physician training and the organization of the hospital on the technical quality of care for episodes that include a hospital stay.

In order to construct the table from which this chart is drawn, Rhee compressed his scales for physician specialty status and type of hospital into two categories for each. Highly trained physicians are those who are either certified or eligible for certification by a specialty board. All others are placed in the category of less highly trained physicians. As to the categorization of hospitals, Rhee was able to show that the more detailed classification described in connection with the preceding chart corresponded well with several indicators of formal organization and control (Rhee 1975, pp. 142–46). Accordingly, the Kaiser Foundation hospital and all the urban teaching hospitals were placed in the more highly organized category, while all other hospitals were considered to have a relatively lower level of formal organization.

The four bars of the chart show the standardized performance scores for physicians in their respective categories, after adjustment for differences in the category of the medical school from which the physicians were graduated (as in Chart 6–16), the duration of practice (as in Chart 6–17), and the organization of office practice (as in Chart 6–18). By comparing the four bars in several combinations one can conclude that (1) each of more training and higher levels of hospital organization contributes to better performance; (2) the effect of hospital organization is the larger of the two; (3) the effect of hospital organization is perhaps somewhat more important for the less well trained physicians; and (4) the level of training is perhaps more important in the less highly organized hospitals.

These findings are not unlike those shown in Chart 6–4 as reported by Morehead et al.

(The reader may be interested to know that the measure of hospital organization used by Rhee to validate his classification included (1) the number of contractual physicians adjusted by the logarithm of the number of beds and weighted according to method of payment and other factors as proposed by Roemer and Friedman, 1971, p. 305; (2) the proportion of physicians who are board eligible or certified; (3) the proportion of operations performed by surgeons practicing within their domains; (4) the proportion of deaths examined postmortem; and (5) the proportion of surgically removed tissue subjected to pathological examination.)

Chart 6–20

Standardized Physician Performance Scores, by Level of the Physician's Formal Training, and by Level of Formal Organization in the Hospitals. Hospital Discharges in Any of 15 Diagnostic Categories, Nonfederal Short-term Hospitals, Hawaii, 1968.

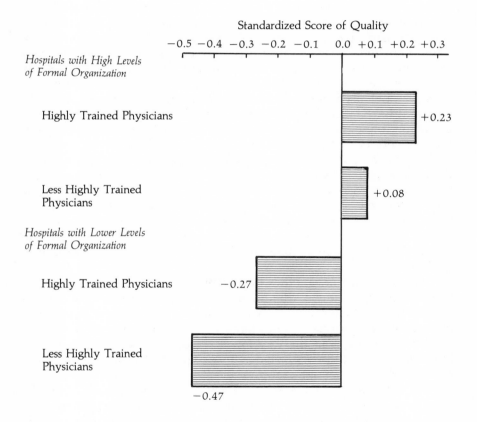

Source: Rhee 1975, Table VII-6, p. 189.

Chart 6–21

This chart and the next are meant to contribute to the second component in the "epidemiology of quality," that which studies the distribution of care, characterized by its quality, according to the attributes of its consumers. This particular chart shows the associations with age.

The information comes from the Hawaiian study which also provided the several preceding charts. The reader will recall that this was a study of episodes of care for a selected set of diagnostic categories, as shown in the chart. The criteria and standards of quality were prespecified by panels of experts. The "physician performance index," which is the measure of quality plotted, is the weighted percent of applicable criteria found to be met, as shown by a perusal of each patient's medical record in the hospital and, where possible, in the physician's office. In this chart, the diagnostic categories for which information from office records was not used are marked with an asterisk. To convey a clearer picture, I have taken the liberty of showing the diagnostic categories as points on a line, rather than as separate bars, which would have been the more orthodox representation.

As to the association between technical quality and the patients' age, the general pattern is the absence of such a relationship. For two diagnoses (cerebrovascular accidents and chronic urinary tract infection) the quality of care is significantly worse among the aged, and for one (bronchitis in adults) it is significantly better. All the other differences observed could very easily have arisen by chance. An overall test of "the entire 15 independent probabilities" showed no statistical significance (p. 927).

There is, however, another important finding which the chart also features through showing the diagnostic categories arranged according to increasingly better average performance in the younger age group. We can, thus, appreciate the differences in performance by diagnostic category, ranging from the very low score of 31.76 for chronic urinary tract infection in those 65 or older, to a high of 74.11 for cancer of the cervix in the younger age group.

In a separate study Lyons and Payne (1974c) show that, with the possible exception of follow-up medical examinations, the quality of office care for several diagnoses is no worse for the aged. One should note, however, that neither study addresses the question of initial access to care.

Chart 6-21

Physician Performance Index, by Diagnostic Category, and by Age of Patients. Discharges from Nonfederal Short-term Hospitals, Hawaii, 1968.

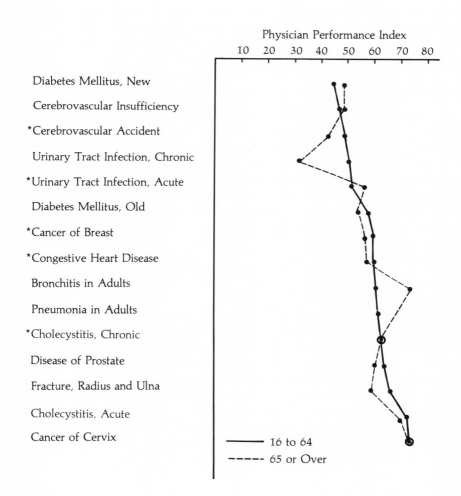

Source and Note: Lyons and Payne 1974a, Table 2, 927. The asterisks are explained in the text.

Chart 6–22

Rhee provides additional information concerning the relationship between patient characteristics and the technical quality of care in the Hawaiian study of Payne et al. This chart shows part of the data about race.
The adjusted standardized scores control for the possible effects of 12
variables including the patient's age and sex; the physician's race and
several attributes of his training and practice; source of payment for
hospital care; and type of hospital (p. 747). The unadjusted scores would
permit any coherent associations of these variables with the patient's
race to express themselves as differences in quality.

Though the chart, because it shows the racial categories in ascending
order of quality, suggests some kind of gradient, the differences observed, whether in the adjusted or unadjusted scores, could very easily
have occurred by chance in samples of the size available for study. The
conclusion is that the patient's race is not related to the quality of care.

Not shown in the chart is the finding that patients in Hawaii are more
likely to receive care from physicians of their own race. The proportions
observed exceed what might have been expected from a random assortment by 1.3 times for whites, 2.2 times for patients of Japanese extrac-
tion, and 2.8 times for both Chinese and Filipino patients. But there
were no "distinct patterns" that would lead one to conclude that receiving care from a physician of similar race would improve or harm the
quality of care (p. 743). It should be remembered, however, that only the
technical aspects of care were assessed in this study; neither patient
satisfaction nor patient cooperation were considered. In fact, the selection of conditions for study included, as one criterion among several,
that they "not require excessive patient participation for good outcomes"
(Payne et al. 1976, p. 7).

Negative findings do not make exciting charts. It is reassuring to
know, however, that at least in Hawaii, neither age (as shown in the
preceding chart) nor race (as shown in this one) affect the quality of
technical care. But we still do not know if there may have been differences in access to care. And Hawaii is not representative of the United
States as a whole, particularly with regard to the cultural and socioeconomic connotations of its racial characteristics.

Chart 6–22

Standardized Physician Performance Scores by Race of Patient. Hospital Discharges in Any of 15 Diagnostic Categories, Nonfederal Short-term Hospitals, Hawaii, 1968.

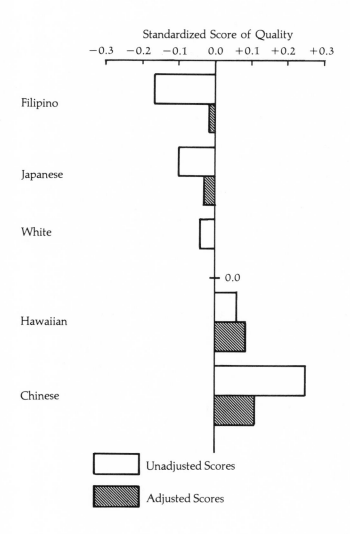

Standardized Score of Quality

Source: Rhee et al. 1979, Table 3, p. 742.

Chart 6–23

The work of Payne and his associates in Hawaii also provides an excellent early example of the use of explicit criteria to assess ambulatory care, with methods very similar to those described in the preceding section. Panels of experts prespecified and weighted criteria for the ambulatory care of selected conditions. The practicing physicians who agreed to participate kept a log of all patients who belonged in each of the categories chosen for study. Samples were drawn from the logs. The medical record of each case was checked for adherence to the criteria. The "physician performance index" was the percent of applicable criteria adhered to, weighted by the rating of importance attached to each criterion item.

The top half of the chart shows the wide range of variation among diagnoses. The lower half shows the very modest differences among sites of care. The most striking feature, however, is the very low level of performance throughout. Overall, there was evidence of adherence to no more than 41 percent of the criteria that the experts judged to be required for "optimal care." We do not know, however, to what extent this disappointing result shows a failure in recording, a failure in practice, or unjustifiably high expectations. We should also remember that the conditions selected for study do not represent the totality of practice. Moreover, because only a third of the physicians who were asked to participate actually did so, the findings may be biased. If, as is likely, more of the better physicians agreed to participate, the situation is, in fact, worse than that shown.

Other findings, not shown in the chart, included the following: (1) specialists performed significantly better than generalists in almost all of the categories chosen for study; (2) board-certified specialists, compared to specialists who were not certified, were about as likely to perform better as worse; and (3) being in practice for 20 years or more was associated with lower levels of performance in most of the categories. These findings are similar to those reported (in the preceding section) for episodes with a large component of hospital care.

Chart 6–23

Physician Performance Index by Specified Diagnostic Categories and by Type of Office Practice. Patients in Any of Eight Diagnostic Categories and Any of Five Types of Periodic Health Assessment, Hawaii, April–May 1970.

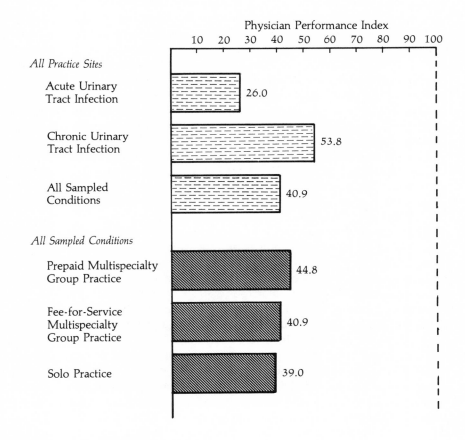

Source: Payne et al. 1976, Table 7, p. 27.

Chart 6–24

More recently, Payne et al. studied the quality of ambulatory care at five different sites in two counties in the Midwest. These were (1) the outpatient clinics of a teaching hospital that is a regional referral center, but also provides care to its locality; (2) a number of clinics at different places which are linked to a medical school; (3) the clinics of a large teaching hospital which are staffed by salaried physicians responsible for both outpatient and inpatient care, with services paid for on a fee-for-service basis; (4) a prepaid group practice based in a medium-sized hospital in the inner city, a small suburban hospital, and several small health centers; and (5) a selection of solo practices, partnerships, and small groups in a county. The sites were chosen as examples of different forms of practice. The findings, therefore, are only illustrative, rather than representative of any identifiable groups of either providers or clients.

The method of quality assessment was very similar to that used earlier in Hawaii, except that there was greater attention to the assessment of therapeutic skills, and a modified method for weighting the criteria resulted in a much wider range of weights. (See Donabedian 1982, pp. 227–31, and 280–83).

By arranging the categories in order of the range of performance among sites, the chart shows differences among sites that are much larger for some categories than others. The less variable the care among sites, the higher the average performance for that category in all sites combined. The comparison between pediatric and adult examinations is particularly interesting. (It will be recalled that Morehead et al. observed something similar to this in their comparison of surgical and medical care in New York Hospitals, as shown in Chart 6–2.)

Though the position of the several sites does vary from condition to condition, some sites are more often near one end or other of the scale. When average standardized scores of performance are computed for all categories at each site, one finds the fee-for-service group practice hospital significantly in the lead, followed by the teaching hospital clinics and the primary care physicians' offices, in that order. The university-affiliated clinics and the prepaid group practice clinics are in last place, at approximately similar levels of performance (Table 3.4, p. 48).

Chart 6–24

Physician Performance Index, by Specified Diagnoses, Conditions, or Clinical Activities, and by Specified Sites of Care. Ambulatory Care at Five Sites in Two Counties in the Midwest, U.S.A., 1974–75.

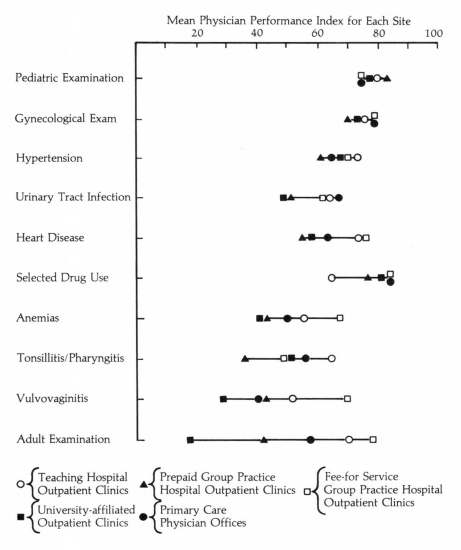

Source: Payne et al. 1978, Table 3.2, pp. 41–42.

Chart 6–25

In this second chart from the study of five Midwestern sites, we see the association between quality ratings and each of several characteristics of the physician or his practice. Also shown are the possible effects of activities carried out between 1975 and 1977 to improve the quality of care.

Because the quality of care was so variable, standardized scores were constructed. The mean score for each category was 500 and the standard deviation 100. The data were also adjusted for relevant differences in certification, domain of practice, and physicians' years in practice. "Modal" care is that provided by a specialist practicing within his field.

The simplest intervention designed to improve quality was to report the findings of each round of assessments to the chief of the service or clinic. More active intervention called, in addition, for a workshop to which selected physicians from each site were invited. The most active intervention added a series of consultations and meetings following the workshop.

The chart confirms some earlier findings from the study of ambulatory care in Hawaii. For example, board certification was not consistently related to quality, whereas restriction of practice to the physician's field of specialization was. The finding that physicians who have been in practice for 20 years or more are less likely to adhere to the criteria of quality is in keeping with earlier findings for hospital and ambulatory care in Hawaii (Chart 6–17 and text of Chart 6–23) and for the office care of general practitioners in North Carolina and Canada (Chart 5–6). Finally, the quality of care is not significantly related to differences in the number of patients seen per hour until a sharp downturn occurs at around six patients per hour.

Roughly speaking, the activities designed to improve quality appear to have a significant effect which is directly proportional to the intensity of the intervention. During the period of observation some clinics made a change in management, such as the hiring of a clinic chief, which increased "the amount of managerial presence" in the clinics. These changes were associated with notable improvements in performance, even in the absence of interventions by the research staff; where such interventions had been instituted, the managerial change added to the improvement associated with the intervention.

Note, however, that the findings of this and similar studies depend heavily on the quality of the medical record.

Chart 6-25

Standardized Physician Performance Scores, by Specified Characteristics of the Physicians' Training and Practice. Ambulatory Care at Five Sites in Two Counties in the Midwest, U.S.A., 1974–1975 and 1977.

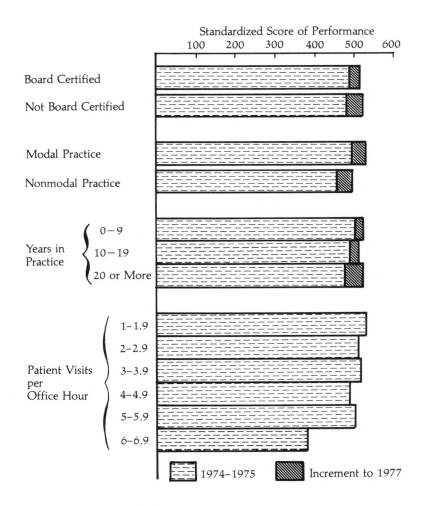

Source: Payne et al. 1978, Tables 4.7 and 6.1, pp. 95 and 183, and Figure 6.2, p. 186.

Chart 6–26

This study is notable for refinements in the methods of formulating and weighting the criteria, for testing the effects of different forms of weighting, for identifying coherent clusters of the criteria, for studying a very large number of variables as possible influences on performance, and for testing the validity of the medical record through direct observation of practice. (For more on these features see Donabedian 1980, pp. 59–62; Donabedian 1982, pp. 169–70, 231–35, and 287–88.)

This chart shows the proportion of unclustered criterion items adhered to. The criteria are weighted equally because this and two alternative forms of weighting gave similar results. Using this method we see that the care in the outpatient department of a hospital is more likely to conform to the criteria than is care in a physician's private office, and that in each of these kinds of places, care by a specialist is more conforming than care by a generalist. (In two instances, indicated by asterisks, no comparisons were possible.)

The place of practice was the most important factor in performance, and specialty the next most important. Board-certified physicians did better than those who were not (p. 181). "Interns, residents and their faculty always received higher scores than attendings" (p. 181). Physicians who worked alone, with few professional contacts, did particularly badly (p. 192). Performance was better when physicians were more likely to delegate tasks to others, said they were comfortable as supervisors, reported knowing more of their patients well, and were judged to be more "patient-oriented" (p. 193). Physicians who spent 15 minutes or more with each patient did better than those who spent less time, particularly in private practice. The best pediatricians had been in practice for either less than 12 years or more than 40. On the whole, the longer a general practitioner had been in practice, the lower the adherence to the criteria (pp. 179, 181).

The credibility of the findings is somewhat weakened by the low response rate (68 percent) in the sample of office practice. The diagnoses selected for study do not necessarily represent all care. The completeness of the record is always an issue, but in this study direct observation of a small sample of pediatricians in private practice showed the record to be almost complete, except that explanations and instructions, when given, were seldom recorded (pp. 114–15).

Chart 6-26

Percent of Preformulated Explicit Criteria of Good Ambulatory Care Adhered to, by Age Group of the Patient, by Diagnostic Category, by Site of Care, and by Physicians' Specialty Status. Metropolitan Areas of New Haven and Hartford, Connecticut, 1974–1975.

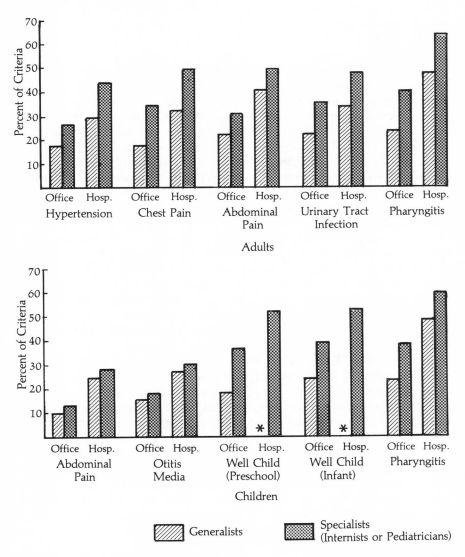

Source: Riedel and Riedel 1979, Tables 7.2a to 7.10a, pp. 130–39. The asterisks indicate missing data.

Chart 6–27

This chart tells us more about the relationship between workload and quality in office practice.

All members of the North Carolina Society of Internal Medicine in four populous areas of the state were invited to participate: only 31 physicians (14 percent of those eligible) participated. The conditions selected for study were diabetes mellitus, hypertension, complaints attributable to urinary tract infection in females, and annual general examinations for adults. The investigators compiled a list of possible criteria for the management of each condition. Each physician was then asked to rate the importance of each item on each list, and to say whether it would be likely to be recorded whenever implemented. The "consensus criteria" were those which a majority of physicians said were both important and subject to recording. (Also see Donabedian 1982, pp. 324–29.)

As we shall see in a subsequent chart, physicians differed widely in their adherence to the criteria. Their workloads were also very different, ranging from 1.6 to 6.4 patients per hour. The chart shows the relationships between the ranks of the 31 physicians, when ordered by each of the two variables.

The investigators found that, on the whole, the busier the physician the less likely was the record to show adherence to the criteria. The chart shows an additional finding: the busier doctors were less likely to adhere to the criteria for the patients' medical history and physical examination while, on the whole, they were more likely to adhere to the criteria for laboratory tests. This suggests that the busier physicians tend to substitute procedures that do not take so much of their own time for those that do.

In Tables 14, 15, and 16 of their report the investigators show the possible effects of other physician characteristics (age, board certification, subspecialty), practice characteristics (group practice, physician extenders, accepting new patients, drop-in patients, laboratory and x-ray facilities, population of site), and patient characteristics (sex, age, race, marital status). There was some reason to infer that adherence to the criteria was greater in group practice, in smaller cities, for the general examinations of males, and for the management of urinary complaints and diabetes in older persons. All other variables, including the race of the patient and the subspecialty of the physician, were unrelated to adherence. But the high selectivity of this study limits the general applicability of its conclusions.

Chart 6-27

Spearman Rank Order Correlation Coefficients for the Relationship Between
Adherence to Preformulated, Explicit "Consensus Criteria" and the Number of
Patients Seen per Hour. Office Care by Selected Internists for Patients with Any
One of Four Conditions, North Carolina, 1975–1977.

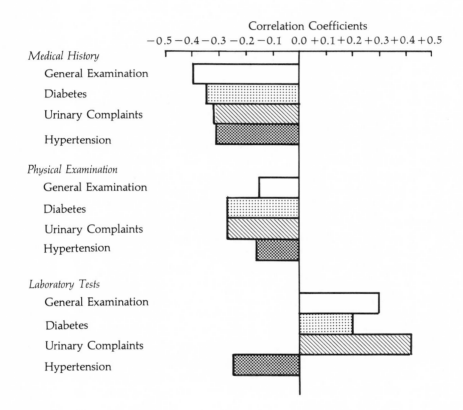

Source: Hulka et al. 1979, Table 27, p. 32.

Chart 6–28

Some of the methods and findings of this study were described in the preceding chart, which dealt with the variation in adherence to explicit criteria of office care associated with how many patients a physician saw per hour. Other sources of variability were described in the comments on the chart. This chart is meant to expand our view of the immense variability, much of it unexplained, that one encounters in this and other studies of the quality of care.

The upper part of the chart shows the distribution of the 31 partici-pating physicians according to the percent of consensus criteria found to be adhered to by each physician when all his sampled records for all four study conditions were considered together. The physicians are seen to differ greatly in performance, even though they are all well-qualified internists. The detailed data show a low of 39 percent recorded adherence for one physician, and a high of 89 percent for another.

The lower part of the chart shows the percent distribution of "batches" of five or more cases of any of the four conditions selected for study managed by any one of the 31 physician participants. The variability is even greater because of added differences by condition among all phy-sicians combined, and the smaller number of cases per unit of analysis. The detailed table shows a range from 28 percent adherence for six hy-pertensives under the care of one physician, to an adherence ratio of 98 percent for three diabetics managed by another physician.

The variability in performance is largely unexplained. Overall, there are significant differences among the several conditions, the adherence ratio being 0.69 for the general medical examination, 0.64 for diabetes, 0.58 for hypertension, and 0.54 for urinary complaints. Though physi-cians varied in their performance according to condition, "there was substantial correlation among the individual physicians' mean adherence scores for the different study conditions" (p.24). The differences ob-served could not be explained by variations in patient characteristics or severity of condition; nor could they be attributed to differences among the criteria espoused by the different practitioners.

We may conclude that though, on the average, some physicians per-form better than others, the reasons for the differences are only partly understood, and that there is still much variability within the practice of any given physician beyond that which can be explained by the mix of his patients. (See Hulka et al. 1979, pp. 29–30 and 60–61.)

Chart 6–28

Percent Distribution of Physicians, and of Physician-Condition Batches, by Percent of Preformulated, Explicit, "Consensus Criteria" Adhered to. Office Care by Selected Internists for Patients with Any One of Four Conditions. North Carolina, 1975–1977.

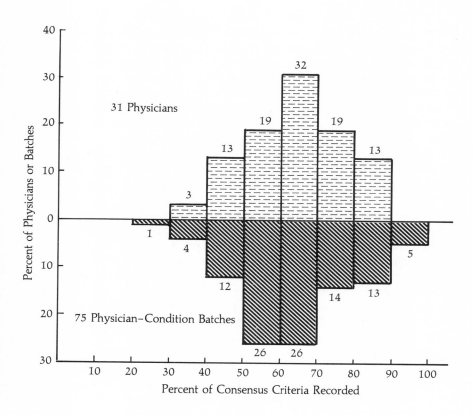

Source: Hulka et al. 1977. Computed from Table 17, pp. 62–63.

Chart 6–29

The study from which this chart is drawn is particularly noted for its exploration of the methods of quality assessment. I shall, therefore, have more to say about it in another section of this book where I deal with the reliability of the criteria and the comparability of different methods of quality assessment. The data shown here are meant to illustrate variability in the quality of care at the most detailed level of analysis: that of individual cases.

Patients with urinary tract infection, hypertension, and ulcer of the stomach or duodenum who were under the care of the outpatient and inpatient facilities of the Baltimore City Hospitals were followed for a period of approximately five months. One of the methods for assessing quality called for the formulation of explicit criteria for care expected to be received during that period, beyond the initial history and physical examination. Criteria were obtained separately from seven specialists for each of the three diagnostic categories. The criteria finally selected were those on which at least five of seven experts agreed. By design, the criteria were finely adapted to subcategories of patients with each diagnosis, for varying according to antecedent clinical events in the course of management, and for paying attention to the timing, frequency, and duration of investigative procedures and treatments.

The chart uses two methods to show the distribution of cases according to the percent of criteria adhered to, one that has class intervals of 10 percentage points each, and another with intervals of one percentage point each. The latter is used to show that care in about 14 percent of cases does not conform to any of the criteria, and that only two percent of cases conform to every applicable criterion. Since care for the median case conforms to about 40 percent of the criteria, one is struck by the immense variation to both sides of the median value, as well as by the low level of performance overall. It is sobering indeed to realize that zero conformance is the single most frequently observed value.

This is care provided primarily by house staff to a disadvantaged population, albeit in a teaching institution under the supervision of distinguished physicians. Lack of cooperation by patients may have contributed to the poor showing. Deficiency of recording may have done so as well, even though the investigator made determined efforts to find and assemble all the available information on each case.

Chart 6-29

Percent Distribution of Patients Whose Care Was Found To Be in Compliance with Specified Percentages of Preformulated Explicit Criteria. Patients in Any One of Three Diagnostic Categories, Baltimore City Hospitals, 1971.

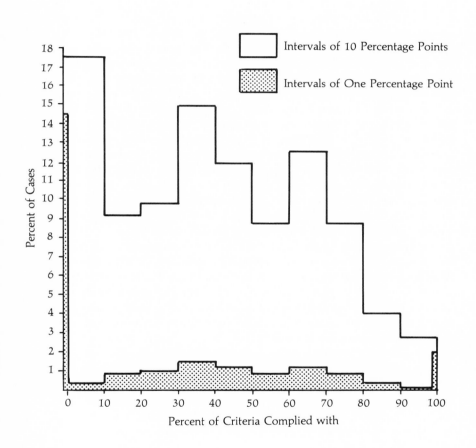

Source: Brook 1973, Table 30, p. 49.

Chart 6–30

As I pointed out in Volume II of these *Explorations* (pp. 50–53), explicit and implicit criteria may be combined in several ways in a method for assessing the quality of care. The work of Fine and Morehead which is illustrated in this chart provides a carefully designed example. The "combined method" or "review pattern," as it is called by its originators, has two parts. The first, which is the "explicit review," consists of questions which can be answered "yes" or "no" by a nonphysician who has reviewed the record. The second part, the "implicit review," also calls for answers to preformulated questions adapted to the diagnostic categories under review, but these questions require expert judgment for their answers. After answering these questions, the reviewer judges the care to be "satisfactory" or "unsatisfactory," and then specifies the deficiencies in care which have been noted. In this way the method attempts to achieve a high degree of consistency in assembling the necessary evidence, while it maintains the flexibility of clinical judgment.

For this test of the method, six voluntary hospitals in New York State were selected, and in each hospital 25 medical records were drawn consecutively from the files of patients with one of six diagnostic categories, some surgical and others medical. For clarity and convenience, the chart shows the types of hospitals as a continuous scale even though, of course, the three categories are discrete.

The chart shows that care is very variable by diagnosis, the percent rated satisfactory ranging, in all the hospitals combined, from 91 percent for prostatectomies to 33 percent for the management of cerebrovascular accidents. With one exception, care was much better in the hospitals affiliated with a medical school. Approval for training interns and residents, in the absence of medical school affiliation, has a much weaker, often equivocal effect. This finding is remarkably similar to that reported earlier by Morehead et al. (Chart 6–3).

Board-certified specialists performed better in some areas of their special competence, but the authors conclude, without giving all the evidence, that "the organization of the hospital has more effect on quality than the individual physician's training" (p. 1968).

Chart 6–30

Percent of Cases in Each of Specified Diagnostic Categories Judged To Have Received Satisfactory Care, by Type of Hospital. Selected Voluntary Hospitals, New York State, circa 1969.

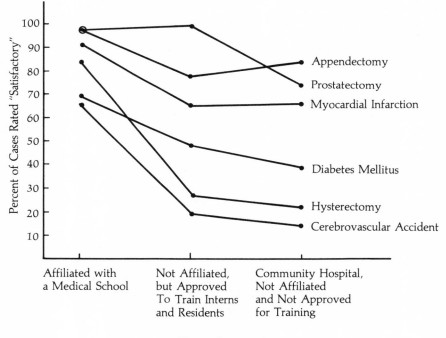

Type of Hospital

Source: Fine and Morehead 1971, Table V, p. 1967.

Chart 6–31

Beginning with her earliest studies of ambulatory care under the auspices of the Health Insurance Plan of Greater New York (HIP) Morehead has distinguished the more routinized diagnostic and preventive services that might be indicated for everyone in a given category of cases from the management of ill patients as dictated by clinical judgment (Daily and Morehead 1956; Morehead 1958, 1967). She has, accordingly, developed a two-pronged approach, using predominantly explicit criteria to assess the former, and implicit criteria, with various degrees of guidance, to assess the latter. The studies of the quality of care in the health centers sponsored by the Office of Economic Opportunity (OEO) applied the method developed at HIP, after some modifications, to a larger number of new sites.

This chart shows the findings of the "baseline surveys" of preventive care for specified categories of patients (adults, infants, and mothers) in different settings: (1) 35 OEO centers, (2) ten outpatient departments (OPD) of hospitals affiliated with medical schools, (3) seven group practices with varying forms of financing, (4) six Maternal and Infant Care (M&I) programs, and (5) four Children and Youth (C&Y) programs. Because the 35 OEO centers studied included the majority of the 50 centers then in operation, the findings may be a true picture of care in this kind of setting; one cannot say the same for the others.

The "baseline survey" uses preformulated, weighted explicit criteria for routine preventive care, first to obtain information from the medical record, and then to construct a numerical score ranging from 0 to 100. Only "ten percent of each case score can be said to contain some element of judgment" (Morehead 1970, p. 121). In the published source the score for outpatient departments was taken to be the empirical standard against which all other scores were compared. The chart uses actual numerical scores kindly supplied by Dr. Morehead. We can see, therefore, that (1) care in almost all settings falls short of the normatively derived standards of the investigators; (2) care in the OEO centers is roughly comparable, on the average, to that in OPDs and group practices; and (3) the more specialized facilities provide better preventive care to pregnant women and infants, respectively.

Chart 6–31

Average Scores of the Quality of Routine Diagnostic and Preventive Services Given to Samples of Cases of Specified Types in Selected Exemplars of Specified Kinds of Sites. U.S.A., circa 1968.

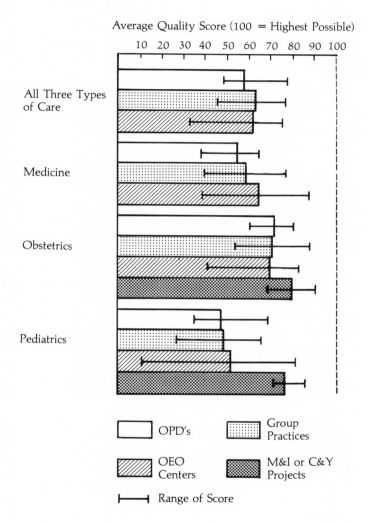

Source: Data supplied by Dr. Morehead to supplement the published description in Morehead et al. 1971.

Chart 6–32

We saw in the preceding chart an application of the first component in Morehead's two-pronged approach to the assessment of ambulatory care. This chart shows some findings from an application of the second component, the one that uses guided implicit criteria to assess the clinical management of patients with a wide range of severe or potentially severe illnesses. This part of the method differs only a little from that already described in connection with Charts 6–7 to 6–12. The construction of the weighted scale has been somewhat modified by the inclusion of a numerically small component designed to reflect the outcomes of care; there is a correspondingly small reduction in the importance attached to treatment and follow-up; and there is an "interlocking of the scoring system," so that overall diagnostic management cannot receive full credit if the history and physical examination are judged to have been inadequate (p. 303). Furthermore, whereas the earlier studies at the Health Insurance Plan of Greater New York were designed to assess the performance of individual physicians, in these more recent studies small samples of cases (five to 35 per center) were used to obtain what can only be a rough indication of each center's performance, including the contributions of administrative support, patient cooperation, and clinical competence.

The findings illustrated in the chart pertain to the possible effects of the continuity of care, a feature that is much lauded and little studied. Medical care for adults was studied in 39, and pediatric care in 36, of about 125 health centers sponsored by the Office of Economic Opportunity. The chart shows that when several primary care physicians see a patient, the quality of care is as good, and may even be better, than when only one physician is involved. One should remember, however, that continuity may also be provided by organizational means, and that the quality of the interpersonal relationship is not assessed, except indirectly as it affects patient cooperation.

Other findings suggest that the quality of care in urban and rural centers is comparable; that it does not seem to be related to the severity of the illness or the duration of care; and that it has only a weak positive association with the strength of the relationship between a center and a hospital. Quality is, however, "consistently higher" in programs that have a majority of physicians who are board eligible or board certified either in medicine or in pediatrics, depending on the type of care in question (p. 308).

Chart 6-32

Average Scores of the Quality of Care for Adults and Children, by Number of Primary Care Physicians Involved in Each Patient's Care. Neighborhood Health Centers, U.S.A., circa 1968–1973.

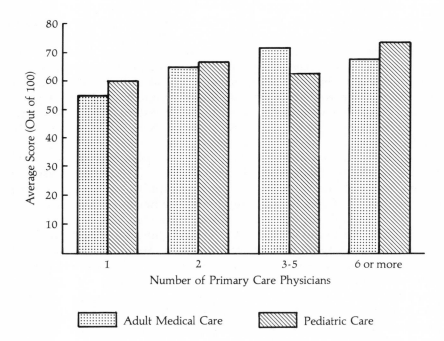

Source: Morehead and Donaldson 1974, Table 3, p. 307.

Chart 6–33

One could argue that the approaches to assessing the quality of ambulatory care illustrated by the two preceding charts are not a two-part method for assessing the same phenomenon, but an assessment of two separate aspects of care using two different methods, each suited to its own subject and purpose. Morehead and Donaldson provide information about the degree to which ratings for the same health centers using both methods of assessment (of course, for two different samples of cases in each center) do or do not correspond.

As described earlier, the scores for each of the two components of the audit range from 0 to 100. To construct the chart, the scores were divided into two segments, 0–60 and 61–100, indicating "unsatisfactory" and "satisfactory" care, respectively. It is interesting to know whether there is an association between the quality of basic diagnostic-preventive services and the quality of clinical management at the several centers. A high degree of correspondence would also enable an auditor (whether internal to the organization or, as in this case, external to it) to use the simpler audit of basic services first, and the more difficult and costly audit of clinical management more selectively.

The chart shows that there is perfect correspondence between the ratings for the two aspects of obstetrical care, but this is because the comparison scale has only two categories (satisfactory, unsatisfactory) and the quality of care is uniformly high. The health centers are somewhat more variable in providing adult medical care. Basic care is satisfactory in 88 percent of centers (81 + 7), and clinical management in 81 percent. There is agreement between the two ratings in 93 percent (81 + 12) of centers. A rating of "unsatisfactory" for basic services always corresponds to a similar rating for clinical management. A rating of "satisfactory" for basic services corresponds to a similar rating for clinical management in 92 percent of cases ($0.81 \div 0.88 = 0.92$). The situation is much less promising with regard to pediatric care; the centers differed more among themselves, and the average level of performance was lower. The ratings were congruent for 67 percent of the centers. Of the centers rated "unsatisfactory" for basic care, only 54 percent [$0.29 \div (0.25 + 0.29)$] would also be rated "unsatisfactory" for clinical management. But of the centers rated "satisfactory" for basic care, 82 percent [$0.38 \div (0.38 + 0.08)$] would also be rated as "satisfactory" for clinical management. Many centers seem to pay more attention to sick children than to preventive care.

Chart 6-33

Percent of Neighborhood Health Centers Rated "Satisfactory" or "Unsatisfactory" with Regard to the Quality of Basic Diagnostic and Preventive
Services, and the Quality of Clinical Management. U.S.A., circa 1968–1973.

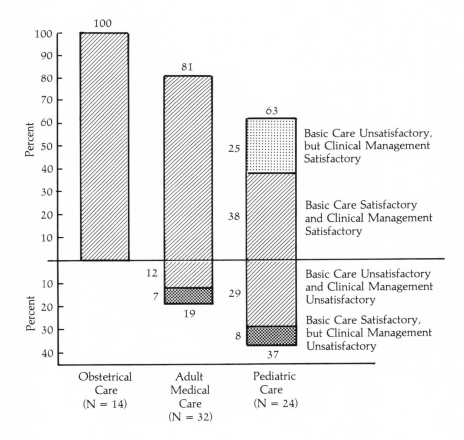

Source: Morehead and Donaldson 1974, Table 5, p. 309.

PART III

The Assessment of Outcomes, Alone or in Conjunction with Process

The Occurrence of
Preventable Adverse Outcomes
or of Achievable Favorable Outcomes

SEVEN

Outcomes are those changes, either favorable or adverse, in the actual or potential health status of persons, groups, or communities that can be attributed to prior or concurrent care. What is included in the category of "outcomes" depends, therefore, on how narrowly or broadly one defines "health" and the corresponding responsibilities of individual practitioners, categories of practitioners, or the health care system as a whole. For example, a restricted concept of health includes only physical and physiological functions, while other concepts go beyond that to include more or less of a range of psychological and social functions as well. Favorable outcomes in these areas could include changes in attitudes, beliefs, knowledge, and behavior that would be expected to contribute to future health. Patient satisfaction occupies a special position in the array of outcomes because it is partly a legitimate objective of current care, partly a factor in improving future care, and partly a judgment by the client on the quality of care, with particular reference to its outcomes and amenities as well as to the nature of the client's relationship with the practitioner.

The choice of one or more kinds of outcomes from the range of possibilities suggested above says something, either explicitly or by implication, about the objectives of care, and therefore about the definition of quality itself. But whether an outcome can tell us anything about the quality of care depends on the strength and exclusivity of the causal relationship between antecedent process and subsequent outcome. It should be possible to improve the outcome through adjustments in care; the improvement should occur regularly and be large; and the influence, good or bad, of factors other than the care under assessment should be relatively small or, if large, should be open to control either through study design or statistical manipulation.

It is difficult to draw confident conclusions about the quality of discrete episodes or elements of care from such "global" measures as overall mortality or longevity, or from indices that combine mortality and functional performance into either a profile or a single measure of health status, because these are so inclusive, reflecting as they do so many influences acting over such long periods of time. These measures are, however, useful indicators of the general environment in a society, and health care is an important ingredient of that environment.

For more detailed information, more specific to health care, the more general measures can be refined by relating them to more specific populations or situations. One would expect maternal and infant mortality, and particularly some segments of the latter, to be more specifically responsive to health care than mortality overall. Fatality, survival, and the more integrative indices of health status tell us more about the quality of care when they pertain to specific conditions, diseases, or procedures.

Another approach is to supplement or replace the more global measures by outcomes that are more discrete, more proximate, more closely related to the aspects of care one wishes to assess. The alleviation of pain in the arthritic, of labored breathing in the asthmatic, and of high blood pressure in the hypertensive, are all more specific and more immediate indicators of successful care than is mortality, important as that is. There is, however, a further important distinction between functions and feelings on the one hand and the subsensory biochemical and physiological phenomena on the other. One valued attribute of many outcomes is that they can be sensed and evaluated by anyone. They help part the veil under which the mysteries of technical care are concealed from public scrutiny.

Whether a good or bad outcome occurs is a matter of probability. It cannot be assumed, when the outcome in any given case is bad, that the antecedent care has been correspondingly deficient. One must observe a succession of cases, until the incidence of adverse outcomes in a sufficiently large number of cases is high enough to confidently say that it exceeds a specified standard. Even then, the judgment on the quality of care is indirect and provisional.

There is another way of using outcomes so as to be more certain of what they have to say about the quality of care, and that is by examining the process of antecedent care whenever the outcomes are undesirable or fall short of professional expectations. When this is done, the outcomes are not so much measures of quality, but rather alarm bells letting us know that care may have fallen below professional standards. This method of using outcomes to assess the quality of care will be described and illustrated in the next chapter, while this one deals with studies that draw conclusions about the quality of care from the mere occurrence of adverse or favorable outcomes.

Chart 7–1

Studies of infant mortality, and some other outcomes of pregnancy, are a time-honored means for comparing the social and economic development of populations in general, and the effectiveness of health care in particular. Pregnancy, childbirth, and the early months of life are highly vulnerable to harmful influences and responsive to corrective intervention. The relevant data are often gathered and reported, even though not always accurately.

This study used several outcomes of pregnancy care to assess the comparative effectiveness of alternative ways of organizing health care. At the time, 80 percent of live births to white residents of New York City were cared for by private physicians, of whom only about a third were certified obstetricians. Only 11 percent of live births to nonwhites were attended by private physicians, and of these only five percent were certified obstetricians. Only obstetricians who were board certified, or had equivalent qualifications, attended to deliveries under the auspices of the Health Insurance Plan of Greater New York (HIP), a plan that, because of prepayment, also reduced the financial barriers to seeking and receiving prenatal care.

The chart shows the late initiation of care as well as mortality during the first 27 days after birth, without implying, however, that a causal relationship between process and outcome is established. We see that membership in HIP makes little difference to the initiation of prenatal care by white mothers, but that it is associated with a significant reduction in neonatal mortality. Nonwhite mothers, most of whom receive care from public sources, are much more likely to be late in initiating prenatal care and to lose their children early in infancy. Membership in HIP is associated with a distinct advantage in both respects, certainly when compared to all forms of care available to this population, and even when compared to their private care. But equally important, membership in HIP does not equalize health care behaviors and outcomes between whites and nonwhites, and it falls far short of eliminating obstacles to early prenatal care even among white mothers.

In this paper and a sequel (Shapiro et al. 1958, 1960) the investigators examine several outcomes of pregnancy care and attempt to disentangle the effects of additional variables, e.g., age of mother, parity, birth weight, and father's occupation. They conclude that the reduction in perinatal mortality associated with HIP membership is real and significant, though the reasons for it can only be conjectured.

Chart 7-1

Percent of Live Births for which Prenatal Care Was Begun During the Second or Third Trimesters of Pregnancy, and Neonatal Mortality per 1,000 Live Births, by Race, for New York City Births, New York City Births Attended by Private Physicians, and Births to Members of the Health Insurance Plan of Greater New York (HIP), 1955.

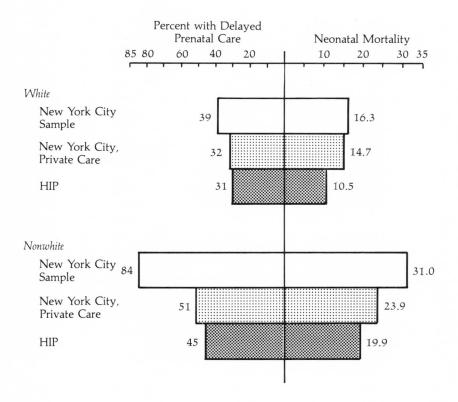

Source and Note: Shapiro et al. 1958, Tables 3 and A, pp. 175 and 185. I computed the neonatal mortality rates from Table A, and the percent with delayed prenatal care from Table 3 by including those with missing information with those who began care after the first trimester.

Chart 7–2

This chart adds to our information on the outcomes of pregnancy by drawing on the findings of a national study of obstetrical services. It is included here mainly to show how difficult it is to understand the relationship between outcomes and the quality of care without knowing more about the factors that may influence the outcomes.

The chart shows the relationship between the size of the obstetrical service (as indicated by the annual number of births) and several indicators of pregnancy outcome: the maternal mortality rate per 100,000 live births, the neonatal mortality rate per 1,000 live births, and the stillbirth ratio per 1,000 live births. Maternal mortality includes death of any woman dying of any cause while pregnant or within 90 days of the termination of pregnancy. Neonatal deaths are those that occur within the first 28 days of being born alive, and a stillbirth is a fetus born dead, either after a pregnancy of 20 weeks or more, or with a birth weight of 500 grams or more. The chart also shows one aspect of the process of care: the proportion of cesarean sections performed by house staff or by "generalists," the latter defined as those who are neither obstetricians nor general surgeons. The source contains much additional information on facilities, equipment, procedures, and staffing.

The maternal mortality rate and the stillbirth ratio show an initial decline as the size of the obstetrical service becomes larger. But the stillbirth ratio soon becomes essentially constant, whereas the maternal mortality rate begins to increase with further increases in service size. Neonatal mortality rates show a distinctly different pattern, increasing as the obstetrical service becomes larger.

It is difficult to interpret these findings, partly because no adjustments have been made for the characteristics of patients cared for in hospitals of different size. Larger hospitals are better staffed and equipped. On the other hand, they also care for more difficult cases, and the largest hospitals also train students and house staff. To take cesarean sections as an example: as the size of the obstetrical service increases, it becomes less likely that the operation will be performed by an untrained surgeon; but with further increases in size, the house staff, another category of possibly less qualified persons, are more likely to perform the operation.

Whatever the cause, all three measures of pregnancy outcome shown in the chart were distinctly and significantly worse in hospitals owned by or affiliated with medical schools.

Chart 7–2

Relative Magnitudes of Specified Outcomes of Pregnancy, and of the Percent
of Cesarean Sections Performed by Generalists or House Staff, by Size of the Hospitals' Obstetrical Services, U.S.A., 1967.

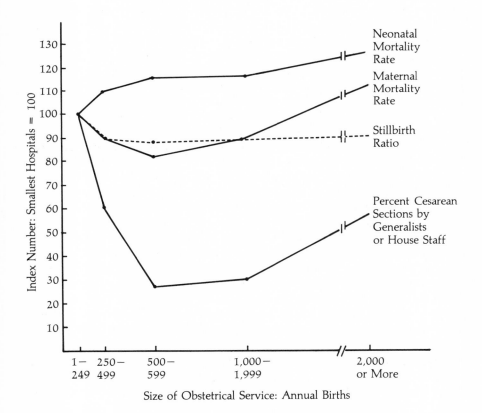

Source: American College of Obstetricians and Gynecologists, Committee on Maternal Health,
1970. I computed the index numbers from Tables IV-1, IV-6, IV-15, and 9-d(1), pp. 11, 13, 17, and
144-45.

Chart 7–3

It is interesting to compare the findings in the preceding chart with those of a recent study. The comparisons are of births to white mothers only; they involve residents in Portland, Oregon, and members of the local Kaiser-Permanente Medical Care Program, a prepaid group practice now included under the rubric of "health maintenance organization" (HMO). Extensive information was collected on the sociodemographic attributes of the mothers, and the characteristics of the current and previous pregnancies. The several categories of risk, as well as the classification of prenatal care according to its adequacy, correspond to categories developed by the Institute of Medicine. Neonatal mortality refers to deaths during the first 28 days of life.

In this study, membership in the group practice was associated with a *lower* level of prenatal care. Partly because of difficulty in obtaining an early appointment, "HMO members began prenatal care an average of one month later and had an average of three fewer prenatal visits . . . " (p. 388). Moreover, neither in private practice, nor in an organization committed to "health maintenance," did women subject to higher risk receive more prenatal care to forestall an adverse outcome.

There is no difference in neonatal mortality between the two populations taken as a whole. Though the chart shows that HMO enrollees experience a distinctly higher mortality in the category with sociodemographic risk, and a lower mortality in the categories that include higher medical-obstetrical risk, multiple regression analysis demonstrated no independent effect of plan membership on neonatal or infant mortality. Rather, the favorable effect of the HMO in some risk categories was associated with somewhat higher birth weight.

The findings of this study suggest that prenatal care is efficacious; other things being equal, more prenatal care was associated with a lower incidence of prematurity (as judged by birth weight) and mortality. Since prepaid group practice achieves a lower incidence of prematurity and a roughly equivalent level of infant mortality, with significantly less prenatal care, it could be argued that it produces health more efficiently. But the multiple regression carried out in this study explained only 10 percent of the variance in birth weight. Many other factors (e.g., smoking, alcohol consumption, diet) were not taken into account, and these may have been partly responsible for the observed differences in the incidence of prematurity and of the higher infant mortality associated with it.

Chart 7–3

Percent of Live Births for which the Mothers Received Prenatal Care Rated as Less than "Adequate," and Neonatal Mortality Rates per 1,000 Live Births, by Specified Risk Categories. Births to White Mothers in Portland, and to White Members of the Kaiser-Permanente Medical Care Program (HMO), Portland, Oregon, 1973–1974.

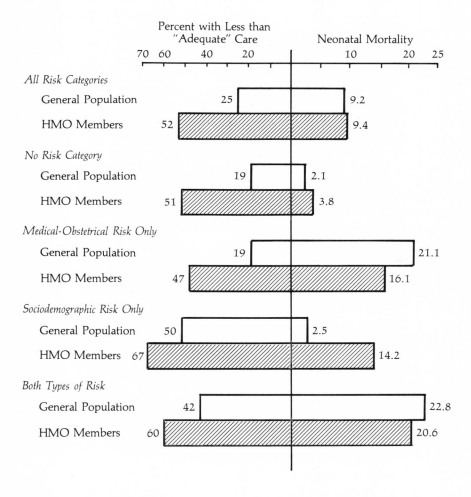

Source and Note: Quick et al. 1981, Table 5, p. 386. I calculated the percent receiving less than "Level 1" (or "Adequate") care from data in the table, excluding those for whom the level of care was "unknown."

Chart 7–4

Fatality from diseases in specified diagnostic categories, with or without surgical intervention, is an outcome very frequently used to assess the quality of care. This chart illustrates an early example of the genre. The data are from "an effectively random" sample of discharges drawn for the Hospital Inpatient Enquiry, an established system of reporting that includes almost all teaching and nonteaching hospitals in England and Wales. The fatalities in the nonteaching hospitals are shown after the composition of their patients by age, and where appropriate also by sex, is made comparable by statistical adjustment to the composition of cases in teaching hospitals. The difference made by this adjustment is also shown.

Although not all the differences observed are statistically significant, there is an intriguing and instructive pattern of findings. We note, first, the wide differences in fatalities among the major diagnoses. It is clear, however, that the broader diagnostic categories conceal large differences among subsets within each category, differences brought about by features that signify different grades of severity and corresponding probabilities of dying.

Teaching hospitals achieve lower fatality rates for the conditions included in this chart, irrespective of the grades of severity identified. Adjustments for age and sex bring the fatalities in the nonteaching hospitals closer to those in the teaching hospitals. This means that part of the adverse results in the nonteaching hospitals is attributable to their having patients exposed to higher risk by virtue of age or sex, or of other factors associated with these variables. In the United States we would expect the teaching hospitals to have more, rather than fewer, of these patients.

How much of the remaining advantage of the teaching hospitals is due to superior skills and facilities is difficult to say, since the patients in the nonteaching hospitals could still be at greater risk because of factors other than those corrected for in this chart. The stage is set, therefore, for still greater refinements in the methods for achieving comparability in case mix, so that ideally, every variable other than the quality of care has been accounted for. It is a difficult, perhaps a hopeless, task. But it is the inescapable burden that the mere observation of differences in outcome must necessarily impose.

Chart 7–4

Fatality per 100 Cases of Specified Diagnostic Categories in Teaching and Nonteaching Hospitals, the Latter with and without Adjustments for Age and Sex. England and Wales, 1956–1959.

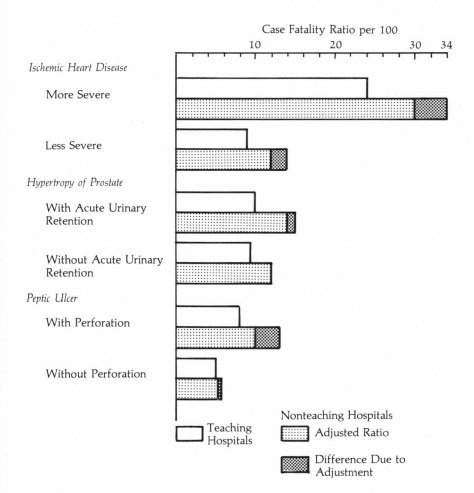

Source: Lipworth et al. 1963, Table A, p. 74.

Chart 7–5

Given the necessary information, much can be done to allow for differences in the case mix of different hospitals. The work illustrated by this chart is an attempt to get the best possible adjustment with very little information. It rests on the assumption that the length of hospital stay is at least a rough indication of case severity. This is especially true when the length of stay is adjusted for differences in the hospital's occupancy ratio, since the level of occupancy influences the hospital's activities in ways unrelated to case severity. Based on this reasoning, Roemer et al. constructed and tested the usefulness of "severity-adjusted" case fatality rates, which are the crude death rates per 100 admissions for all cases (regardless of diagnosis, but excluding deaths in the newborn) adjusted for the difference between each hospital's mean length of stay and mean occupancy ratio, on the one hand, and the mean values for length of stay and occupancy ratio for all the comparable hospitals in a community on the other. The detailed computations are shown in the source.

As evidence in support of their measure, Roemer et al. showed, in a sample of hospitals in Los Angeles, that the differences in occupancy-adjusted mean lengths of stay among hospitals explained as much as 59 percent of the observed variation in crude (unadjusted) fatality rates. They then demonstrated that the use of the severity-adjusted rates would lead to judgments of quality that correspond reasonably well with what one would expect, knowing the hospitals' other characteristics. The chart shows this part of the evidence. Briefly, the crude fatality rates vary directly with characteristics expected to be positively related to quality, whereas the adjusted ratios, in general, conform to expectations. (The construction of the technical adequacy score is a particularly interesting feature fully explained in the source.)

The limitations of the method are known to its proponents. Some hospitals discharge or transfer patients who are likely to die; some receive more patients who are "dead on arrival," or die soon after; some keep patients longer for teaching or research. The length of stay can be either prolonged or shortened by bad care as well as good. The findings of Roemer et al. suggest that the method is useful, nevertheless. But a replication in New York City by Goss and Reed (1974) suggests that the measure does not permit inferences about quality from comparisons across regions, and that even within one area, the adjusted fatality rates do not rank categories of hospitals according to their expected quality.

Chart 7–5

Crude and "Severity-Adjusted" Case Fatality Rates, by Ownership, Accreditation Status, and Technical Adequacy Scores, in a Representative Sample of 32 General Hospitals, Los Angeles County, California, 1964.

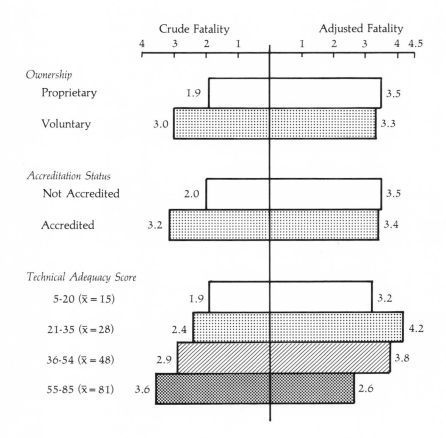

Source and Note: Roemer et al. 1968, Tables 4 and 5, pp. 109 and 113, and text tables on pp. 114 and 115. I computed the mean ($\bar{x}$) for the technical adequacy score interval 36-54 from data in Tables 4 and 5, knowing that the difference is caused by the omission of one hospital in Table 5.

Chart 7–6

The hope that some simple adjustment for differences in patient characteristics will sweep away enough of their influence to uncover the consequences of differences in quality is perhaps doomed to disappointment. The study illustrated by this chart is an important milestone on the road toward greater complexity.

Soon after the introduction of halothane as a general anesthetic, there were reports of deaths from liver damage possibly related to its use. Consequently, a cooperative study of postoperative deaths was undertaken to determine whether the anesthetic was associated with a higher probability of death, especially from liver damage. Thirty-four medical centers volunteered for the study, which required information about all deaths occurring within six weeks of the administration of anesthesia, and about a random sample of all cases receiving anesthesia during a four-year period. Nearly a million operations and about 17,000 deaths were studied.

In order to see whether different anesthetic agents were associated with different probabilities of death it was necessary to correct for the effects of other patient characteristics that might influence the risk of dying. Operations were coded into 100 categories, which were sometimes condensed to 25, and at other times to three subgroups with high, intermediate ("middle"), and low death rates, respectively. Other variables included physical status (seven categories), age (eleven categories), sex, prior surgery, the duration of surgery, and the probability of the operation being associated with surgical shock.

Almost incidentally, it was observed that there were very large differences in postoperative fatality among institutions which were all associated with medical schools and which, presumably, were all capable of providing the highest levels of care. The chart shows nearly a 24-fold difference in the crude fatality ratio (deaths over operations plus deaths). It also shows that the range of differences in fatality ratios can be reduced by correcting for differences in patient characteristics. This was first done for one variable at a time and then for several variables simultaneously. The relative influence of each variable, or group of variables, is shown by the reduction in the variability in fatality ratios. Important though these adjustments are, large unexplained differences remain. The investigators hesitate to attribute these to differences in quality, partly because we do not know the consequences of not operating.

Chart 7–6

Relative Postoperative Fatality Ratios, without Adjustment and after Adjustment for Specified Case Mix Characteristics, One Variable at a Time, and for Several Variables Simultaneously. Thirty-four Medical Centers in the Collaborative National Halothane Study. U.S.A., 1959–1962.

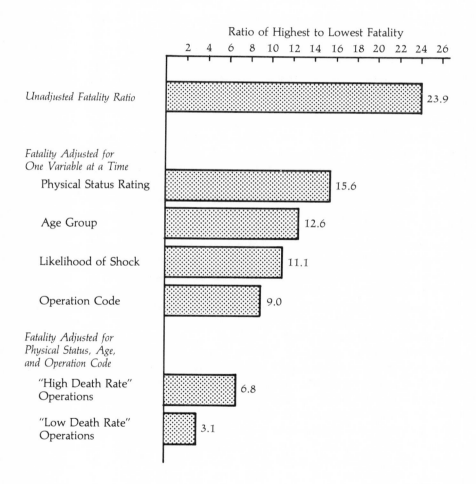

Source: Bunker et al. 1969, Tables 5 and 12, pp. 196 and 334, and text on p. 342.

Chart 7–7

The observation of large unexplained differences in postoperative fatality among medical centers led to the Institutional Differences Study. The first ("extensive") part of the study used data routinely collected by all 1,224 short-term, U.S. hospitals in the Professional Activities Study (PAS) of the Commission on Professional and Hospital Activities during 1972. All surgical patients in any one of 14 diagnostic categories were included. The case abstract (the basis for PAS) shows whether the patient died in the hospital and provides much additional information. The probable effect on fatality of concurrent trauma, additional diagnoses, and additional surgical interventions was recognized by an elaborate system of weights. These were used partly to subdivide the original diagnoses into 33 more homogeneous "analytic categories," and partly to standardize for differences within each analytic category. Patients were also classified by age, sex, race, and other demographic attributes. Status on admission was characterized by the findings of laboratory and other examinations. In all, there were up to 75 descriptors to choose from. Of these, sets of only 15 were used, the variables included differing somewhat according to analytic category. But after the first few variables entered each stepwise linear regression there was little further effect on explaining differences in fatality. About ten variables would have been sufficient.

The measure of outcome is the ratio of observed deaths during hospitalization to expected deaths, the latter being computed on the assumption that the probability of dying in each hospital is the same as that of dying in all hospitals combined, after adjusting for the effect of differences in patient characteristics. The chart shows that in spite of these adjustments a great deal of variability remains, at least for some of the diagnoses studied. Although the standardization method may have been inadequate, some of the remaining variability may be due to differences in the quality of care. But preliminary analyses have shown relatively few significant relationships between hospital characteristics and the fatality ratio; when present, these relationships vary according to diagnosis, are weak, and taken as a whole, are refractory to coherent interpretation. Particularly notable is the absence of consistent positive associations with hospital size, medical school affiliation, residency training, and accreditation. The small number of deaths in many hospitals may be partly responsible for these disappointingly inconclusive results.

Chart 7-7

Percent Distribution of Hospitals by Standardized Postoperative Fatality Ratio for Each of Two Diagnostic Categories. Short-term Hospitals Subscribing to the Professional Activities Study (PAS) of the Commission on Professional and Hospital Activities, U.S.A., 1972.

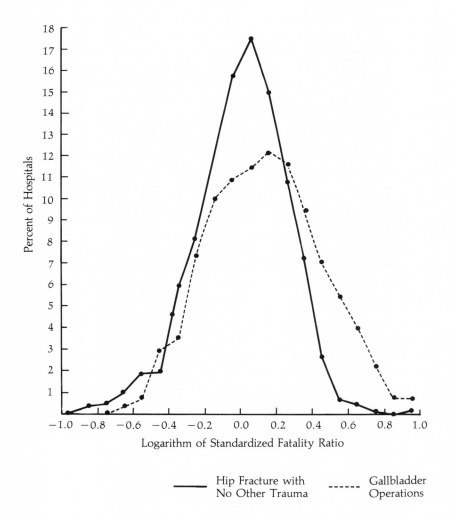

Source and Note: Staff of the Stanford Center for Health Care Research, 1974, Appendix I.B, Exhibit 13, pp. 365 and 367. The findings of the "extensive study" are described on pp. 57-76 and shown in subsequent tables.

Chart 7–8

The second ("intensive") part of the Institutional Differences Study uses a subsample of 17 hospitals and a selection of 15 diagnostic categories partly to replicate the more "extensive" study, and partly to break new ground. As for new ground: this part of the study uses more complete information obtained expressly to achieve more rigorous standardization of case mix, to develop a wider range of outcome measures, and to examine the organizational characteristics of the hospital in remarkable detail. For example, the anesthetist rated each case according to physical status and cardiovascular function. The surgeon reported findings during the operation that could be used to characterize preoperative status. Nurses provided information about the severity of physiologic disturbances and continued use of monitors, drains, or catheters on the seventh postoperative day. Patients reported whether 40 days after the operation they were better or worse than they had been a month before their hospitalization. These measures of status, plus the occurrence of death within 40 days of surgery, either in the hospital or outside, were used in a variety of combinations, and using several weighting schemes, to indicate the outcomes of care.

As to hospital characteristics, in addition to the more usual attributes, information from a variety of personnel was used to construct measures of "differentiation," "coordination," "power," and "staff qualifications". There were several measures of each, and at several levels: the hospital, the medical staff, the ancillary service units, the surgical wards, and the operating room.

The chart shows the 17 hospitals ranked according to the ratio of observed to expected fatality, the latter corrected for case mix. It also shows the corresponding ratios for the presence of severe or moderate morbidity on the seventh postoperative day. The two measures are known to be highly correlated by diagnosis, but the apparent lack of correlation at the hospital level suggests that one can add information as well as statistical stability by combining the two. The relative weighting of the several components remains a problem.

Expenditures per patient day, a larger ratio of registered nurses to other nurses, greater control over surgical privileges, and greater concentration of a surgeon's practice to one hospital were each associated with better outcomes. The hospital's size and teaching status, and the surgeon's degree of specialization, were not. Seemingly, the attributes of the settings are more influential than those of each surgeon.

Chart 7–8

Standardized Postoperative Fatality Ratios and Standardized Ratios for Severe or Moderate Morbidity (Physiologic Difficulty) on the Seventh Postoperative Day, for Each of 17 Hospitals. Sample of Hospitals Subscribing to the Professional Activities Study (PAS) of the Commission on Professional and Hospital Activities, U.S.A., May 1973–February 1974.

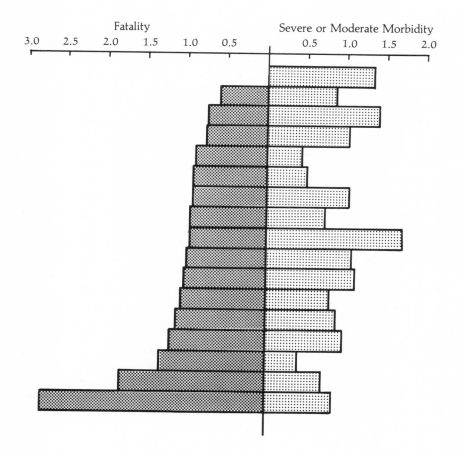

Source and Note: Staff of the Stanford Center for Health Care Research, 1974, Tables 8 and 10, pp. 160 and 162. I computed the morbidity ratios. Other information in the text comes from Scott et al. 1976, Flood and Scott 1978, and Flood et al. 1979.

Chart 7–9

This chart represents the culmination of a progression whose earliest steps are illustrated in this book by the "severity-adjusted" fatality index of Roemer et al. (Chart 7–5). Now, over 40 characteristics of patients are used to correct for differences in case mix among hospitals. These include several demographic characteristics (such as age and sex), the major diagnosis explaining admission (in 332 groups), the presence of additional diagnoses, admission test findings, the number and severity of surgical interventions, the occurrence of hospital complications, discharge status, and much more. All this information can be obtained from case abstracts, but only if the hospital subscribes to a service such as that of the Commission on Professional and Hospital Activities. One can then determine, using appropriate statistical techniques, to what extent the observed case fatality in any one hospital differs from what would have been expected, given the case mix of that hospital, and the relationship between case mix variables and fatality in a set of hospitals to which the study hospital belongs.

The hospitals studied are the 17 used in the more detailed of the investigations of institutional differences in surgical fatality. These hospitals were divided into four subsets, according to whether the average length of stay and the "service intensity" (a measure of the quantity, variety, and cost of special services), were more or less than expected, given the case mix of each hospital, and given the relationship between case mix and each of the two dependent variables (length of stay and service intensity) in the set of 17 hospitals. The chart shows that both shorter stays and more services are associated with lower-than-expected fatality rates. Further analysis showed, however, that the association with length of stay was caused mostly by regional differences in length of stay among hospitals, while within each region more-than-expected care continued to be positively associated with less-than-expected fatality. This is a welcome confirmation of the expected (though often debated) relationship between quantity and quality, at least when the entire hospital's experience is the unit of analysis. It also shows the importance of regional variations in the patterns of care, after correcting for differences in case mix.

In two related papers, Scott et al. (1979) and Flood et al. (1982) tell us more about some expected and unexpected relationships between hospital characteristics and the adjusted fatality rates.

Chart 7-9

Observed Case Fatality Relative to Expected Fatality in Four Sets of Patients after Adjustment for Differences in Patient Characteristics. A sample of 17 Hospitals Classified by Whether They Keep Patients Longer or Shorter, and Provide More or Less Service than Would Be Expected Given Their Case Mix. U.S.A., 1970–1973.

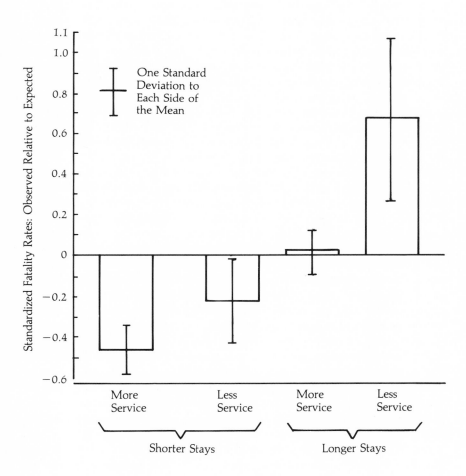

Source: Flood et al. 1979, Table 3, p. 1097.

Chart 7–10

The question asked by this study is whether doing more of a particular surgical procedure is associated with higher quality, as indicated by differences in postoperative fatality during the hospital stay. Data for 12 selected procedures were obtained from almost all short-term, general hospitals in the United States which subscribed to the Professional Activities Study (PAS) of the Commission on Professional and Hospital Activities during 1974 and 1975. Cases were classified by sex, by whether or not there was more than one diagnosis, and by five age groups. Expected postoperative fatality ratios were computed for each hospital, assuming that the relationship between fatality and these variables for the patients of all the hospitals combined also holds for the patients of each hospital.

The investigators found that the 12 procedures studied fell into three categories. For some procedures, typified in the chart by open heart surgery, there was a regular decline in excess fatality as the yearly number of such operations increased. For others, represented by total hip replacement, there was an initial rapid decline followed by insensitivity to further increases in the number of operations performed. In the third category were operations like cholecystectomy (not shown in the chart), for which there was no relation between the yearly number performed and excess fatality. The inference is that some operations should be restricted to high-volume hospitals.

For some operations, the inverse association between volume and excess fatality is partly due to referral to hospitals known to obtain better results. Moreover, doing an operation more frequently also results in greater skill. For some procedures the relationship between outcome and volume is highly specific to the procedure, whereas for others the number of procedures in an interrelated set also counts. But all the findings are for hospitals taken as a whole; we still need to examine the relationship between volume and outcome for individual surgeons.

The investigators also report that several measures of hospital size have little effect on surgical outcome, apart from the number of procedures performed, and that teaching status (interns and residents per bed) may increase excess fatality a little. Hospitals in the West have clearly lower excess fatality, but this could be due to the lower length of stay, and the consequent exclusion of some postdischarge deaths, in this region. Also, remember that neither the outcomes of not operating, nor outcomes other than death, are included in this study.

Chart 7-10

Excess of Observed over Expected Postoperative Fatality Rates per 1,000 Operations, by Type of Operation and by Yearly Number of Operations of Each Type. Short-term General Hospitals Subscribing to the Professional Activities Study (PAS) of the Commission on Professional and Hospital Activities, U.S.A, 1974 and 1975.

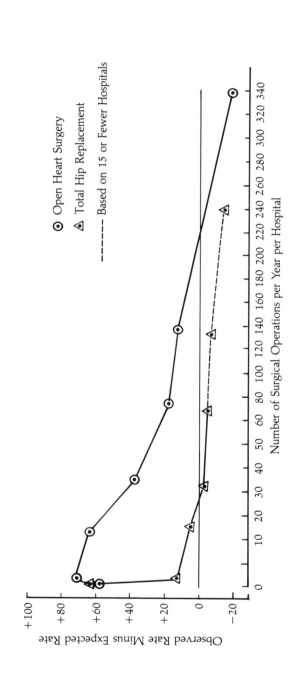

Source and Note: Luft et al. 1979, based on estimates made from Figure 1, p. 1366. To allow for easier charting, I have varied the scale on the abscissa, causing some distortion of which the viewer should be aware. Additional information in the text is from Luft 1980b.

Chart 7–11

Survival is only the opposite of dying, but survival does have the dimension of finite duration which death lacks, unless the occurrence of death is converted to the number of years of expected life lost. Moreover, the measurement of survival opens the way to a consideration of the quality of life as well as of its duration. But overall longevity has to be cut into finer slivers of survival if it is to be used as a reasonably sensitive and specific measure of the quality of defined bundles of medical care. That has been done in this case by selecting cancer of the cervix as the subject of study, and by also differentiating stages of the cancer that influence survival. Unfortunately, age, which was also found to influence survival, was not corrected for, nor is there any information about the quality of life. Nevertheless, the study illustrated by the chart tells us a great deal of unusual interest.

Using the New York State Tumor Registry, supplemented with their own search of hospital records, the authors identified one group of cases of cancer of the cervix that had been first recorded in 1949, and another group first recorded during 1959–1962. They were able to obtain almost complete information about whether each person was or was not alive five years later. Independent checks showed a high accuracy in diagnosis and staging.

The chart shows that during the period studied there was relatively little improvement in survival with cancer of the cervix for women treated in hospitals affiliated with the medical schools of Albany, Buffalo, Rochester, and Syracuse. By contrast, there was a great deal of improvement in the results obtained by other hospitals. This suggests that the science of caring for this cancer advanced relatively little during this period, but that the skills and knowledge formerly more restricted to the major medical centers later became more widely available. (For example, the number of board-certified surgeons, gynecologists, and radiologists in the area had increased from 320 in 1949 to 814 in 1962.) Earlier diagnosis and more discriminating referral of the more difficult cases to the medical centers may have contributed to the findings. Other hospital attributes, such as sponsorship, size, number of cases of cervical cancer seen, number of house staff, and number of board-certified specialists relevant to the management of cancer, were unrelated to survival. Socioeconomic status of urban dwellers (measured by median rental in the census tract of residence) was also irrelevant.

Chart 7–11

Percent of Persons with Cancer of the Cervix Who Survived for at Least Five Years, by the Year in which the Cases Were First Recorded in the Tumor Registry, and by Type of Hospital. New York State, Excluding New York City and Adjacent Counties, 1949 and 1959–1962.

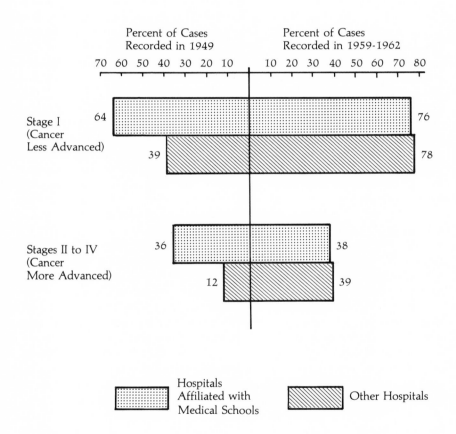

Source: Graham and Paloucek 1963, Tables III and IV, pp. 407 and 408, with additional information supplied by Dr. Graham.

Chart 7–12

When specified kinds of morbidity can be prevented or substantially reduced by proper medical care, the occurrence of such morbidity can serve as an index of quality, assuming that other factors that either contribute to or reduce the incidence of the illness have been taken into account. Access to care, institutional support, professional performance, and patient cooperation are all necessary to success. Quality is therefore rather broadly defined in investigations such as the one illustrated by this chart. In this case, the incidence of first attacks of rheumatic fever in children between the ages of five and fourteen was used as the measure of quality because these attacks "are known to be preventable by prompt and adequate treatment of streptococcal infections" (p. 331). Rutstein et al. (1976) have compiled lists of other phenomena, each a "sentinel health event," that could be used to monitor the health and health care of a community.

During 1968–1970, the census tracts of Baltimore that were predominantly populated by black residents could be divided into two groups. In one, children were eligible for care at one of four "comprehensive-care programs": three Children and Youth projects and one neighborhood health center. In the other group of tracts, the population had access only to the more traditional sources of care. The period between 1960 and 1964, which preceded the establishment of the comprehensive care programs, is used for comparison.

Information about first attacks of rheumatic fever was obtained by a search of hospital charts. Diagnostic accuracy was reconfirmed by the investigators. Census data were used to estimate the population of children. Further standardization for age did not alter the findings.

The chart shows that the incidence of rheumatic fever was significantly reduced in the census tracts which became eligible for comprehensive care, whereas in the other tracts there was no reduction, and there may even have been an increase. The conclusion that the difference is due to the superiority of comprehensive care is strengthened by the observation that the reduction in rheumatic fever occurred only in the subset of cases who, according to the hospital chart, had a history of "clinical upper respiratory infection." But conclusions based on purely epidemiological observations can only be tentative. It is ironical that Gordis himself was unable to confirm the advantages of "comprehensive, continuous pediatric care" in a controlled, randomized trial (Gordis and Markowitz 1971).

Chart 7–12

Incidence of First Attacks of Rheumatic Fever in Persons Eligible and Not Eligible for Care by One of Several Comprehensive Care Programs, before and after the Establishment of These Programs. Children between the Ages of 5 and 14 in Census Tracts Predominantly Populated by Blacks, Baltimore, 1960–1964 and 1968–1970.

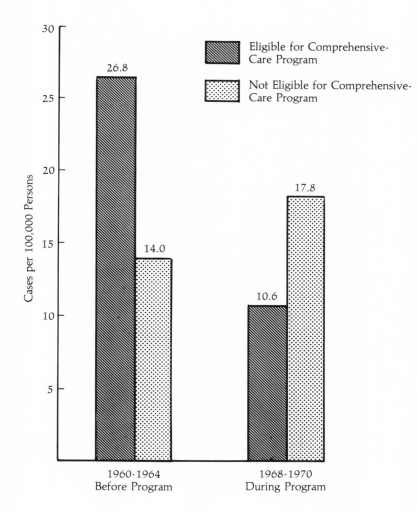

Source: Gordis 1973, Table 4, p. 333.

The Study of "Preventability" in Adverse Outcomes

EIGHT

The studies that investigate the "preventability" of adverse outcomes may be classified into two categories. In one, the outcome is so serious and unusual that it deserves investigation every time it occurs. The studies in this category may be described as "retrospective," since there is no specification of precise standards in advance, unless it is the expectation that if the event occurs, there is a high probability that the care has been deficient. In the second category of studies, rather precise standards are specified in advance, and the care provided is reviewed, either selectively or for an entire category of cases, only if the standards are not met. These studies may be thought of as "prospective" in orientation, since they depend so heavily on the occurrence of a deviation from pre-specified outcomes.

The category of "restrospective" studies is illustrated in this chapter by investigations of maternal, perinatal, and infant mortality. The studies of maternal and perinatal mortality conducted under the auspices of the New York Academy of Medicine are notable landmarks, not only as studies of the quality of care, but also as the initial steps in a movement to control the needless loss of precious life that they showed to be occurring. The report on maternal mortality merits particular attention for being the first in the series, for exploring with such sensitivity and insight the social and medical contributions to needless death, and for being so well written. It is at once a social document of the first rank and one of the literary treasures of our field.

A notable feature of the studies in the first category is the attention they give to identifying the factors that may have contributed to the probably preventable death. They often reveal the role played by the medical attendants, the patient, and the institution in which care was provided. By pointing to precisely what may have gone wrong, these studies can suggest the appropriate action needed to avoid a repetition of the error. Another advantage is that this method takes account of all the other characteristics of the subjects and their conditions which may have influenced the outcome, but which are extraneous to the quality of care received. Thus, clinical assessment replaces epidemiological analysis.

John Williamson is the major proponent of the category of studies that rely on deviations from predetermined outcomes to prompt the review of antecedent care, and of the system characteristics that influence the care (Williamson 1978). The method of "health accounting" advocated by him requires that the health professionals responsible for a program begin by selecting conditions that require attention because they believe that care may be deficient, and because improvements in care are feasible and would produce large benefits to health. The principle of "achievable benefits" occupies an important position in Williamson's method.

Next, it is necessary to specify the outcomes to be studied and to set the standards of performance expected to be achieved. If the standards are met, antecedent care is not reviewed. If performance falls short of the standards by a margin that cannot easily be explained by chance, antecedent care is reviewed for the entire group of patients. Williamson believes his method provides information the practitioners want, consider relevant, and are motivated to act upon.

Williamson puts a large variety of phenomena under his heading of "outcomes," including the accuracy of diagnosis as a "diagnostic outcome," and changes in the patients' knowledge, health behavior, and health status as "therapeutic outcomes." Some of the measures of health status are specific to each condition, examples being the lowering of blood pressure in hypertension, or the relief of respiratory distress in asthma. But Williamson's method is distinctive in also offering a measure of "overall health and functional status" that can be used to assess the outcomes for any condition, as shown in the chart included in this section.

The "problem status" measure of Mushlin and Appel, the second of the two methods that study deviations from prespecified outcomes, builds on Williamson's work, but differs in setting the standards so that 100 percent of cases must meet them by a given deadline. It is possible to set the standards for patients with a given condition as a group. It is also possible for each patient's physician to set a standard of outcome which that patient is expected to meet by a specified deadline. In either case, the "problem status" method is oriented to assessing the care of individual cases, whereas "health accounting" is oriented to assessing performance only when the outcomes fall below expectations in *groups* of cases.

Chart 8–1

The mere observation of the occurrence of favorable or adverse events, no matter how carefully done, almost always leaves doubts about the contribution of the quality of care to the outcome, as compared to the influence of other factors, known or unsuspected. Even if, as a result of meticulous adjustment for extraneous variables, one is reasonably confident that the quality of care is at fault, one does not know how the failure has occurred, or what is needed to correct it. There is, therefore, the inevitable pressure to study the antecedent process of care. Thus, careful clinical assessment, case by case, using implicit or explicit criteria, supplements or supplants statistical manipulation. The study that I have chosen to begin our exploration of this method deserves to be cherished as one of the classics of our literature.

Based on weekly reports by the N. Y. C. Department of Health, all deaths accompanied by pregnancy were investigated by a thorough review of the hospital chart, including nursing notes, and by interviewing as many as necessary of those who provided care at any time during the pregnancy. The information obtained in this way was then reviewed by a committee of obstetricians who judged whether the death could have been prevented and, if so, what was responsible for the death.

The chart shows that an astounding 64 percent of maternal deaths were judged to be "preventable," even though whenever information was incomplete, or the members of the committee could not agree or had doubts, the death was called "nonpreventable." The chart also shows the relative contributions of the patients and the medical attendants to total deaths, and to the subset of preventable deaths. The failures of medical care were clearly the more important of the two, being responsible for almost half the deaths. In turn, these failures were equally divided between errors of technique and errors of judgment. (When, as was often the case, both kinds of error occurred together, the case was assigned to the more important of the two.) Though it may have been due to circumstances beyond her control, the patient's behavior was responsible for 17 percent of deaths, because the patient either "failed to obtain medical advice," or "failed to cooperate with her attendant" (p. 31).

Chart 8–1

Percent Distribution of All Maternal Deaths, by Whether Preventable or Not, and the Percent Distribution of Preventable Deaths, by the Kinds of Factors Responsible for the Death. New York City, 1930–1932.

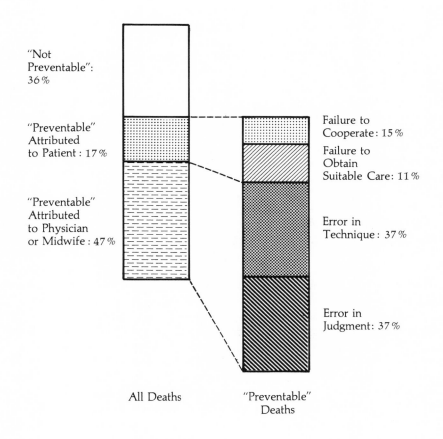

"Not Preventable": 36%

"Preventable" Attributed to Patient : 17%

"Preventable" Attributed to Physician or Midwife : 47%

Failure to Cooperate: 15%

Failure to Obtain Suitable Care: 11%

Error in Technique : 37%

Error in Judgment: 37%

All Deaths

"Preventable" Deaths

Source: New York Academy of Medicine, Committee on Public Health Relations, 1933. Computed from Tables 5B, 6, 7 and 8, pp. 33, 37 and 43.

Chart 8–2

The second chart drawn from the study of preventable maternal mortality shows associations with the qualification of the attendant at delivery. We see, on the right-hand side, a steep progression in the rates of overall mortality and of mortality attributed to errors by the attendant. By contrast, we see on the left-hand side of the chart that no matter what the qualifications of the attendant, about half of the deaths under the care of each category of attendants is attributable to "lack of judgment, lack of skill, or careless inattention to the demands of the case" (p. 49).

The author attributes the larger mortality rates in the case loads of the more qualified physicians to the higher proportion of more difficult cases they handle, including the more frequent cesarean sections performed especially by surgeons. He also points out that the classification of physicians is imperfect, and that some physicians who are included as specialists may lack the requisite knowledge and skill. It is not inconceivable, however, that certain risky procedures thought to be medically justifiable could, in fact, be unjustified. These are, in other words, findings that might throw doubt on the normative standards of care themselves. The virtually invariant proportion of cases found to be poorly handled irrespective of type of attendant could also lead one to question the method of the study. Another, more plausible, explanation is that there is a remarkably fine adjustment between the complexity of the case load and the capacity of each category of practitioner, so that though the practitioners differ widely in competence, the quality of their care is relatively the same. In particular, this study shows that midwives, who cared for about nine percent of deliveries, obtained comparable results, so that for selected cases home delivery would be an appropriate option.

In arriving at these judgments, the Committee had considerable information about each case. It used as a standard "the best possible skill, both in diagnosis and treatment, which the community could make available" (p. 19). Its criteria were implicit, but guided by an explicit set of considerations described in the report and illustrated by case abstracts. All judgments were made without knowing the attendant's identity, and whenever in doubt the Committee exonerated patients and attendants. Nevertheless, the reliability of judgments has not been tested. It is also interesting to speculate on how the validity of the method might be verified.

Chart 8–2

Maternal Mortality Among those Under the Care of Specified Types of Attendants at Delivery, by Responsibility for the Death and Percent of Deaths in Each Category Attributed to the Attendant. New York City, 1930–1932.

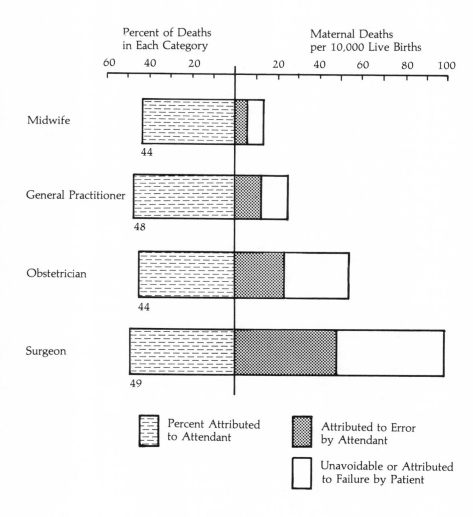

Source and Note: New York Academy of Medicine, Committee on Public Health Relations, 1933, Tables 79 and 80, pp. 184 and 188. The data exclude deaths following abortion and ectopic gestation.

Chart 8–3

When the New York Academy of Medicine conducted its study of maternal mortality, about 29 percent of births took place at home and only 71 percent in the hospital. The maternal death rate per 10,000 live births was 19 for the former and 45 for the latter (Table 55, p. 140), the difference being attributed mainly to the greater complexity of the cases admitted to the hospital. But, as this chart illustrates in part, the hospitals were very different from each other in the rates of maternal mortality and the proportion of maternal deaths judged to be preventable.

The information in the chart comes from 67 hospitals that reported about 75 percent of all the hospital deliveries during 1930–1932. It includes all cases delivered in each hospital, regardless of the place of subsequent death, and all pregnant women who died in the hospital, irrespective of whether they were delivered or not.

The left-hand panel of the chart was constructed by excluding all 14 hospitals that reported less than 1,000 deliveries during 1930–1932. Even though variability due to exceptionally small numbers is thus removed, we see how greatly the remaining hospitals differed from each other in the proportion of deaths judged to have been preventable. The range was from 14.3 in one hospital that reported seven deaths, to 81.8 in another that reported 11 deaths.

The right-hand panel of the chart shows the rates for overall mortality and preventable mortality, each according to the size of the hospital's obstetrical service as indicated by the number of deliveries during the period of the study. Because no corrections for case mix have been made, one cannot accept the total mortality rate as a measure of a hospital's performance. But the preventable mortality rate includes a clinical judgment taking account of all known attributes of each case, including its severity. One can use it, therefore, to conclude that performance tends to improve as the obstetrical service grows larger in size, but only up to a point. Part of this improvement could be due to other attributes related to size. We are told, for example, that the mortality rate (defined as in the chart) was 98 for municipal hospitals, 59 for voluntary hospitals, and 49 for hospitals devoted to obstetrics and gynecology. The corresponding rates of preventable mortality were 34, 29, and 25 (p. 181); but we are not told how much of the preventable mortality is attributed to medical error and how much to failure of the patient to seek and maintain care. The rates for proprietary hospitals could not be determined accurately.

Chart 8–3

Percent Distribution of Hospitals by Percent of Maternal Deaths Judged To Be Preventable; and Total Preventable Maternal Mortality Rates, by Size of the Hospital's Obstetrical Service. New York City, 1930–1932.

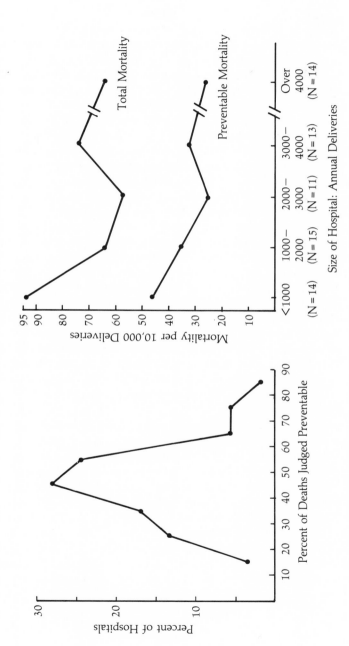

Source: New York Academy of Medicine, Committee on Public Health Relations, 1933. Computed from tables on pp. 251-54.

Chart 8–4

The last chart in this series on preventable maternal mortality presents a part of the findings on factors such as the mother's place of residence, place of birth, and race.

To construct the chart, socioeconomic status was determined, rather crudely, by grouping the "health areas" of New York City into four groups, depending on the average rents of houses in each area. The chart shows that the overall maternal mortality rate tends to decline with improvements in socioeconomic status. Much more marked is the decline in the rate of preventable maternal deaths, but this is due very largely to a reduction in the deaths attributed to the failure of pregnant women to initiate care or to adhere to the medical regimen.

The corresponding reduction in mortality attributed to medical error is relatively small, so that as socioeconomic status improves, the relative importance of patient cooperation as a factor in preventing maternal deaths decreases, and that of medical performance increases. In the highest economic group, 90 percent of all *preventable* deaths are attributed to physician error. But the proportion of *all* maternal deaths attributed to medical error is essentially constant across groups, at about 45 percent. The Committee attributes this relative invariance to a tendency for women in the higher economic groups to get care from private physicians who are not always more qualified than those who provide care in the public and quasi-public institutions that serve the less advantaged. There is another factor: as socioeconomic status improves, the rate of nonpreventable deaths actually increases, from 14.6 per 10,000 live births in the lowest economic group to 19.5 in the highest, perhaps due to differences in other maternal attributes.

The gradients in preventable mortality shown in this chart are a good illustration of the "social definition of quality," as described in Donabedian 1980, pp. 15–16 and in Donabedian et al. 1982. One might debate how responsible society should be for the more equal distribution of quality, especially when client behavior is at fault. The Committee recognized that "in many, if not most, instances where the patient has been held responsible, . . . she is, in fact, helpless by reason of circumstances which are beyond her control. She may be, and very often is, the victim of poverty or ignorance and, in such eventualities, it is manifestly the failure of society to provide proper and effective education, assistance and care, which have forced her, unwittingly and surely unwillingly, to become the deciding factor in her own death" (p. 31).

Chart 8–4

Total Maternal Mortality Subdivided According to Whether Preventable or Not, and if Preventable, According to Who Is at Fault, in Each of Four Socioeconomic Groups. New York City, 1930–1932.

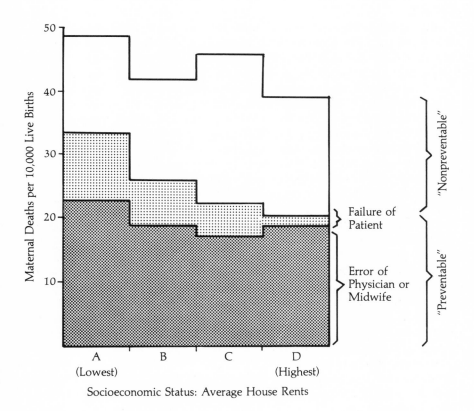

Source: New York Academy of Medicine, Committee on Public Health Relations, 1933. Computed from Tables 62 and 68, pp. 151 and 161.

Chart 8–5

The fate of the mother, whether marked by health, death, or morbidity, is only one part of the outcome of pregnancy; what happens to the child, in utero, during birth, and soon afterward is another cause for concern. Accordingly, the New York Academy of Medicine, about 20 years after its classic study of maternal mortality, returned for a look at the second half of the picture, using some of the methods that had earlier served it so well.

Beginning with a sample of stillbirths and deaths during the first 30 days after birth, information about each case was obtained from hospital records, supplemented by interviews with nurses, house staff, private physicians, and members of the family. The purpose was to determine what caused the death, what factors contributed to it, and whether it was preventable. Partly by accident, the procedure for making these determinations was tortuous, involving (1) a determination by an obstetrician, (2) a review of doubtful cases by a committee, (3) a second review of all cases by another obstetrician, and (4) a review of still doubtful cases by yet another committee. At the end, each case had two designations: one as to whether it was preventable, and another as to what "responsibility factors" were present. More than one "responsibility factor" could be present in each case, "unavoidable disaster" being included as one such factor. Unfortunately, the relation between the two classifications is not fully clear, especially since the author tells us that the panel had trouble in determining preventability, only being able to decide "whether or not there was mishandling of the case or that the patient did or did not receive optimal care" (p. 25). My interpretation is that, excluding an "unavoidable disaster," a "responsibility factor" is an error that may or may not have contributed substantially to the death, and that a "preventable death" is one in which one or more errors have made a substantial contribution to the outcome.

Keeping this interpretation in mind, the top part of the chart is taken to show that the deaths were "preventable" in 42 percent of mature infants, were due to an "unavoidable disaster" in 48 percent, and were associated with error, but not substantially so, in the remaining 10 percent. The remainder of the chart shows the percentages of mature deaths associated with specified "responsibility factors." While the information cannot be synthesized into a coherent, nonoverlapping whole, it is clear that medical management is often faulty and that the errors are often at least partially responsible for the death.

Chart 8–5

Percent Distribution of All Perinatal Deaths of Mature Infants, by Whether Due to an "Unavoidable Disaster" or "Preventable"; and Percent of Perinatal Deaths of Mature Infants with Specified "Responsibility Factors," Partitioned by Whether "Preventable" or Not. New York City, 1950–1951.

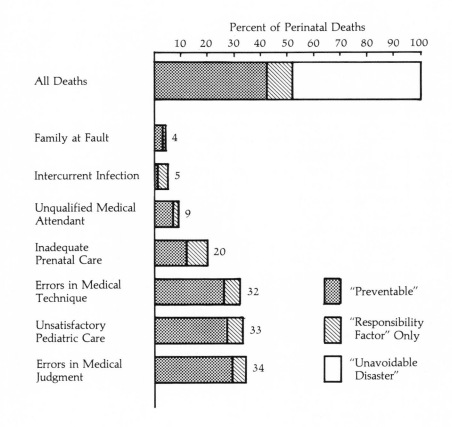

Source and Note: Kohl 1955, Tables XIV, XV, and XVI, pp. 18, 24, and 27. Perinatal deaths are stillbirths and deaths during the first 30 days, of infants beyond 28 weeks of gestation or weighing more than 1,000 grams at birth.

Chart 8–6

This second chart based on the study of perinatal deaths under the auspices of the New York Academy of Medicine shows some of the associations between "type of professional service" and some deficiencies of medical care that may or may not have rendered the death "preventable." Perinatal deaths are stillbirths and deaths during the first 30 days following birth in children beyond 28 weeks of gestation or weighing more than 1,000 grams at birth. "Preventability" is not a clearly defined concept. While it was possible to determine whether or not the case was "mishandled" or received "optimal care," the additional judgment as to whether or not the death could have been averted was often a difficult one. In this study (unlike the procedure for the earlier study of maternal mortality) doubtful cases have been reported as "preventable."

In the absence of clear information in the report, I assume that the categories of "professional service" used in the chart refer to the practitioners who were in charge of prenatal care and delivery, and that the errors of medical judgment and technique shown are attributable to these practitioners. I have, therefore, also included information about pediatric care which may have been provided partly by the attendants at the birth and, I suppose, partly by others. The reader should also know that a death may have more than one error of management associated with it, and that the presence of an error without associated preventability of the death has not been explained in the report. It may mean the error was not serious enough to contribute to the death, but I cannot exclude the possibility that some of the deaths may have been unavoidable.

In spite of these ambiguities, the chart does show that errors which may have fatal consequences are quite frequent, even under the care of specialists. As one might expect, errors of medical judgment are most frequent under the care of the less experienced house staff.

Corresponding data for premature births (not shown in the chart) reveal that these are less often "preventable," and more often due to "unavoidable disaster," in 29 and 62 percent of cases, respectively. The differences introduced by variations in the qualifications of the practitioners are correspondingly smaller.

The author cautions us that the patterns of errors associated with deaths may or may not correspond to their incidence among those who survive. A parallel study in a sample of survivors might have taught us a great deal about the validity of the method and about the quality of obstetrical and pediatric care.

Chart 8–6

Percent of Perinatal Deaths in Mature Infants, Under the Care of Specified Types of Practitioners, Judged To Be Associated with Specified Deficiencies in Care, and To Be "Preventable" or Not. New York City, 1950–1951.

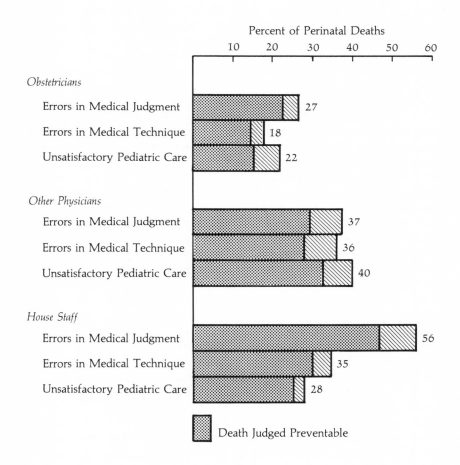

Source: Kohl 1955, Tables XXV and XXVI, pp. 35 and 37, with some computation.

Chart 8–7

In this last chart on "preventable" perinatal mortality we see the relationships between the "preventability" of death and characteristics of the place of birth. The definitions of perinatal mortality and the meaning of "preventability" were described in connection with the preceding chart. Unfortunately, the report does not separate the contributions of the two factors: staff qualifications and institutional attributes. We also do not know if the distinction between "teaching" and "nonteaching" hospitals refers to affiliation with a medical school, or only to the presence or absence of residency training programs.

By including the 100 percent limit, the chart conveys a fair image of possible reductions in the deaths of mature infants. We also see the hospitals arrayed in the expected order of quality, except for the proprietary hospitals, which perform better than expected. Also surprising (if we are to be guided by the findings of the earlier study of maternal mortality) is the very high percentage of preventability when the delivery was at home. But this finding is based on fewer than 20 deaths.

The effect of case mix has been excluded by the judgment of "preventability," except for the influence of client behavior. We know, however, that "family at fault" was a "responsibility factor," either alone or in association with other factors, in only four percent of perinatal deaths in mature infants (Chart 8–5). But this factor may play a relatively much larger role in some settings, such as municipal hospitals and the ward services of voluntary hospitals. For example, I estimate that "family at fault" may add up to five percentage points to the already high percentage of "preventable" deaths of mature infants under the care of house staff in all hospitals.

The observed differences between teaching and nonteaching hospitals (which are statistically significant), and among voluntary, municipal, and proprietary hospitals, no doubt also reflect the qualifications of the attending staff as well as the role, quality, and supervision of house staff. The proprietary hospitals may also have improved their performance by limiting care to the cases that they can handle well.

The data for premature infants (not included in the chart) closely replicate those for mature infants, except that the preventability is lower by anywhere from 18 to 42 percent, depending on the category shown in the chart.

Chart 8–7

Percent of Perinatal Deaths of Mature Infants Judged To Have Been "Preventable," by Place of Birth and by Hospital Service. New York City, 1950–1951.

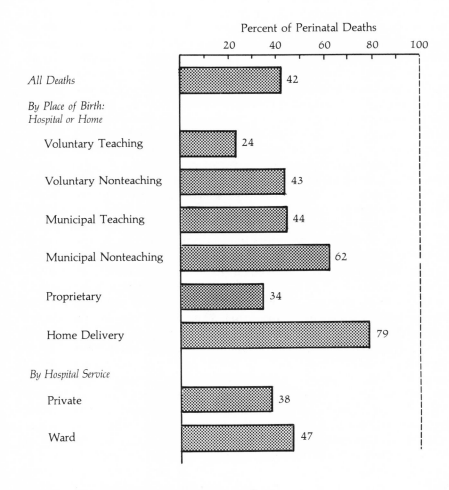

Source: Kohl 1955, Tables XX and XXVIII, pp. 31 and 39.

Chart 8–8

By including a longer period of infancy, and by showing the findings in another country under a different system of care in more recent times, this study of preventable deaths suggests the pervasiveness of the problem and the wider applicability of the method.

Of all the deaths studied, 37 percent occurred in the hospital, without the newborn infant ever having gone home. Only a few of these deaths were judged to have been possibly preventable. The remaining 63 percent of deaths were in infants who left the hospital alive, only to become ill later, to be readmitted to the hospital, and to die there. A substantial number of these deaths were judged to have been "possibly avoidable," some through family initiative, some through more competent care by the general practitioner, and still others through more effective hospital care. To summarize, 25.9 percent of all deaths were considered possibly preventable, with part of the responsibility for the unhappy event being attributed to hospital care in 7.4 percent of cases, to the general practitioner outside the hospital in 8.6 percent, and to the family in 9.9 percent.

Beyond these stark statistics, the anecdotal accounts of the investigators illustrate almost every possible pitfall on the tragic journey to unnecessary death. In one case the parents did not know the child was so desperately ill. In three cases the parents waited too long to call the doctor because they did not want to disturb him. In one case the doctor was called, but the parent could not explain how seriously ill the child was; in another case, a mother too illiterate to use the telephone directory took her child directly to the doctor, only to be turned back by the receptionist because she had not first called for an appointment. In two instances the parents actually failed to follow advice, but more frequently the practitioner's expectations that he would be kept informed of the patient's progress were simply too much for the parents to meet. In about as many cases, it was the practitioner who did not seem to realize that the patient was very ill, even though he had seen the patient several times before the decision to hospitalize was finally made. And even after admission to the hospital, the care was sometimes sufficiently inadequate to contribute to the death.

The importance of the client-physician relationship to successful care is amply demonstrated by these accounts. In several cases the parents said they were not getting along with their doctors even before the events that led to their bereavement.

Chart 8-8

Percent Distribution of Deaths in Children Between the Ages of One Week and Two Years, by Whether or Not the Children Were Ever Discharged from the Hospital, and the Factors Contributing to the Death. Deaths in All Hospitals, Sheffield, England, January 1, 1973–July 31, 1975.

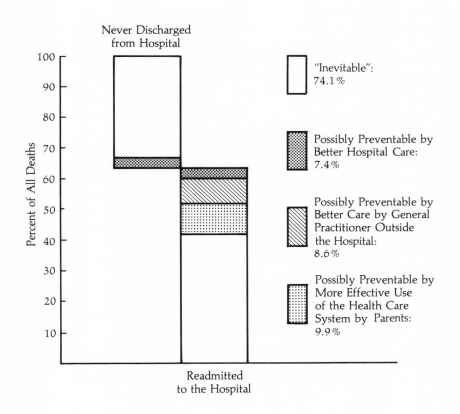

Source: Oakley et al. 1976, figure on p. 770 and text on p. 772.

Chart 8–9

Williamson's method of "health accounting" begins when, in any given program, a properly constituted committee, using a carefully designed procedure, identifies those aspects of care which are most probably deficient, most amenable to improvement, and most likely to provide the greatest benefit to the largest number of people, when improved. Next, those responsible for care specify the standards of outcome that they would consider acceptable for their program, within a specified period of the initiation of a given activity. To what extent the standard has been met is verified by mailed questionnaires, interviews, and actual examinations. If the findings reveal statistically significant and substantively important failures, the program is expected to find out the reasons for the deficiencies, to take corrective action, and to verify its success by reassessing the outcome.

The study selected as an illustration used two kinds of outcomes. The outcomes of treatment ("therapeutic outcomes") were measured by the frequency distribution of patients among the categories of an ordinal scale proposed by Williamson (p. 126). Other outcomes, more precisely tailored to the physiological or functional consequences of specific conditions, can also be used. Patient behavior, knowledge, and satisfaction may also be included. The accuracy of diagnosis ("diagnostic outcomes") was studied by reviewing the medical records of all the patients of the group to see if tests for diabetes were done when they were not indicated ("false positives"), or were not done when they should have been ("false negatives").

The chart shows a larger frequency of erroneous screening ("diagnostic") decisions than the group was willing to accept. Too many patients who should have been tested for diabetes were not, and too many others who should not have been tested, were. The distribution of actual therapeutic outcomes was also significantly different from the standard. In this case it is clear that, except for the smaller number of deaths, the results are worse than expected. The difference may not always be so obvious, and because the several categories of the scale are not weighted, it is not possible to obtain a single, overall measure of the difference.

We are not sure what can be done to improve the health status of diabetics. In this case, the group did not act to improve care.

Chart 8-9

Percent of All Patients Tested for Diabetes Unnecessarily (False Positives) and Percent Erroneously Not Tested (False Negatives), and Percent Distribution of Diabetics by Health Status Categories, as Specified by Maximum Acceptable Standards and as Observed. A Multispecialty Prepaid Group Practice, U.S.A., Undated.

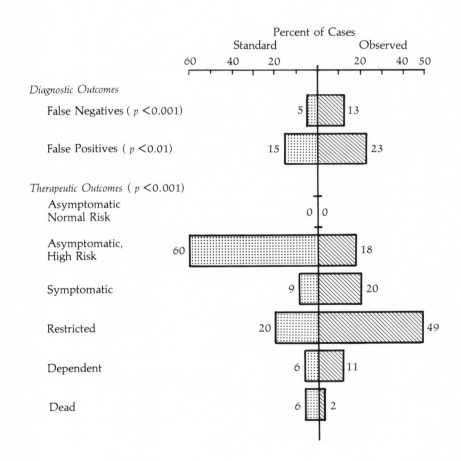

Source: Williamson 1978, Table 8.16, p. 205.

Chart 8–10

In 1969 the Johns Hopkins University Medical School sponsored the formation of a prepaid group practice plan, staffed by its faculty members, in the "new city" of Columbia, Maryland, "a suburban middle-class community in the Baltimore–Washington corridor." Williamson used this plan as one of the sites for testing the method of health accounting described in the preceding chart. Later, Daniel Barr (1973, 1974), working in the same place, developed a Problem-Status Index of ten items, which was meant to characterize both the patient's reason for seeking care and the patient's condition subsequent to care. After testing an index similar to Barr's, and finding that many of its components were intercorrelated, Mushlin and Appel developed the measure of "problem-status" shown in this chart, and tested its usefulness in quality assessment.

When an episode of care begins, the patient is asked to give "the principal reason" for the visit and, if the visit is due to a "problem," to answer the questions meant to show how troubling the problem is. At a preselected later date, the patient is contacted by phone or letter, reminded of the problem that occasioned the first visit, and asked to indicate its "status" in the same way. The chart shows the findings of one such study. Obviously, a great deal of improvement has taken place during the month, but this is not surprising, since many of the patients had self-limiting conditions.

The standards of improvement in problem-status could be set in a number of ways. One way is to select diagnostic categories or conditions and ask a group of physicians to specify the expected status below which no patient should be at a specified period after care is begun. (Mushlin and Appel give examples on p. 20.) Another method is to ask each physician to specify for each patient, at the first visit, what the status should be at a specified subsequent time. This does not require a preselection of conditions, though it does not preclude it. Using either method, any patient who fails to achieve any part of the standard could be suspected of having had less than acceptable care, and could be called in for further study.

The "problem-status" index is a set of criteria analogous to Williamson's scale of "therapeutic outcomes." But the standards of the former are expressed as a minimum that every case must meet, rather than as a frequency distribution of all cases. Mushlin and Appel judge the care of individuals; Williamson judges the care of groups.

Chart 8–10

Percent Distribution of Patients by Reported Severity of Each of Three Consequences Attributed to a "Problem" Responsible for Obtaining Care, at the First
Visit, and One Month Later. Columbia Medical Plan, Columbia, Maryland,
1974.

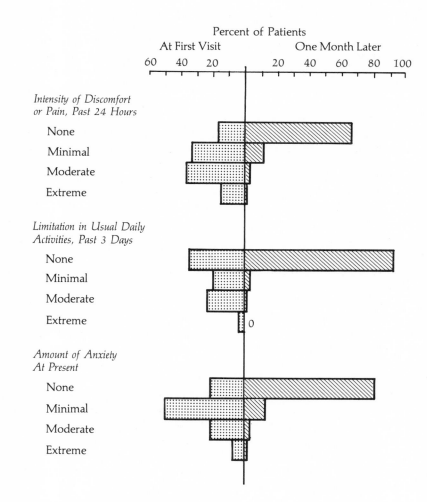

Source: Mushlin and Appel 1980, Table 3-3, p. 19.

Chart 8–11

The preceding chart displayed the components of the "Problem-Status Index" and showed evidence of changes in status associated with, though not necessarily caused by, medical care. In this second chart we see an example of what may happen when the standards of acceptable outcomes are applied, and the deficiencies in outcome are investigated.

The standards for vaginitis (the most frequent condition in the office practice of gynecology) specified that there should be no symptoms, activity limitation, or anxiety one month after starting care (p. 20). In the sample of 47 patients studied, 38 percent failed to meet the standards because they had at least "minimal" deficiencies in at least one of these three functional areas. In practice, only those who failed to meet the standards would be called back, but because this was an investigation of the usefulness of the method, all patients were studied further.

First, without knowing the outcomes, the record was assessed using explicit criteria which specified the "critical . . . elements of the process of care which should be done for every patient [with vaginitis] and recorded" (p. 7). Then, the reviewers used their own judgments to assess the recorded management of care, thus combining explicit and implicit criteria to reach a final opinion. The top third of the chart shows the findings of record review for those who met the standards (acceptable problem-status) and those who did not (substandard problem-status). "Possible errors" are omissions in diagnostic workup that could have been only failures to record what was done. "Definite errors" include mistaken diagnosis and incorrect or incomplete treatment. Because so few were studied, the differences between "acceptable" and "substandard" cases were not statistically significant.

The remainder of the chart, based on information obtained from the patients, shows that those who have "substandard" outcomes are more likely not to have taken their medications as prescribed, and to be dissatisfied with their care and its results. They also seem to know more about their problem, perhaps because it has troubled them for so long.

The investigators conclude that the assessment of "technical" care by chart review is insufficient, because it does not show the frequent deficiencies in the management of the interpersonal aspects of care which the follow-up of "substandard" outcomes will reveal.

There will be more on "health accounting" and "problem-status" assessment in subsequent sections of this book.

Chart 8–11

Percent of Patients with Vaginitis Whose Care Was Judged To Have Specified
Deficiencies, by Whether the Outcome of Their Care ("Problem-Status") Was
"Acceptable" or "Substandard." Columbia Medical Plan, Columbia, Maryland,
1974.

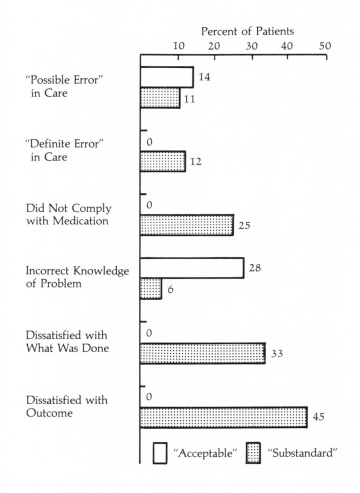

Source: Mushlin and Appel 1980, Tables 4-9 and 4-10, pp. 32 and 33.

Exploration of System Properties through Combinations of Process and Outcome Assessment

NINE

This chapter presents three assessment methods which are hard to classify, but which do have some shared characteristics. First, they are capable of using various combinations of processes and outcomes. Second, they are usually meant to throw some light on the performance of a system of health care, rather than on the management of individual conditions by individual practitioners.

Of the three methods, the first offers itself most modestly. It is not the pet brainchild of any one investigator, though the recent interest in it may be attributed to the report by Brook and Stevenson which is the basis for the opening chart of the chapter. It also has no name, though I think it could very well be described as the "trajectory" method. This is an apt description because the method of assessment begins with selecting a cohort of persons who share a distinguishing characteristic, such as a diagnosis, a laboratory finding, or a set of signs and symptoms. It then follows the path of this company of people through the health care system, noting what happens at important junctures along the way, and what outcomes are achieved by the end of the journey.

The clear identification of the succession of steps, and the inclusion of a measure of performance at each step, are the distinctive characteristics of the method, characteristics that set it apart, for example, from a method that provides an overall quality score for the management of patients in a given category. Provided the stepwise design is maintained, both the starting point and the end point of the "trajectory" may vary from study to study. One study may begin with a group of people only some of whom enter the system of care and end with long-term changes in health status. Another may begin with patients who are already diagnosed and follow them for a few steps, perhaps until they are discharged, assessing the steps in the process of care, but without measuring the outcomes. The chapter offers several examples, illustrating trajectories of various descriptions and lengths.

The second method has both a sponsor and a name. It is the "tracer method" developed by Kessner and his associates (1973) for a study of health care in Washington, D.C. The method has two essential components. The first is some kind of formulation, usually a tabular matrix, that identifies the aspects or components of the health care system to be assessed. Kessner et al., for example, wished to assess the following aspects of the system's performance: prevention, screening, evaluation, and follow-up care. Under "evaluation" they distinguished the history and physical examination, laboratory tests, and other diagnostic procedures; under "management" they detailed chemotherapy, health counseling, and specialty referral. They further subdivided the population by sex and by age groups. The tracer method does not, of course, prescribe this particular format. It does, however, require some kind of prior specification analogous to this.

The second essential component of the method is the set of "tracers" that are meant to obtain information about the performance within each cell of the two-dimensional matrix defined as described above, by function and by age-sex group. Each of the tracers is a condition (such as anemia, hearing loss, or cervical cancer) which, by the way it is handled by the health care system, provides information on how one or more of the functions prespecified by the matrix are performed. It is essential that a number of tracers be used, and that they be selected carefully so as to obtain information about each component of the matrix. Thus, the entire system being studied is subjected to multiple soundings, under the assumption, still unproven, that the information provided by the tracers also holds for other similar conditions which have not been directly studied.

The "staging concept" described by Gonnella and Goran (1975), the third method included in this chapter, is little more than the measurement of an adverse outcome (in this instance the preventable progression of disease) and the investigation of its antecedents. Gonnella and his coworkers have made a useful contribution, however, by calling attention to how easy it is to obtain information about the stage of illness when the patient is first admitted to hospital, and then for offering methods for the staging of many illnesses (Gonnella 1982).

The argument behind the "staging concept" is that if a patient is first admitted to the hospital with a disease which has progressed beyond what is considered appropriate, one may suspect either a barrier to access or inadequate prior care. The nature of the barriers or of the inadequacy requires further investigation, however.

Chart 9–1

As patients journey through the health care system, they encounter successive obstacles which produce an accumulation of failures in access, compliance, and quality, all leading to poor results.

This chart reconstructs what I have called the "trajectory" of one such journey: that of patients with "nonemergency gastrointestinal symptoms" who came to the emergency room of a teaching hospital to get care, mainly from interns and residents educated in the United States. One sees the cumulative effect of successive failures at each important step in this progression. Of 141 patients referred for X-ray examination, only 67 percent showed up, and only 55 percent also had an examination considered to be "adequate." Moreover, though 27 percent of the original 141 patients had an abnormal finding (through adequate or inadequate X-ray examination), only 10 percent received treatment that was rated at least minimally adequate.

The overall impact of these events can be shown in two ways. The outcomes of care were determined by interviewing 131 patients an average of 3.5 months after their first visit. As the chart shows, 31 percent said that their symptoms had disappeared or were better. But we cannot use this finding to judge the performance of this system because we do not know what the best care can accomplish, and because many patients received care from other sources as well.

A summary of the process of care shows more precisely another aspect of performance. In only 38 percent of cases was performance at least potentially "effective," because cases with abnormal findings were treated at least minimally well (though we do not know with what results), and those without abnormalities were not treated. The investigators estimate, "by combining the results of diagnostic and therapeutic outcomes," that "the health system exerted a positive effective action in only 38 out of 141 patients (27 percent)" (p. 907). They also report that the interpersonal process of care was often at fault. Many patients were not given an appointment slip, were not told why X-ray examination was needed, or could not remember being told the results.

Chart 9-1

Percent of Patients Referred for X-Ray Examination for Gastrointestinal Symptoms Who Experienced Specified Subsequent Events or States. Emergency Service, Baltimore City Hospitals, April–June 1969.

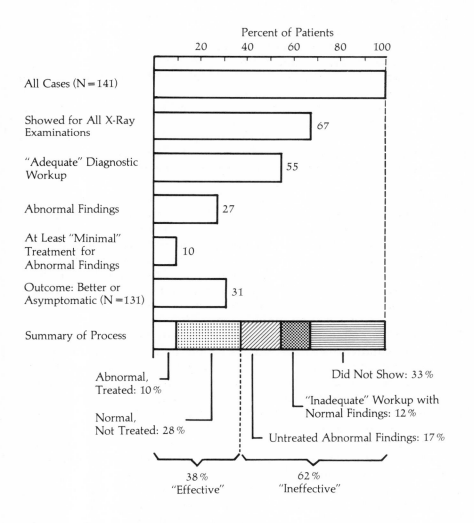

Source: Brook and Stevenson 1970, Figures 1 and 2, and Table 2, p. 906.

Chart 9–2

This chart summarizes some of the findings of another study that reconstructs the "trajectory" of a cohort of patients as it passes through a medical care system, one in which care happens to be provided by interns, residents, and fellows in pediatric training. Besides providing another example of the method, the chart raises additional questions by contrasting the outcome of care for adequately treated cases with that for cases treated inadequately or not at all.

The investigators examined a file of laboratory reports to identify a sample of children, aged six months or older, who were newly found to have anemia, as judged by a blood hemoglobin level under 10 gm/100ml. The medical record of each case was reviewed, and about six months later the mother was interviewed and the blood hemoglobin measured again. The outcome was considered "adequate" if this final hemoglobin reading was 10 gm or above. The study owes a great deal to the relative precision and specificity of this measure of outcome in iron-deficiency anemia.

The chart documents the cumulative succession of failures, in one component of the system or another, that the "trajectory" is designed to reveal. The very first step is a stumble, since in only 81 percent of cases is there evidence that the physician was told that the hemoglobin was low. There was then, as judged by the record, a frequent failure of the physician to "recognize" the problem. Not all the cases recognized to have a low hemoglobin level were treated, and many cases were judged to have had inadequate treatment because the children did not take an iron preparation for at least one month, often because the mother did not follow recommendations. In the end, only 12 percent of the original group of children had traversed the system to a successful conclusion. But even this modest degree of success cannot be totally attributed to the program being assessed. Though, as the chart shows, adequate treatment is significantly associated with the desired outcome, the blood hemoglobin can also improve without specific treatment or when the treatment is less than adequate.

This chart excludes cases with undetermined outcome, those known not to have iron deficiency, and those cared for elsewhere. One could question the reliability of hemoglobin determinations and the choice of the level that signifies anemia. The investigators report that physicians were more likely to "recognize" the presence of anemia when the child had symptoms and the reading was particularly low. But the test was never repeated to verify a suspicious laboratory finding.

Chart 9–2

Percent of Children with Newly-found Low Blood Hemoglobin Levels Who Experienced Specified Events or States. Two University-affiliated Outpatient Facilities, Baltimore, 1969–1970.

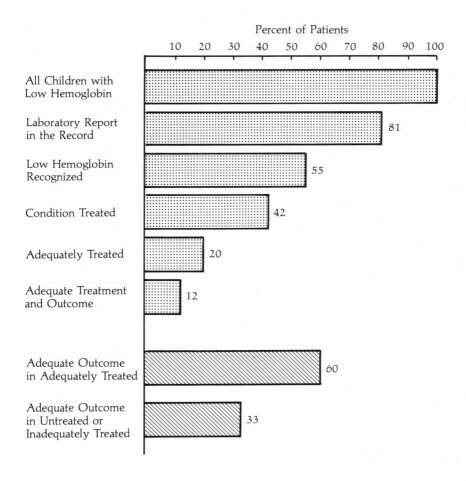

Source: Starfield and Scheff 1972, Figures 1, 2, and 3, pp. 548 and 549.

Chart 9–3

The "trajectory" used to assess performance may begin at different points in the progress of care, and need not continue to its final outcome. The study portrayed in this chart starts with an undifferentiated cohort of patients (as contrasted to those with an already demonstrated laboratory abnormality), and includes only the steps leading to a diagnosis, a juncture which some regard as a "diagnostic outcome" in its own right (Williamson 1978, pp. 153–55, and elsewhere). This study is also notable for including as a standard for comparison the performance of an expert, the "criterion physician."

The study begins with a group of new patients at a general medical clinic. Using a questionnaire that embodied the most recent authoritative medical knowledge, the criterion physician obtained the medical history of each patient so as to identify those who were likely to have a urinary tract infection. All these patients had a microscopic examination of the urine, as well as a urine culture and colony count, in order to verify the presence of an infection. The results of this diagnostic strategy were compared with those of the procedure used by the regular team (composed of a senior medical student and an attending physician) responsible for the care of the same patients. In general, the team ignored historical information suggesting urinary tract infection, relied on a routine urine examination to identify cases with many white blood cells in the urine, and requested a urine culture only for these.

The chart shows that the team regularly responsible for patient care was less likely to elicit information suggesting the possible presence of urinary tract infection, and to perform investigations beyond the routine urine examination in order to confirm or reject the diagnosis. As a result, only 43 percent (6/14 × 100) of the urinary infections known to be present in this group of patients were discovered in the regular course of care. Lacking information about ultimate health status, we can accept this as an interim measure of the relative effectiveness of the two strategies of care.

To show another aspect of performance I have added a measure of yield relative to effort, which tells us how often more complete investigation identified a confirmed case of infection. By this criterion, the diagnostic strategy used by the clinic team is more efficient than that of the criterion physician. The optimal strategy is one that balances these two considerations: effectiveness and efficiency.

Chart 9–3

Percent of Patients Accepted for Clinic Care Who Had Specified Evidence of Urinary Tract Infection, as Determined by a Criterion Physician and by the Regular Treatment Team of the Clinic Respectively, and the Relationship of Yield to Effort in the Two Alternative Strategies of Management. General Medical Clinic, Outpatient Department of a University Hospital, U.S.A., Spring, 1965.

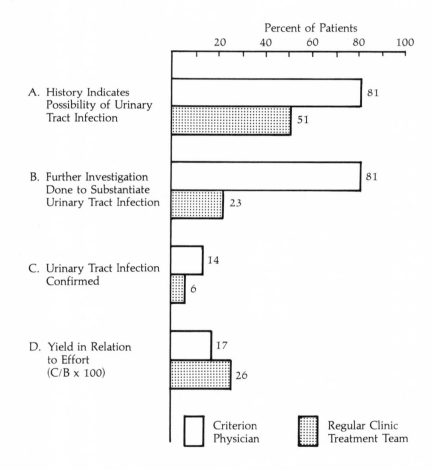

Source: Gonnella et al. 1970, figure and text, p. 2041.

Chart 9–4

This chart is similar to the preceding one in beginning with a population of patients, but it portrays a longer trajectory in the process of care, which is still, however, short of a measure of improvement in health. The data were obtained by reviewing the medical records of patients who received health care almost exclusively from a "service unit" of the Indian Health Service. The records showed, assuming they were to be trusted, what proportion of patients between the ages of 35 and 70 were screened for the presence of hypertension and were then, upon returning to the clinic, recognized to need further investigation to confirm or reject the diagnosis within one year of the first visit, at the latest. The likelihood of the subsequent milestones in the progression of care could be determined in the same way.

From these data the investigators reconstructed the course of a hypothetical cohort of patients who *have* hypertension, making two assumptions: (1) that the probability of screening for hypertension would be the same for these patients as for all patients in the comparable age range who visited the clinic, and (2) that if a person has hypertension, the screening tests would give a positive result in every case. Except for these assumptions, the chart is based on the actual experience of patients in this particular clinic.

The chart shows the cumulative erosion of system performance as one proceeds from step to step. It indicates at which steps the largest deficiencies occur, and whether the fault lies with the patients, because they do not return to the clinic, or with the practitioners who do not do what is needed when the patients do return. In the end, only 12 percent proceed successfully to the point of follow-up subsequent to receiving antihypertensive therapy.

Because the investigators used only minimal criteria of acceptable performance at each step in the course of care, they offer their findings not as a measure of *quality*, but as a measure of the *continuity of the process* of care, irrespective of whether the care is provided by one or by several practitioners in the clinic. But it is difficult to disentangle "quality" from "continuity" in this case: something that needs to be done cannot be done well unless it is done.

The investigators report the findings for six other conditions whose trajectories, with some significant variations, also follow the pattern shown in the chart; taken together, these might represent reasonably well the total care of this population.

Chart 9–4

Percent of Adults with Hypertension Who Would Be Expected to Encounter Specified Milestones in the Course of Care. Ambulatory Care Clinic, Sells Service Unit, Indian Health Service, Papago Indian Reservation, Southern Arizona, 1967–1973.

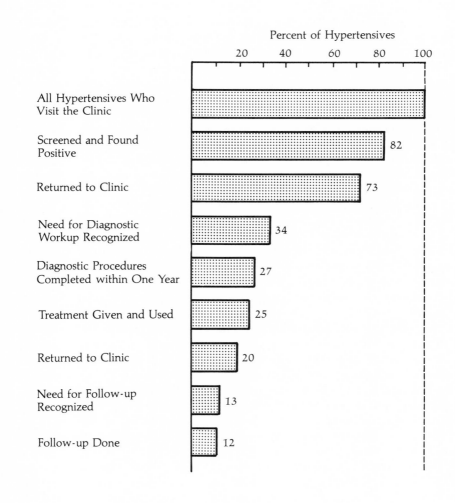

Source: Shorr and Nutting 1977. Computed from Tables 4 and 5, pp. 462 and 463.

Chart 9–5

We see here a further extension of the application of the assessment method called the "trajectory." The extension consists, first, in beginning with a group of persons who may or may not become patients, and then, in using an actual experiment to assess the relative merits of two ways of organizing health care.

Persons who applied for public assistance in the Yorkville Welfare District of Manhattan were randomly assigned to one of two groups: those who continued to receive care in the ordinary way, and those who were invited to receive care from an experimental program at the New York Hospital–Cornell Medical Center. Among other things, this program centralized care in the general medical and pediatric clinics; co-ordinated this care with that provided in the home, the hospital, and the nursing home; and assured continuous access to care irrespective of fluctuations in the eligibility for public assistance. To compare the costs and effects of the experimental program with those of the more established system of care, information about the presence of symptoms and illnesses, about attitudes and beliefs, and about the sources and volume of care was obtained at the start, a year later, and at the end of the second year, when the study terminated. Medical and other records were also reviewed.

The chart shows only a fragment of the many findings of this remarkable study. We see, moreover, only selected milestones in the progression of those adults who, during the very first interview, reported that they had trouble with urination, some reporting blood in the urine as well.

Access of care, the first step in the progression, was achieved by almost everyone with urinary symptoms, though the group invited to participate in the experimental program ("study group") has a small edge. After that, there are progressively compounded deficiencies in performance due to failures to note, diagnose, and treat the urinary problem. Though this occurs in both the study and control groups, the first fares better in all respects. It is the more disappointing, therefore, to see that in the end the proportions of those with no trouble in urinating is the same in both groups.

The differences shown in the chart do not represent the full potential of the experimental program, since only about two-thirds of those invited to participate did so, and even those who participated often received care from other sources as well. The chart also does not show the striking improvement in satisfaction among those who did use the program.

Chart 9–5

Percent of Persons with Urinary Symptoms Who Experienced Specified Events or States During Two Subsequent Years. Recipients of Public Assistance Invited to Receive Care in a Hospital-based, Comprehensive Care Project Compared to those Who Continued as Usual. Yorkville Welfare District, New York City, 1961–1964.

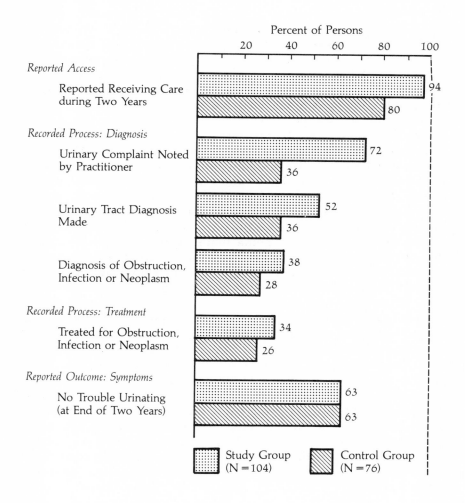

Source: Goodrich et al. 1970, Tables 87, 89, 91, 93, and 94, pp. 180–85, and text on pp. 184, 185, and 186.

Chart 9–6

The "tracer method" developed by Kessner et al. (1973) may be seen as a more systematized investigation of the trajectories of several cohorts of persons or patients. The most fundamental feature of the method is an initial mapping of the parts of the health care system, for example, as categories of health care functions, of population groups, and of classes of providers. Next, one selects the "tracers," each tracer being a condition expected to provide information about performance in one or more segments of the conceptual map or matrix that represents the system to be assessed. Either lengthy trajectories or only selected milestones may be assessed. But because performance at each milestone, for each tracer, is expected to be similar to analogous aspects of performance for other comparable conditions, a relatively few measurements are expected to portray, in microcosm, performance over a broader field.

This chart shows selected findings from a partial application of the tracer method by its originators. The investigation is limited to certain aspects of pediatric practice, including prevention, screening, diagnosis, treatment, and follow-up. The tracers expected to explore one or more of these aspects of care were anemia in children six months through three years of age, ear infections and abnormalities in children six months through 11 years of age, and hearing loss and visual defects in children four through 11 years of age. Population samples were drawn from two areas in Washington, D.C., chosen to include a broad range of social and economic characteristics, and from the membership roster of a neighborhood health center. Information was obtained by household interview, questionnaires mailed to physicians, medical examinations of children to determine the prevalence of health problems in the population, and review of records at the neighborhood health center, a prepaid group practice, and hospital-based clinics used by the people sampled.

The chart documents the frequent failures in case finding and treatment, to which may be attributed the high prevalence of these largely preventable conditions. An important finding not shown in the chart was the great similarity of performance among many different sources of care, including solo practice, prepaid group practice, hospital-based ambulatory care clinics, and a neighborhood health center. But because of the local nature of the study, as well as its many peculiarities in sampling, these findings should be considered only as illustrative and preliminary.

Chart 9–6

The Percent of Incidence or Prevalence of Specified Indicators of Health and Health Care in Samples of Children Who Received Care from Selected Organizations, and/or Resided in Selected Geographic Areas. Washington, D.C., 1972 and 1971, Respectively.

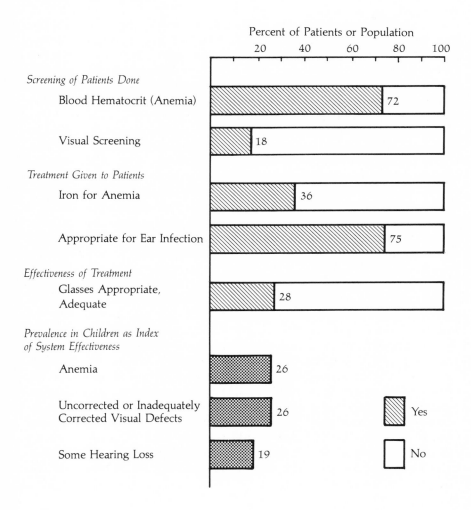

Source and Note: Kessner et al. 1974, Figures 3-2, 3-4, and 3-10, pp. 77, 80, and 89, and text on pp. 27, 34, and 43. The providers of care and the ages of the children with each tracer condition are given in the text.

Chart 9–7

Most studies that purport to use "tracers" are not examples of the "tracer method"; they simply show the more or less complete trajectories of one or more conditions. By contrast, the study illustrated by this chart meets all the basic requirements of the "tracer method" as it was originally proposed.

First, attention was focused on ambulatory care, excluding conditions requiring specialized management. Next, health care was subdivided into its major "functions": prevention, screening, health-status monitoring, diagnostic evaluation, treatment, follow-up, and ongoing management. The tracer conditions were then selected so that the management of each condition would reflect performance with respect to one or more functions, and so that any one function would be represented by the management of two or more conditions. In addition to the further subdivisions according to the patients' age and sex implied by the choice of the tracers, the care to be assessed was also subdivided according to its site and to the category of the practitioner responsible for it.

Information concerning the care provided was obtained from samples of medical records; it is, therefore, influenced by the completeness and veracity of these records. The criteria and standards used to judge the process of care were meant to signify a level of basic health care which most physicians would endorse and consider achievable. Information about health outcomes was also collected, knowing full well that outcomes could be only partly attributed to the adequacy of antecedent health care.

This chart shows only a small corner of the domain assessed by this method. It is concerned only with the function of follow-up, it does not show subdivisions by site of care or by type of practitioner, and it includes information garnered by only three tracers. We see, nevertheless, that the failure to institute indicated follow-up procedures when the patient was available in the clinic was a more frequent cause of inadequate follow-up than was the failure of the patient to make a visit in the first place, though there was much room for improvement in patient compliance as well. The particularly poor showing for iron-deficiency anemia is also apparent. The original report cites several additional examples of how the method could detect particular weaknesses localized by function, site of care, category of practitioner, and tracer condition.

Chart 9–7

Degree of Success in Performing the Follow-up Function, According to Minimal Standards and within Prescribed Periods of Time, as Indicated by Specified Measures for Each of Three Specified Tracer Conditions. Twenty "Service Units" of the Indian Health Service, U.S.A., Undated.

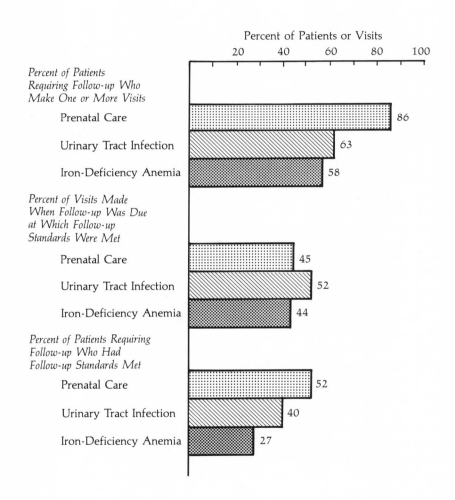

Source: Nutting et al. 1981, Table 2, p. 288.

Chart 9–8

This chapter ends with an application of the "staging concept" as a research tool used to determine whether those who enroll in a comprehensive health center receive better care than persons who are not clients of such a facility. Better care, it was argued, would lead to early diagnosis, and to a correspondingly early admission to the hospital, before a disease progresses to stages of successively greater severity.

The study design was to select four comprehensive health centers in communities of different types, to identify the one hospital used by a large majority of the enrollees of each center, to determine the stages at which enrollees with one of 21 diagnoses were admitted to the hospital, and to compare the distribution of these stages with the corresponding distribution for a sample of all other patients admitted to each hospital. The chart shows the findings for one hospital, the only one in which it was possible to match the two sets of patients (enrollees and others) by age, sex, and income.

The first pair of bars shows that when the findings for all 21 diagnoses are combined, a somewhat higher percentage of the enrollees of the health center are admitted to the hospital at the earliest of stages. The difference is statistically significant. When patients with each of the diseases were compared, the differences between the enrollees and the others were more than "minimal" in only seven. For three of the seven diagnoses, a higher percentage of the nonenrollees was admitted earlier. Only for four diagnoses was the proportion of enrollees admitted at an early stage larger than the proportion of other patients admitted early, and the difference was significant for only one diagnosis: pancreatitis.

The differences noted in the other hospitals were neither in a consistent direction nor statistically significant. Either there are only small differences in quality attributable to health centers, or this method of quality assessment is insensitive to the differences.

In using the "staging concept" for quality assessment one should be able to control for differences in population characteristics; to exclude diseases for which ambulatory treatment in the early stages is preferred or acceptable; to exclude cases who are in their advanced stages due not to faulty care but to success in achieving longevity; and to specify the stages at which admission is appropriate, being neither too early nor too late. Only some of these adjustments were made, to some extent, in parts of this study.

Chart 9-8

Percent of Patients Admitted to a Hospital with Stage I of Their Disease, according to Whether or Not They Were Enrolled in a Comprehensive Health Center. Patients with Any of 21 Diagnoses, and Those with Specified Diagnoses, a "Large Urban Setting," U.S.A., 1971–1975.

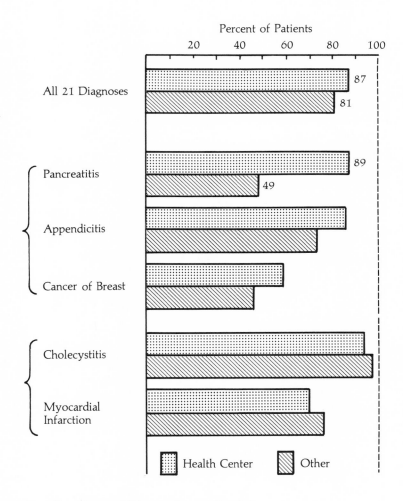

Source: Gonnella et al. 1977, Tables 2 and 3, pp. 17 and 18.

The Optimal Strategies of Care

TEN

In attempting to assess the technical quality of care, our primary purpose is to determine whether what we already know is appropriately used. But in the course of doing so, we often discover how uncertain some of that knowledge is. Thus quality assessment provides the impetus, not only to the elucidation of current knowledge, but also to more fundamental epidemiological and clinical research. That research, in its own turn, provides the new knowledge for the quality assessments of the future.

The proper formulation of current and future knowledge for the purpose of quality assessment requires a model of the clinical task. This task can be conceptualized as a strategy designed to deal with the patient's problem. The search for a solution is a progression of steps, each influenced by the findings of the preceding step and by the range of possibilities still ahead. The immediate objective is to establish a diagnosis and devise a plan of treatment; the ultimate purpose is to improve the patient's health.

In plotting his course of action, the practitioner almost always has a choice among alternatives, even if it is only between doing something and doing nothing. The choice should depend on the expected contribution of each of the alternatives to the immediate and ultimate purposes of care, taking into account the expected dangers inherent in almost any clinical intervention. Clinical virtuosity is evident in the use of the most parsimonious course of action consistent with the objectives of care. It is also important to reduce the monetary cost of care, provided this does not diminish the expected net benefits of care. When the benefits are diminished, the reduction in the cost of care must be weighed against the reduction in expected benefit, a matter that is not only technically difficult but ethically questionable as well.

The "criteria maps" devised by Greenfield et al. (1975), based on previous work on clinical "protocols" and "algorithms" by many investigators, are one way of specifying a strategy of care. Each map plots an extensive set of pathways, meant to accommodate the many causes and manifestations of a given problem as well as the variety of equally acceptable approaches to its solution. Thus the map can be adapted very precisely to the requirements of any given case, through selecting the relatively small part of the map corresponding to that case.

A logic-flow diagram such as the criteria map embodies the considered opinions of recognized experts, perhaps supplemented by a search of the relevant literature. In that sense, it is only a codification of current norms. But the validity of the strategy it represents can be tested more formally by decision analysis. This requires those responsible for constructing the algorithm to assign probabilities to the events on its several branches, and values to its objectives, so that alternative courses of action may be more rigorously compared. There is nothing more that can be done, beyond making certain that all reasonable alternatives have been identified and accurately portrayed. Only new knowledge can confirm or modify the recommended strategy.

Two kinds of research can provide the new information that may form the basis for more valid and more efficient strategies of care: epidemiological studies and clinical trials. Epidemiological studies are carefully designed observations of existing experience from which one can draw reasonably valid inferences, in this case about the events in the clinical algorithm. There may be, for example, information about the incidence and prevalence of pathological conditions in specified populations, about the association between the findings of diagnostic procedures and the conditions that they purport to discover, and about the probabilities of the consequences to health, both good and bad, of therapeutic and diagnostic procedures. Clinical trials differ in being true experiments. They benefit, therefore, from the greater assurance of validity conferred by random allocation of subjects to study and control groups, and by other features of experimental design. Traditionally, both epidemiological studies and clinical trials have ignored monetary costs and benefits, but this information can be added if it is considered to be relevant.

A complete exploration of these issues and methods is much beyond the intended scope of this book. Here I will only illustrate some steps in defining a strategy for managing cases with suspected acute appendicitis, using data derived from epidemiological studies. An example of a clinical trial will be cited for comparison. The reader is referred to the introductory section of the book for an example of decision analysis applied to screening for cancer of the colon, and to the next section for more on criteria maps.

Chart 10–1

It is customary, in assessing the quality of care, to begin with diagnoses already made or therapeutic procedures already performed. But this approach to assessment tells us nothing about the cases in which the diagnosis under study should have been made, but was not, or in which the procedure was not performed when it should have been. This omission is remedied when a representative sample of all cases is studied, so that missed diagnoses or procedures in one part of the sample are discovered as unjustified diagnoses or procedures in another part.

Another remedy is to begin, not with diagnoses or procedures, but with undifferentiated clinical problems which may be resolved in one of several different ways. The strategy used to handle the problem can then be assessed through a study of its component features, and of its outcomes as well. This chart begins an exploration of the strategies used to deal with one such problem: acute abdominal pain that suggests the possible presence of appendicitis.

As part of an extensive study of appendectomies in Scotland, Howie collected information about 533 patients between 12 and 29 years of age admitted to the Western Infirmary of Glasgow during 1963 with a diagnosis of possible appendicitis. He found that approximately 70 percent of these had an appendectomy performed, whereas 30 percent were not operated on. Among those who had been operated on, a considerable number, amounting to 25 percent of the total, and 36 percent of those operated on, could be judged, in retrospect, not to have needed the operation, since the tissue removed was not clearly diseased. We may consider the removal of a normal appendix an "error of commission," but only provisionally.

As to the patients who had been discharged without an operation, about a third, amounting to approximately 10 percent of the total, had "recurrent symptoms" within the next two years. Howie seems to have thought that many of these cases should have had an appendectomy at the initial hospital admission. If this is true, the "error of omission," which is the nonremoval of an abnormal appendix, could be as high as 10 percent.

There is no need to argue about the validity of the inferences based on these data, since the purpose of this chart is only to demonstrate the possible presence of two kinds of error, and to emphasize that only through a study of the entire cohort of cases can these errors be identified and measured.

Chart 10–1

Percent Distribution of Patients Admitted as an Emergency Because of Possible Appendicitis, According to Whether an Appendectomy Was or Was Not Performed, and According to the Results of Each Course of Action during the Subsequent Two Years. Patients 12 to 29 Years Old, Western Infirmary of Glasgow, Scotland, 1963.

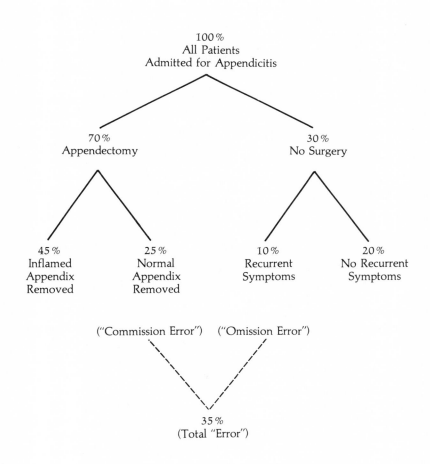

Source: Howie 1968, Table 1, p. 1366.

Chart 10–2

The story of appendectomies at the Western Infirmary of Glasgow continues with the observation that patients were assigned, in rotation, to one of five surgical teams. Three of the teams were "conservative"; they operated on only 60 percent of cases admitted with acute abdominal pain suggesting an inflamed appendix. The other two teams were more "radical"; they operated on 80 percent of such patients. Judging by the proportion of operations in which normal tissue was removed, the conservative surgeons are clearly ahead. Only by knowing the fate of the two cohorts of patients do we find out that the "conservative" surgeons also removed fewer abnormal appendices, and that within two years a larger proportion of their patients suffered from recurrent symptoms, requiring an appendectomy in an unspecified number of cases.

It looks as if, when in doubt, the "conservative" surgeons preferred to err on the side of not operating, whereas an equally competent group of "radical" surgeons, treating a presumably similar group of patients, preferred to take the risk of operating unnecessarily. Only a study of outcomes can tell us which of the two propensities to operate and to err is to be preferred.

Based on a more extensive study of appendectomies in Scotland, Howie estimated that the fatality ratio for surgical removal of a normal appendix is 0.02, and for not removing an inflamed appendix the ratio is 0.04. Assuming the two groups of patients at the Western Infirmary were comparable, Howie concluded that the "conservative" surgeons failed to remove an inflamed appendix in eight percent of their cases (49–41 = 8). Under these assumptions, the "avoidable mortality" for the "conservative" approach is $0.19(0.02) + 0.08(0.04) = 0.0070$. The "avoidable mortality" for the "radical" approach is $0.33(0.02) + 0(0.04) = 0.0066$. Analogous computations showed that the "conservative" strategy could be expected to be followed by "potentially serious" morbidity in 19.3 percent of cases, compared to 16.6 percent for the "radical" strategy. Thus, on the grounds of morbidity as well as mortality, the "radical" approach is to be preferred.

This chart does not pretend to offer a proven strategy for the management of abdominal pain. It is only intended to illustrate the properties of a method for identifying the preferred strategy. Even in that respect the method is incomplete, since it does not include information about monetary costs and does not tell us how to combine morbidity and mortality when these two point in different directions.

Chart 10-2

Percent Distribution of Patients Admitted as an Emergency Because of Possible Appendicitis, and Cared for by "Conservative" and "Radical" Surgeons, Respectively, According to Whether an Appendectomy Was or Was Not Performed, and According to the Results of Each Course of Action during the Subsequent Two Years. Patients 12 to 29 Years Old, Western Infirmary of Glasgow, Scotland, 1963.

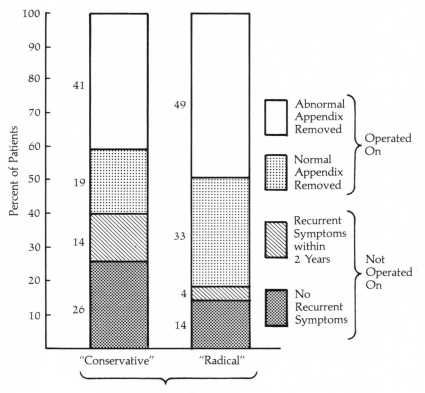

Source: Howie 1968, Table 1, p. 1366.

Chart 10–3

One of the almost incidental findings of Howie's study of the management of suspected appendicitis at the Western Infirmary of Glasgow was
a fascinating difference in the way both "conservative" and "radical"
surgeons treated patients who were in, or had connections with, the
medical or nursing professions. As shown in the chart, both "conservative" and "radical" surgeons were more likely to operate on these
patients, presumably acting upon a lesser suspicion of the presence of
an inflamed appendix than when dealing with their other patients. The
conservative surgeons adopted a stance more characteristic of the usual
practice of their more "radical" colleagues, and these latter went a step
beyond even their more usually suspicious selves.

These observations correspond to reports about the incidence of surgery in professional families in California, as illustrated in an earlier
section of this book by a chart (4–15) showing the cumulative risk of
hysterectomies among the wives of physicians, as compared to other
women in the United States and abroad. Howie does, however, give us
the additional information on the consequences of surgery, so that we
may speculate about whether the greater susceptibility to surgery experienced by health care professionals is good or bad.

The experience of the more radical surgeons, as shown in the chart,
suggests that the true incidence of appendicitis is closer to 30 percent
among patients connected with the health care professions, and to 50
percent among all the others. This difference could reflect undocumented
differences in age and sex; it could also show that persons connected
with medicine or nursing seek advice earlier, and with milder symptoms
that are, therefore, more often unrelated to appendicitis. Beginning with
these baselines of incidence, and using the method and estimates offered
by Howie and shown in connection with the preceding chart, we can
compute "avoidable mortalities" as follows:

Conservative Surgeons
  Patients Connected with Health Care $0.50(0.02) + (0.30 - 0.29)(0.04) = 0.0104$
  Other Patients $\qquad 0.17(0.02) + (0.51 - 0.42)(0.04) = 0.0007$
Radical Surgeons
  Patients Connected with Health Care $0.60(0.02) \qquad\qquad\qquad = 0.0120$
  Other Patients $\qquad\qquad 0.30(0.02) \qquad\qquad\qquad = 0.0060$

If this model and these assumptions are correct, patients connected with
medicine and surgery suffer from the oversolicitude of their surgical
colleagues!

Chart 10-3

Percent Distribution of Patients Admitted as an Emergency Because of Possible Appendicitis (Subclassified by Type of Surgeon and by Whether or Not the Patient Had "Connections with the Medical or Nursing Professions") Who Had an Appendectomy or Not, and in Whom the Appendix Removed Was Normal or Abnormal. Patients 12 to 29 Years Old, Western Infirmary of Glasgow, Scotland, 1963.

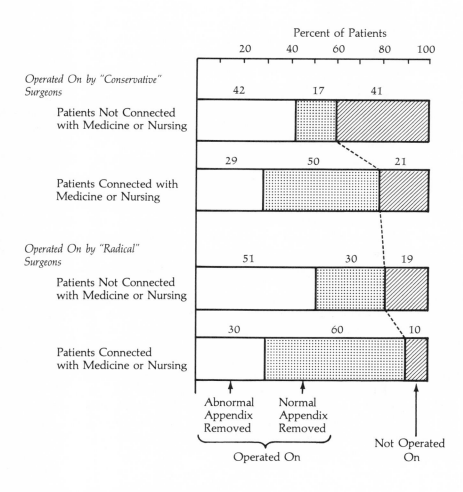

Source: Howie 1968, Table 1, p. 1366, and text on p. 1367.

Chart 10–4

The next step in our study of appendectomies is to define more precisely the concept of "the propensity to operate."

Generally, information is available about the frequency of specified signs and symptoms in those patients who prove to have an inflamed appendix, and in those who appear to have had "nonspecific abdominal pain." Given this information, and the estimated frequency of acute appendicitis among the group of patients who come to the surgeon with suspected appendicitis, it is possible, using Bayes' Theorem, to compute the probability that, when a particular set of signs and symptoms is present, the patient will either have or not have an inflamed appendix.

Neutra used information reported by Staniland et al. (1972) and de Dombal et al. (1972) to compute such probabilities for each of 24 combinations of an illustrative set of signs and symptoms, under highly simplifying assumptions. These 24 combinations of signs and symptoms, when arranged in ascending order of the likelihood that each connotes the presence of true appendicitis, are in effect a scale of explicit criteria which corresponds to a range of propensities to operate. For example, position number 24 denotes rebound tenderness and severe pain in the right lower quadrant of the abdomen, together with rectal tenderness. A surgeon who will not operate except in the presence of this rather compelling stimulus would, as shown by Curve B in the upper panel of the chart, find a diseased appendix in 96.6 percent of cases. But he also would, as shown by Curve A, remove only 11.8 percent of the inflamed appendices in those who seek his advice because of acute abdominal pain. By contrast, position number one on the scale denotes only mild, nondescript abdominal pain. A surgeon who regularly used even this as a signal to intervene would operate on every patient, and would remove every inflamed appendix. At the same time, only 36 percent of the operations would reveal a diseased organ, since this is the estimated frequency of acute appendicitis in this population.

The lower part of the chart shows what is, in effect, the balance of the two errors of omission and commission. According to the assumptions of this model, a surgeon would be most often correct if an appendectomy were done only in the presence of criteria 16 through 24. In 87.9 percent of cases either the operation would reveal a diseased appendix, or the decision not to operate would be made when the appendix is not inflamed.

Chart 10–4

Predicted Diagnostic Accuracy of Performing an Appendectomy When the Requirements of Each Specified Level of Criteria and All Levels Above It Are Met, the Criteria Being Arranged in Ascending Order of the Probability that the Patient Has Appendicitis. Simulation, with Data from Various Sources, Representing Various Time Periods.

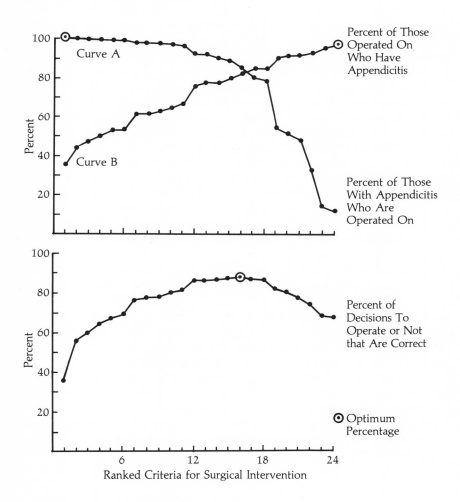

Source: Neutra 1977, computed from Table 18-2, p. 281.

Chart 10–5

The preceding chart defines an optimum propensity to operate, but only if the errors of omission and commission were equally serious, which is not the case, since the failure to remove a diseased appendix is much more dangerous than the mistaken removal of a normal one.

This chart is constructed assuming that in 6.4 percent of cases an inflamed appendix will perforate unavoidably before surgical care is available, and that if surgical intervention is further delayed another 30 percent will perforate, but that the rest will not, so that the operation can be done some days later at no greater risk. Based on data reported earlier by Howie (1966), the case fatality ratio for removing a normal appendix was taken to be 0.00065, that for a timely operation for a diseased organ to be 0.0012, and that for a delayed operation with perforation to be 0.027. Estimating that there are approximately 700,000 candidates for appendectomy each year in the United States, one could expect 2,505 deaths if *none* of these candidates were operated on. The top panel of the chart shows the percent of these expected deaths that would still occur if surgery were guided by each of the points on the scale of criteria. Clearly, in order to minimize expected deaths one must intervene if any criterion at position eight or above is satisfied.

Additional information and assumptions about the days of convalescence and the direct cost of hospital care associated with the decisions to operate or not were used to compute the consequences shown in the lower panel of the chart, the maximum expected days of convalescence and expected cost of hospital care being the result of operating on *every* case.

It is clear that to minimize deaths one must be prepared to operate even when the likelihood of true appendicitis is rather low, but that to minimize direct and indirect costs one must be less ready to operate, awaiting the clearer indications of a higher probability that the appendix is inflamed. There is no way of reconciling these two opposing considerations (of minimizing deaths and of minimizing costs) unless one is willing to put a money value on human life. The model does tell us, however, what our quality standards cost. For example, to move from position nine to position eight would save one life nationwide, but at a price of over $8 million in direct hospital costs alone.

Chart 10-5

Predicted Outcomes of Performing an Appendectomy When the Requirements of Each Specified Level of Criteria and All Levels Above It Are Met, the Criteria Being Arranged in Ascending Order of the Probability that the Patient Has Appendicitis. Simulation, with Data from Various Sources, Representing Various Time Periods.

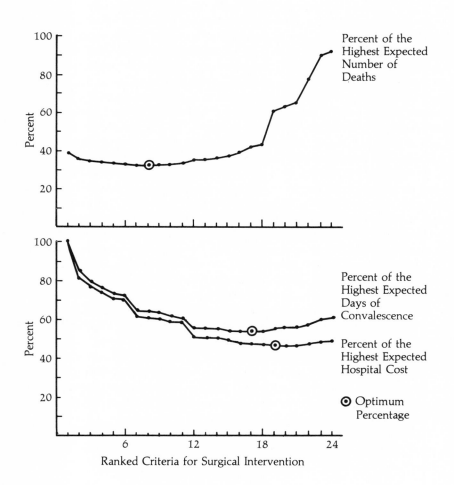

Source: Neutra 1977, computed from Tables 18-2 and 18-6, pp. 281 and 292.

Chart 10–6

The preceding review of the strategies for managing suspected appendicitis showed that the surgeon always faces two errors, one of commission and another of omission, so related to one another that any attempt to reduce one inevitably causes an increase in the other. To improve the ability of the strategy to "discriminate," both of these errors must be reduced, or one reduced without an increase in the other.

The discriminatory power of any strategy depends, of course, on the accuracy of the information obtained and used by the surgeon. The strategy itself can be improved, first by more skillful incorporation of existing knowledge, and later by the inclusion of new knowledge from advances in the medical sciences. The model developed by Neutra, for example, was meant only to illustrate some issues of decision anaylsis; it was not meant as a guide to clinical practice. Neutra points out that the model does not subclassify patients, for example, by age or sex; includes only a small number of the more obvious signs and symptoms; and does not consider the later evolution of these findings during the course of care.

This chart illustrates the improvement that can occur with a rather simple modification in the strategy of caring for children with suspected appendicitis admitted to a teaching hospital. During the six years between 1965 and 1970, the guiding strategy ("Strategy A") was to operate whenever the diagnosis was "uncertain." The first bar shows the consequences: 92 percent of children had an operation, and 14 percent of them (15 percent of operations) had a normal appendix removed.

More recently, a different "philosophy" of care ("Strategy B") was in force. When the diagnosis was uncertain, surgery was postponed. Instead, the child's condition was assessed every few hours until the diagnosis of appendicitis could either be excluded or made more confidently. As shown in the second bar of the chart, only 75 percent of children were operated on, and only one percent had a normal appendix removed. At the same time there were no perforations of the appendix during the course of care, the case fatality rate was no higher, and no children discharged without an operation returned later with recurrent symptoms of appendicitis.

Though this more recent strategy has been tested and justified by actual observation, this "natural experiment" falls somewhat short of a rigorously controlled clinical trial.

Chart 10–6

Percent Distribution of Children under 14 Years of Age Admitted with a Diagnosis of Possible Appendicitis, by Whether Operated On or Not, and by the Findings in Operated Cases. Child Care Program, the Johns Hopkins Hospital, Baltimore, Maryland, 1965–1970 and 1971–1974.

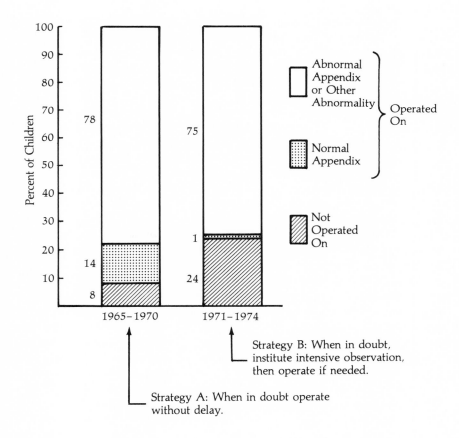

Source: White et al. 1975, Tables 1 and 2, p. 794.

Chart 10–7

Decision-making models, documented by careful epidemiological observations, can provide a much firmer basis for both clinical practice and
quality assessment. Often, more rigorous clinical trials are either not
permissible or not feasible. Thus our progression of appendectomy studies ends with a clinical trial of treatment for varicose veins, and not for
appendicitis.

In this clinical trial, suitable patients were assigned at random to one
of two forms of treatment: conventional surgery, or injections of the vein,
which caused them to be blocked. The clinical results, in what proved
to be two comparable groups, were evaluated by a single observer who
was not told what form of treatment was used, though in some cases he
could see the surgical scars.

The chart shows that, three years later, a slightly smaller percentage
of those who had had injections did not need more treatment and were
therefore classified as improved, but the difference was not "significant."
Complications were more frequent among the injected group, but the
excess was mainly of discoloration at the site of the injection; the incidence of more serious complications was comparable. The respective
case fatality ratios could not be compared in this small trial. Other studies
suggest that the fatality is somewhat lower for injection therapy, but not
certainly enough to make this an important consideration. The choice
must depend, therefore, on a comparison of costs—and here, injection
therapy is clearly preferred.

The chart shows several measures of cost. Patients who were referred
for injections were more likely to receive treatment and therefore less
likely to forgo the net benefits of care. The direct monetary costs of
injection therapy were less. The indirect costs were also less, in that less
time was lost for treatment and travel and, if the patient was employed
full-time, the losses in time away from work or in wages were smaller.

One can point out some limitations of this study without, however,
judging the clinical relevance of the findings. Capital costs could not be
measured. Loss of time by the nongainfully employed was not included.
We are not told how the losses from death and from several grades of
disability can be combined together, or with the direct and indirect
monetary losses. All this and more is needed for more complete assessments of the cost–benefit consequences of alternative strategies of care.

Chart 10-7

Degree to which Specified Measures of Outcomes and Costs for the Treatment
of Varicose Veins with Injection-compression Sclerotherapy Are More or Less
than Those for Surgical Treatment. Clinical Trial, London, England, February
1967–February 1968.

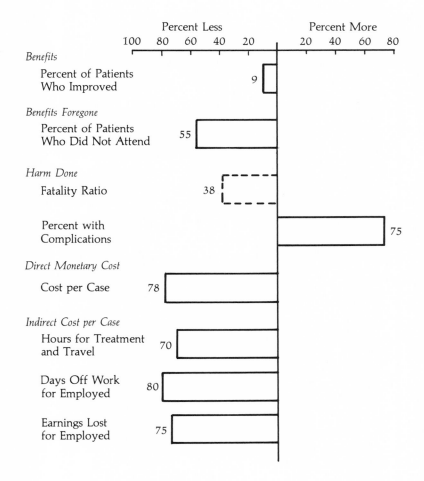

Source: Piachaud and Weddell 1972, Tables II, III, and IV, p. 289, 290, and 292, and text on
pp. 290 and 291.

PART IV

Some Problems of Method

ELEVEN

The Information

ELEVEN

Assuming that one knows something of the causal relationships among structure, process, and outcome, access to valid information about these elements is the next most important requirement for quality assessment.

The possible sources of information include the medical record, written or electronically registered and available in full or as a summary or abstract; the claims for payment submitted by the providers of care; the service statistics of operating agencies, often incorporating data from claims or record abstracts; official vital statistics reports; interviews with, or questionnaires submitted to, practitioners, patients, or others; and, most ambitious of all, the observation of practice, either in person or by audiovisual recording, and the direct examination of the health status of individuals.

Quality assessment and monitoring are shaped and limited by the properties of the medical record, including the kinds of information to be found there, the completeness and accuracy of that information, and the ability of the record to communicate the objectives and management strategies of the practitioners responsible for care. In spite of what is known about the remarkable unreliability of most forms of information, the veracity of the record has attracted little attention in the literature of quality assessment. By contrast, the disorganization and incompleteness of the record, especially in ambulatory care, have led many to say that, based on the record, one can judge only the quality of recording and not the quality of the care itself.

There are several ways of responding to this sometimes self-serving evaluational nihilism. For one, the quality of recording is worthy of assessment in its own right because the record, besides being an educational and research tool, is a necessary vehicle for ensuring continuity and coordination of care, and the legal protection of patient and practitioner. There must be, moreover, an association between good recording and good care, since the conditions that encourage the first should also contribute to the second. Finally, even with its present deficiencies, the record is often complete enough to provide a reasonably accurate picture of the quality of care, at least for some purposes.

Assessments of the quality of care have adapted to the deficiencies of the medical record so as to reduce their disabling effect. This adaptation is evident in the choice of those criteria most likely to be adhered to, and in the selection of diagnostic categories which most heavily depend on such criteria. Beyond such adaptations, the available information can be augmented by adding outpatient to inpatient records, and including the nursing notes in the latter. Supplementation and interpretation can also be obtained by interviewing physicians and practitioners. In some studies, practitioners have been asked to keep records designed particularly for these studies. However, one might question the veracity of information obtained by such interviews, and the representativeness of records kept expressly for a research study.

A more definitive response to the current deficiencies of recording is to improve the record itself. This seems to happen, to some extent, when special preprinted forms are used, or when management by clinical algorithm is introduced (Schmidt et al. 1974, Grimm et al. 1975, Grover and Greenberg 1976). The "problem-oriented" record (Weed 1971) should make it easier to assess the completeness and the rationale of the practitioner's care. But more research is needed to discover how the record can be best adapted to the requirements of quality assessment, rather than, as is the case now, adapting the assessment to the limitations of the record. The assessment of the interpersonal process of care would be a particular beneficiary of this change in orientation.

The charts in this section will deal mainly with the completeness of the medical record and its implications for quality assessment. The veracity of recorded information will only be touched upon. Those interested in studies of "observer error" are referred to the reviews by Kilpatrick (1963) and Koran (1975).

There will be more on the relevance of recording to quality assessment in subsequent chapters on criteria formulation and the comparison of assessment methods.

Chart 11–1

We begin our assessment of medical records with the findings of two studies described earlier in Chapter Five, "Observation of the Process of Care." The physicians who observed each practitioner at work were guided in their assessments by a schedule that specified the aspects of care to be noted, and assigned numerical scores to described levels of performance for each category included in the schedule. Clinical recording was one of these categories.

In both studies, a score of zero was assigned if no records were kept, or if the only information recorded was medications, fees, or isolated data such as blood pressure readings. A score of 1 was awarded if the record provided only "minimal" information about positive findings. A score of 2 was reserved for "very good records" which included all positive findings of the medical history, physical examination, and laboratory investigations. These ratings described the usual practice of each physician, rather than each record separately.

The chart shows the remarkable prevalence of poor recording. It also suggests the immense variability of recording practices; some physicians kept excellent records, while others kept very poor records or none at all. For example, about 12 percent of general practitioners in rural North Carolina kept no medical records, noting only the patient's name and the fee charged in a daily ledger. Twenty percent of the practitioners studied in Ontario, and 38 percent of those in Nova Scotia, kept only lists of the names and addresses of those patients who did not pay cash at the time of the visit.

Many other studies since these have also suggested that poor performance continues to be prevalent, especially in office practice. But in most of these studies, because the record is the only source of information, it is not easy to disentangle poor performance from poor recording. An exception is a description of the office records of a selection of internists in New York State who agreed to participate in a study by Kroeger et al. (1965). In these records, there was information about the physical examination in 84.5 percent of cases, about the treatment in 83.7 percent, about the diagnosis in 76.4 percent, about the systems review in 66.5 percent, and about the family history in 58.8 percent. Only 67 percent of this self-selected group of unusually well-qualified internists kept office records that were complete and legible enough to be abstracted by nonphysicians in preparation for a study of the quality of care.

Chart 11-1

Percent Distribution of General Practitioners by the Observed Quality of Their Medical Records. North Carolina, and the Canadian Provinces of Ontario and Nova Scotia, 1953–1954, July 1956–October 1957, and December 1958–February 1960, Respectively.

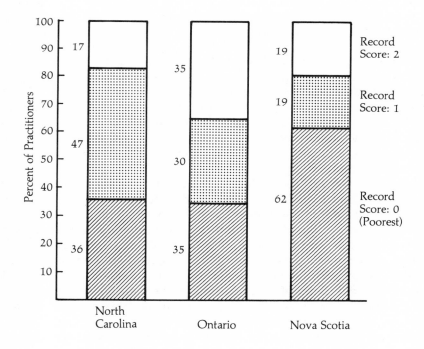

Sources: Peterson et al. 1956, p. 46, and Clute 1963, p. 304.

Chart 11–2

There has been a recent flurry of interest in how accurately the written medical record reflects what actually transpires between the practitioner and the patient. This chart is the first of three dealing with that topic.

The study includes all physicians at a general medical clinic, these being either faculty members or second-year residents. But the patients are not a representative sample, since about half were too illiterate to be suitable and some others refused to take part. In all, 55 patient–physician encounters were recorded on tape, of course with the knowledge of the participants. The tapes were transcribed and the information abstracted. The corresponding medical records were also abstracted, by the same investigator, using the same conventions. The two abstracts were then compared.

The comparison was between "units of information," each "unit" being an item such as the diagnosis, or several interrelated items, such as the symptoms pertaining to an organ system, or some groupings of treatments or tests. Using such groupings raises the level of concordance between taped and recorded information, since it means acceptance of summary methods of recording, such as an entry that there were "no pulmonary symptoms" when the tape shows a much more detailed form of questioning.

The chart shows the frequency distribution of the units of information in six categories according to whether the information was found (1) in both the record and the transcript of the tape; (2) only in the record, which means that the physician either wrote something he was not told, or something he did not tell the patient about; or (3) only in the transcript, which means that the record is incomplete. The categories shown in the chart are arranged in descending order of completeness of recording, from a deficiency of seven percent for the patient's chief complaint, to a deficiency of 64 percent for units of medical history pertaining to systems not related to the present illness.

Errors in recording, and the failure to communicate information, reflect on the quality of current care. The failure to record information may affect future care, but it also shows that the record underrepresents the quality of current care. We do not know, however, how important the omissions from the record are, nor what discrepancies exist between the sum of information obtained and the standards of good care.

Chart 11-2

Percent of Units of Information of Specified Kinds Found Only in the Medical Record, Only in a Transcript of the Physician-Patient Encounter, or in Both. General Medicine Clinic, North Carolina Memorial Hospital, Chapel Hill, North Carolina, 1976 and 1978.

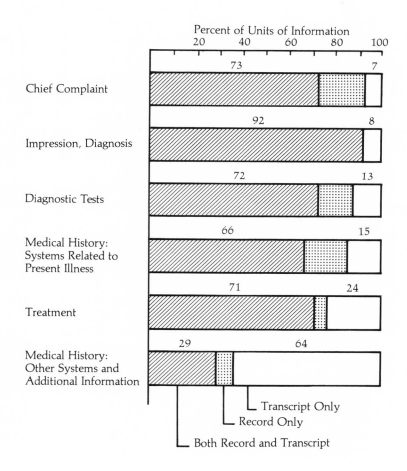

Source: Romm and Putnam, 1981, Table 3, p. 313.

Chart 11–3

This short series on the completeness of the medical record continues
with a second, and earlier, study which used methods very similar to
those of the study portrayed in the preceding chart. Tape recordings of
the patient–physician encounter were made with the knowledge and
consent of the participants, followed by a comparison of the tape with
the medical record. The "coding was generous, giving credit for partial
or minimal entries. The basis for coding regulations was whether the
data in the record or patient interview were adequate for a subsequent
physician to determine accurately the nature of the care given or to carry
out a medical audit" (p. 408).

The patients were children under 13, cared for in a Children and Youth
Project of a University Medical Center. All three full-time staff physicians
participated. In all, 51 visits were studied. It is difficult, therefore, to
generalize on the basis either of these findings or the findings of the
study summarized in the preceding chart.

This chart shows only a selection of the findings, and these are arrayed
under three headings: diagnostic information, drug therapy, and follow-
up. The items under each of these are shown in descending order of the
completeness of information elicited, irrespective of whether the information was in the medical record or on the tape. If, as the investigators
imply, the information should have been present in all of the instances
tabulated, we have here a measure of quality that was not present in the
preceding chart. We see for example how infrequently, even in this
teaching center, the physician tells the patient about the studies to be
performed, the indications for follow-up, or the actions and side effects
of drugs.

The second kind of deficiency is in recording, as shown by the percent
of information found on the tape but not in the record. A review of the
medical record would, therefore, underestimate performance, but much
more so in some aspects of care than in others. Nonrecording also reduces the record's efficacy as a means for fostering the coordination and
continuity of care. The authors also report that the older person who
accompanied each child was more likely to have understood the diagnosis and treatment regimen when these had been both recorded and
verbally communicated by the physician (p. 410).

Chart 11–3

Percent of Instances in Which Specified Items of Information Are Found Only in the Medical Record, Only in a Tape Recording of the Physician-Patient Encounter, or in Both. Children and Youth Project of a University Medical Center, U.S.A., August 1973.

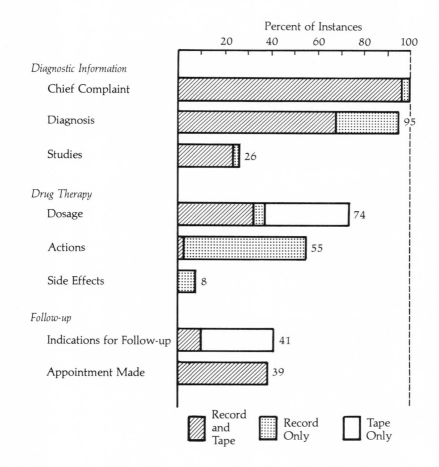

Source and Note: Zuckerman et al. 1975, Tables I and II, pp. 408–9. The number against each bar is the percent of instances in which the information was elicited as judged by the record and tape, the record only, or the tape only.

Chart 11–4

This chart shows that the perceived importance of the information contributes to variability in the completeness of its recording.

This is one of several reports on a study of the continuity of care, continuity being defined as the recognition at a subsequent visit of medical problems and other elements of care identified at a previous visit. An important finding of the study was that the likelihood of subsequent recognition depended on the perceived importance of the information and the clarity or specificity of its documentation at the initial visit. This particular chart, however, is not concerned with the likelihood of subsequent recognition, but with whether or not, when recognition does occur, there is evidence of it in the medical record.

The elements of care that merit subsequent recognition, if care is to have "continuity," were determined by an examination of the record, supplemented by two listings of the patient's problems, one by the practitioner and another by the patient. At the next visit, a member of the research team was allowed to observe what went on between the practitioner and the patient. The notes of the observer were later compared with the medical record of that visit.

The chart shows the percent of all recognized items of information (recognition being judged by what the practitioner told the patient or wrote in the record) that were found in the record. It is clear that the completeness of recording varies according to the "importance" or saliency of the original information. Problems that had been listed at the previous visit by both patient and practitioner were more likely to be recorded, if recognized, at the subsequent visit, than were problems listed only by the practitioner or the patient, or only inferred with greater or lesser certainty from the record. Recognition of information about drugs with important effects was more likely to be documented than recognition of information about lesser drugs or treatment other than drugs. Similarly, recognition of diagnostic tests with abnormal findings was more likely to be documented than recognition of other tests. The investigators conclude that the record is suitable as a source of information on continuity, particularly if one focuses on the more important aspects of care.

The recording of information was not related either to the type of practitioner or to the practitioner being the same person at both the initial and subsequent visits. The possible effect of the presence of an observer will be shown in a subsequent chart.

Chart 11–4

Percent of Instances of Recognition by the Health Care Practitioner of Specified Problems, Therapies, and Tests in which the Medical Record Contained Evidence of Such Recognition. The East Baltimore Plan, Baltimore, Maryland, July and August 1977.

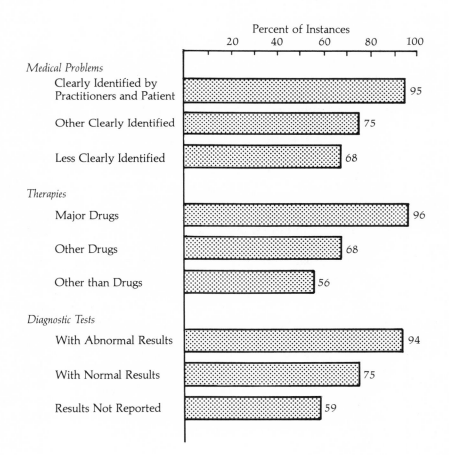

Source: Starfield et al. 1979a, Table 5, p. 763.

Chart 11–5

The organized ambulatory care programs which provided the information shown in the preceding three charts are hardly representative of office practice in general. Also, some of the information missing from the medical records, even in these programs, may not be important to assessing the quality of technical care. The study illustrated by this chart meets both these objections, first by observing the performance of physicians in private practice, and then by tying the observations to explicit criteria for assessing that performance.

This study of the quality of ambulatory care, as described earlier in this book (see Chapter 6, p. 236), used preformulated explicit criteria to assess the quality of care for selected conditions, based on information in the record. Unfortunately, an ambitious plan to assess the completeness of the information in the record could not be implemented fully, partly for lack of funds and partly because the sampled physicians were reluctant to participate in this phase of the study. It was possible, however, to observe nine pediatricians at work, to note their adherence to the criterion items, and to compare what was directly observed with what later appeared in the record. There were 135 cases, in one of four categories of patients (pharyngitis; otitis media; well-child examination, infant; well-child examination, preschool), with 13 to 16 criterion items for each condition.

The chart shows that, with the very striking exception of the criteria for instructions and explanations to the patient, there was a very high degree of agreement between the observations and the record, for all physicians and conditions combined. The chart also shows the range of agreement when the four conditions are taken separately.

The obvious conclusion that the medical record is a suitable means for assessing many aspects of the quality of care, at least when physicians and patients in a category are grouped, must be tempered by some limitations of the study. The samples of physicians and conditions were small and highly selected. The criteria pertained mainly to technical care and included only a modest number of items considered, by large majorities on panels of local physicians, to be "essential" to good care. Finally, we are not told precisely what is meant by what the investigators call "the overlap between activities and behaviors observed and notations in the patient record" (p. 114).

Chart 11-5

Percent of Preformulated Explicit Criteria of Good Ambulatory Care Observed
To Be Adhered to that Were Also Documented in the Medical Record, by Type
of Criteria, and Among Four Categories of Patients. Selected Pediatricians in
Private Practice, Metropolitan Areas of New Haven and Hartford, Connecticut,
1974-1975.

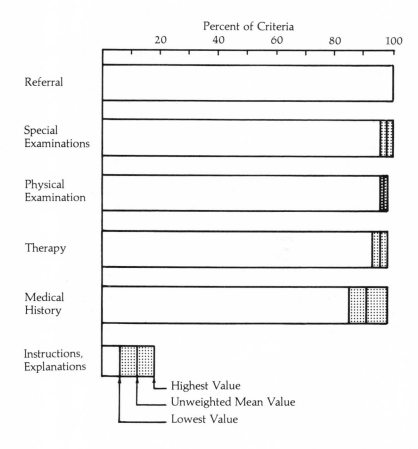

Source: Riedel and Riedel 1979, Table 7.1, p. 115.

Chart 11–6

As we saw in the introduction to this section of the book, one argument in favor of using the medical record for assessing the quality of care is a presumed association between good recording and good care, because the personal or institutional attributes conducive to good recording are thought to be, at the same time and in the same way, conducive to good care. While this is a reasonable hypothesis, evidence to support it is difficult to find.

We saw in an earlier chart based on the work of Morehead et al. (Chart 6–12) that even something as simple as the physical dimensions of the medical record may be related to the ratings of the quality of care—the larger the sheet, the better the quality! There may be a circularity, however, in this kind of association, since recording is itself awarded 30 points out of a total quality score of 100, and the remaining 70 points are also awarded on the basis of information contained in the record.

The data reported in this chart are virtually free of this circularity, since recording was awarded a rating that ranges only from zero to two based on criteria described earlier in this chapter (Chart 11–1). The remaining 78 points, out of a total of 80, were awarded on the basis of information obtained by direct observation of the general practitioner at work.

The chart shows a direct association between the quality of recording and the observed quality of care, an association which Lyons and Payne (1974b) have tested and found to be statistically significant. Clute alerts us, however, that "lack of adequate records is not incompatible with practice of a good, or even an excellent, quality, inasmuch as a considerable number of the doctors who were given 0 for records had overall scores of 61 percent or more and a few had overall scores that were above 80 percent" (p. 305).

Chart 11-6

Average Numerical Scores of the Quality of Performance of General Practitioners Categorized by Scores of the Quality of Their Medical Records. Ontario and
Nova Scotia, Canada, July 1956–October 1957, and December 1958–February
1960, Respectively.

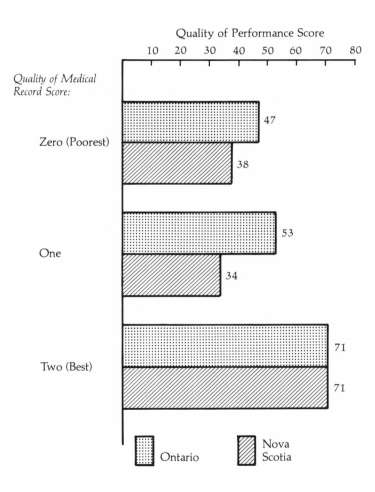

Source: Clute 1963, p. 303.

Chart 11–7

Direct observation of practice, in order to assess either the quality of performance or the completeness of the medical record, may itself influence both practice and recording, very probably improving both, and in similar or different degrees. The users of observation as a method for assessing the quality of care have recognized this possibility, but have believed that, perhaps after an initial period of unusual vigilance, the practitioner probably reverts to his accustomed routines (Peterson et al. 1956, p. 16; Clute 1963, p. 18). This chart addresses the issue more directly.

The investigators were primarily interested in studying the continuity of care, which they defined as the practitioner's recognition of medical problems and other pertinent information identified at a previous visit. The items that deserved subsequent recognition were found in lists of problems obtained separately from the practitioner and the patient, and from entries in the record. To test the validity of the medical record as a source of information on subsequent recognition, arrangements were made to have an observer present at some visits, so that what was seen and heard to occur could be later compared to what was written in the record. But it was not possible to complete these arrangements about half the time. As a result, by happenstance rather than design, there were two groups of reasonably comparable cases, some observed and some not. The chart compares the two, based on evidence in the record alone.

As was seen in Chart 11–4, information that could be considered more important or more salient was more likely to be recognized. We now see that this was true irrespective of whether the visit was observed or not. More importantly, it looks as if, in general, the records contained evidence of recognition more often when the visit was observed.

Observation does appear to stimulate better performance, but we do not know whether or not the effect would wear off with repeated or prolonged observation, and whether recorded performance is as much affected as the unrecorded part.

One should keep in mind that only one of the differences observed (that for problems listed by both practitioners and patients) was statistically significant, that the comparison group was not generated by design, and that a small prepaid group practice serving low income patients is not a typical site for care.

Chart 11-7

Percent of Medical Problems Identified at One Visit which Were Also Recognized at the Next Visit, by Type of Problem, and by Whether the Subsequent Visit Was or Was Not Observed by a Third Person. The East Baltimore Plan, Baltimore, Maryland, July and August 1977.

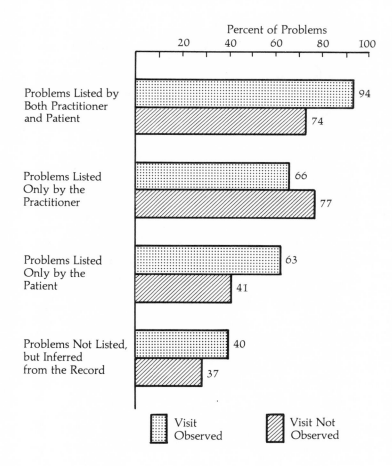

Source: Starfield et al. 1979b, Table 2, p. 1023.

Chart 11–8

There is a less direct, but also much less obtrusive, method than observation to verify the validity of the record as a means for assessing the quality of care. This rather ingenious method was used by Rosenfeld in a study of the quality of care for selected medical, surgical, and obstetrical-gynecological conditions in four Boston hospitals, the hospitals being exemplars of the kinds of institutions present in a large urban community. Each sampled medical record was rated independently by two judges who used implicit criteria, but in a carefully organized fashion, as described in Volume II of this series, pp. 26–29. Specified components (or "items") of management were rated "good," "fair," or "poor," and these judgments were then combined, using defined rules, to arrive at an overall rating.

Rosenfeld noted that the components of management were sometimes rated "poor" based on evidence that was very unlikely to be dependent on the recording practices of individual physicians. This he called "substantial" evidence. At other times, the evidence for the "poor" rating could have been either a failure in practice or only a failure to record. This he called "presumptive" evidence. The chart shows how the four hospitals were distributed when simultaneously classified by the percent of the components of care rated "poor" based on each of the two forms of evidence. The chart suggests a positive correlation. (Incidentally, it also shows that the two hospitals affiliated with a medical school, those in the upper right hand corner of the chart, do better than the remaining two community hospitals.)

In a review of the literature on the relationship between recording and quality, Lyons and Payne (1974b) noted that Rosenfeld's findings could conceal much variation among cases and physicians, since only hospitals were compared. They went on to use the same method to verify the findings of their own study of hospital care in Hawaii. To do so they divided the items on their lists of explicit criteria into two categories analogous to Rosenfeld's "presumptive" and "substantial" classification, and computed the percent of adherence to the criteria in each sublist for each of their cases. A comparison of the two ratings for the cases in each of eight diagnostic categories showed positive correlations in seven, the correlations being clearly significant in four. The average correlation coefficient of 0.23, though not large, was also significant statistically.

Chart 11–8

Four Hospitals Classified Simultaneously by the Percent of "Items of Management" Rated "Poor" Based on "Presumptive" Evidence, and on "Substantial" Evidence, of Deficient Care. Metropolitan Boston, Massachusetts, 1956.

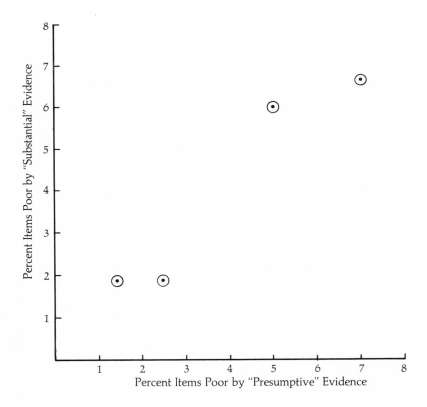

Source: Rosenfeld 1957, Table 4, p. 862.

Chart 11–9

We have seen that the information in the medical record is usually in-complete, but that it is often sufficient to allow a reasonably valid judg-ment of the quality of care to be made, though perhaps only roughly, only for groups of cases, and only about the technical aspects of care. Some have hoped that it may also be possible to supplement the record by interviewing patients, practitioners, or both. This chart shows some of the findings of one study that adopted this approach.

This is the study of hospital care in Michigan which was reviewed rather extensively in Chapter Three, on "The Justification of Resource Use." It will be recalled that explicit criteria were used to assess the appropriateness of admission and length of stay for samples of cases in any one of 18 primary discharge diagnoses. Whenever the initial judg-ment was that the stay was inappropriate, the physician responsible for the case was interviewed and given an opportunity to explain. As a check, the same procedure was followed in a representative sample of cases initially judged to have had an appropriate stay. The additional information was used to revise the initial judgment of appropriateness, but only if unrecorded medical information was obtained; "extramedical factors" were often reported, but were not accepted as a justification for relaxing the criteria.

The top pair of bars in the chart shows the initial judgments. The middle pair of bars shows the actual or (because of sampling) projected changes brought about by the additional information obtained from the physicians. An initial judgment of appropriate stay is seldom altered, whereas an initial judgment that the stay was inappropriate is quite often changed. The net result, shown in the lowermost pair of bars, is a marked proportional diminution in the percent of cases with inappro-priate stay, a category which includes stays that are shorter or longer than required. When judgments on the appropriateness of admissions (not shown in the chart) are also included, the additional information is found to reclassify 12.6 percent of all cases.

Physician interviews were used to supplement the record in the earlier studies of the quality of ambulatory care at the Health Insurance Plan of Greater New York, but they were found not to "elucidate further under-standing of the clinical handling of the case" (Morehead 1967, p. 1646).

Chart 11–9

Percent of Cases in which the Length of Stay Was Judged To Have Been Inappropriate, Before and After Supplementation of Recorded Information by Information Obtained by Interviewing the Physician Primarily Responsible for Care. Cases with One of 18 Primary Discharge Diagnoses, Short-term Nonfederal Hospitals, Michigan, 1958.

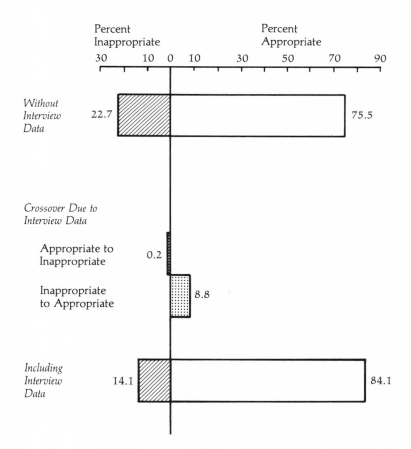

Source: Fitzpatrick et al. 1962 , computed from Table 232, p. 501.

Chart 11–10

The medical record may be defective in not including information needed for quality assessment. But, in addition, the information that *is* there could conceivably be inaccurate or false. Faulty information may lead, in turn, to conclusions and actions which are justifiable in the light of that information, but which are in fact wrong, since they are based on erroneous premises. This being the case, it is surprising how little attention has been paid to the measurement of "observer error" in assessments of the quality of care, even though such error is known to be frequent and pervasive (Kilpatrick 1963; Koran 1975). It is almost as if the attribute being tested in assessments of the process of care were merely the capacity to reason correctly, rather than that of being correct. Assessments of the outcomes of care would, of course, not suffer from this deficiency.

The work of Lembcke is a notable exception, in that it included verification of diagnostic information. In one study, duplicate microscopic examinations of tissue showed that "the true incidence of endometrial hyperplasia, which was being diagnosed in 60 to 65 percent of all uterine curettages, was only five to eight percent" (Lembcke 1956, p. 654).

The study illustrated by this chart should not have qualified for inclusion in this book. It is old; it reports the performance of medical students, not doctors; it is not based on medical records; it is not part of the literature of quality assessment. I have selected it, nevertheless, because it shows the several levels of error into which the eliciting of physical signs may fall.

In this experiment, medical students listened to recordings of heart murmurs. They were then asked to describe the timing and intensity of the murmur and the regularity of the heartbeat. Based on these perceptions, and knowing the location on the chest from which the recording was made, the students were then asked to make a diagnosis, which meant naming the murmur. The chart shows three levels of error: first of perception, then of "reasoning" based on medical knowledge, and finally, as a result of the preceding faults, an error in diagnosis. Narrowing (stenosis) of the mitral valve of the heart accompanied by an irregularity of the heartbeat posed a greater problem than did the narrowing of the aortic valve without a disturbance in rhythm.

How often, one wonders, do such errors find their way to the medical records on which quality assessment may rest?

Chart 11-10

Percent of Second-year Medical Students Who Correctly Identified Specified Attributes of Two Recorded Heart Murmurs. Ohio State University College of Medicine, 1964.

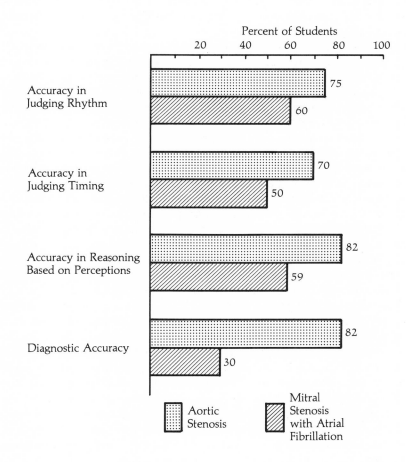

Source: Evans and Bybee 1965, Tables 1, 2, and 3, pp. 200 and 201.

Chart 11–11

This chart illustrates the probable effects of faulty laboratory findings on clinical practice in one hospital. On May 9, 1956 (near the start of the two-month period indicated by arrow A on the chart), the hospital adopted a new method for measuring blood hemoglobin. The immediate effect was a rise in the average hemoglobin readings, and a fall in the amount of blood used for transfusions, relative to the corresponding values for July–August 1955.

Blood use practices during six months soon after the change in laboratory procedure were compared with those during the preceding six months when, most of the time, the old method was in use. The proportion of admitted patients who were suspected to need transfusion, and who therefore had a blood cross-match test, had not changed. But a smaller proportion of the cross-matched patients were transfused, apparently because a much smaller proportion of them had hemoglobin values in the "borderline range." In this range, where the clinical indications are not compelling, small changes in the frequency of questionable hemoglobin readings seem to tip the balance for or against prescribing a transfusion. The investigators looked for other explanations, but found none. Blood use was less in the practices of over 80 percent of the doctors who used transfusions frequently, and within all major diagnostic categories.

On January 1, 1957 (arrow B on the chart), the hospital's hemoglobin apparatus was recalibrated. There was another rise in the average level of hemoglobin values, and a further fall in blood use, though this is not so clear. One aberration, the peak in blood use during January–February 1958, is attributed to a temporary reduction in hemoglobin readings caused by a contaminated reagent.

It is estimated that the elimination of laboratory bias produced a yearly reduction of $25,000 in the then current costs of care in this hospital (Commission on Professional and Hospital Activities 1959b). And there is reason to believe that this was only one instance of a pervasive problem. A study of hemoglobin values in 66 hospitals showed a degree of variability that could not be fully explained by interhospital differences in age or sex of patients, types of cases treated, or geographic altitude. Laboratory bias was the remaining most reasonable explanation (Commission on Professional and Hospital Activities 1959a).

Chart 11–11

Relative Hemoglobin Values per Patient Tested, and Relative Quantities of Blood Used per 100 Discharges, Before and After Changes in the Method of Determining Hemoglobin Values. Butterworth Hospital, Grand Rapids, Michigan, July 1955–August 1958, Inclusive.

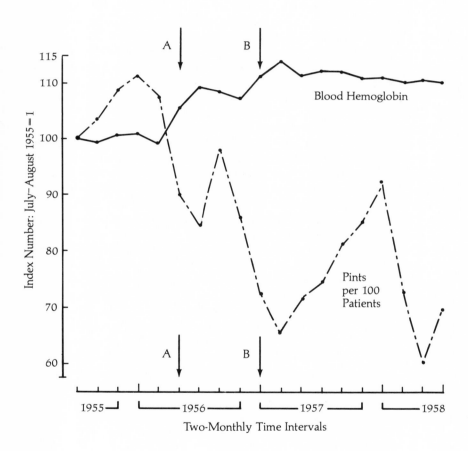

Source and Note: Mann et al. 1959, computed from Table 1, p. 227. The method for measuring hemoglobin was changed at A and B.

Chart 11–12

This chart shows the findings of three studies of the reliability of coding diagnostic information in abstracts of medical records. All three were conducted under the auspices of the Institute of Medicine of the National Academy of Sciences. Study A assessed the performance of several private organizations that offer statistical services based on record abstracts prepared by client hospitals, but included only that part of their work which involved Medicaid and Medicare patients during 1974. Study B tested the coding of Medicare data done at the central office of the Health Care Financing Administration, based on case reports submitted by hospitals. Study C verified the coding done at a facility of the National Center for Health Statistics based on information obtained mainly from the face sheet of the medical record. This information is submitted by or on behalf of the hospitals that participate in the National Hospital Discharge Survey, and it is meant to represent the entire case load of these hospitals. The data studied were for discharges during 1977.

The first step in each study was to draw a sample of the relevant universe of hospitals, and then a sample of cases in a reasonably large variety of diagnostic categories, many of which were chosen for all three studies. The research staff abstracted and coded the information in the sampled records and compared the results with the reports of the several organizations under study. There are three steps that influence the degree of agreement: (1) finding the most valid information in the record; (2) identifying which of several diagnoses is the one most responsible for the hospital admission, or which of several procedures is the most important; and (3) coding the diagnosis and the procedure selected.

The chart shows the percent of cases in which the code assigned by the research staff corresponds to the one originally reported. There is a considerable amount of disagreement; the magnitude of the disagreement is roughly similar in all studies; and, as expected, disagreement is more frequent when more detailed (four-digit) coding is attempted.

The statistical compilations that contain these probable errors are used to compute "norms" for length of stay and other clinical activities, and also to construct "profiles" to characterize and compare the performance of physicians and hospitals. These errors may either trigger unnecessary review or conceal deficient care.

Chart 11-12

Percent of Cases in which There Is Agreement Between Two Codings of Each of the Principal Procedure and the Principal Diagnosis. Three Studies of Record Abstracts, U.S.A., 1974, 1974, and 1977, Respectively.

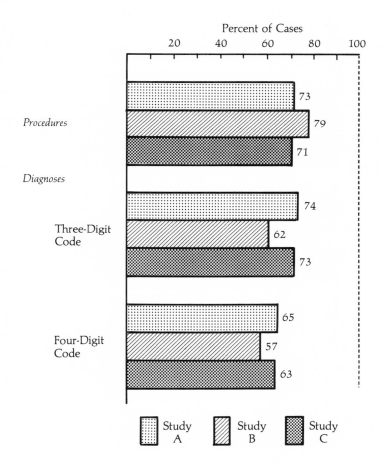

Source: Demlo et al. 1981, Tables 3 and 6, pp. 1033 and 1036, supplemented by information from Professor Demlo.

The Formulation
of Criteria and Standards

TWELVE

Before the quality of care can be assessed or monitored, the abstract formulations of quality need to be translated into more specific criteria and standards which can serve as reliable and valid measuring devices. In some methods of assessment, this transition from concepts to measurement tools is hidden; it takes place in the judge's mind, as each case is reviewed without benefit of external guidance. We get a glimpse of the criteria when a judge of quality is asked why some cases were rated worse than others. But, increasingly, the criteria and standards of care are being formulated in explicit detail prior to assessing the care itself. In this way, the definition of quality and the manner of its assessment are controlled by those who set and propagate the criteria.

As I tried to show in Volume II of this series, the criteria and standards used to assess the quality of care are themselves subject to assessment as to whether or not they possess a variety of desirable attributes. To begin with, we need to see what components of the abstract formulations of quality are included or excluded by the more specific criteria. Do the criteria pertain primarily to cost containment, for example, or do they take a broader view of the quality of care? If quality, more broadly defined, is the focus, are the criteria confined to technical care, or are the interpersonal aspects of care also subject to assessment? Technical care itself can be viewed narrowly, as being concerned only with diagnosis and treatment, or broadly, as reaching out to include preventive, anticipatory, and rehabilitative care. The relationship between the cost and the quality of care can be ignored, as when all the procedures are listed that can possibly do some good; or it can be included in the assessment, through attention to redundancy and to the relation between cost and expected benefits.

Scientific validity, based on a demonstrated causal relationship between process and outcome, is the key attribute of the criteria as measurement devices. Then comes reliability, which is the ability of the criteria to lead to the same results when the same care is assessed more than once by the same person, or when it is assessed by more than one person at the same time or at different times.

Sponsorship by the leadership of a profession confers legitimacy on the criteria. But for the criteria to be acceptable to the majority of practitioners, they must not only be scientifically valid and professionally endorsed, but also relevant to the peculiarities and limitations of everyday practice in whatever settings the criteria are to be applied. The degree of professional consensus on the criteria is, therefore, a key issue in their assessment.

Sometimes, the criteria and standards of quality are "empirically derived," which means that they are obtained by the observation of good, acceptable, or average practice. More often the criteria are "normatively derived," which means that they represent published scientific knowledge as interpreted, and perhaps added to, by its leading students and practitioners.

Arriving at a manageable set of criteria can be a long and arduous process. It usually begins with the forming of a panel of experts. The panel may start without preparation, or it may be aided by the findings of earlier staff work, including reviews of the scientific literature, samples of preexisting criteria, and summaries of the opinions and the practices prevalent in the professional community.

The task of the expert panel is to winnow down a potentially large and rather incoherent assemblage of candidate criteria into a smaller more manageable set. To do so it includes only the more valid, the more widely relevant, the more readily measured, and the more important items. Sometimes the individual items are weighted differentially, presumably to reflect different degrees of usefulness in arriving at a diagnosis, or different contributions to the outcomes.

As described in Volume II of this series (pp. 153–93), the composition of the panel and its procedures can vary a great deal. In some cases the Delphi technique is used, and in others the "nominal group process." Most of the time, however, the panel members do all their work in open discussion under the leadership of a chairman.

This brief section cannot hope to encompass the full variety of criteria and the many issues they raise. It will deal with only some of the methods used to formulate lists of explicit criteria, with emphasis on the selection of important criteria subject to documentation in the medical record, and on the degree of agreement on such items. Some other issues will receive only passing mention.

Chart 12–1

Explicit criteria are usually developed for the management of specific diagnostic categories, though what I have called the "referent" for the criteria may also be a still undiagnosed health condition or some other situation requiring care (Vol. II, pp. 65–86). The chosen referents may then be presented to a group of experts who are asked to specify the criteria, such as those for establishing a diagnosis (through medical history, physical examination, and diagnostic tests), and for providing appropriate preventive, therapeutic, and rehabilitative care. The physicians who are given this charge may begin anew, or they may have before them a proposed set of criteria which is purposely too large, so that they can select a smaller subset, though they may add items as well.

In this case, the researcher selected three diagnostic categories. For each he prepared a lengthy questionnaire that embodied detailed criteria for follow-up care, assuming the diagnosis had already been made. All three questionnaires were submitted to ten internists who practiced general medicine. In addition, seven physicians in each of three groups of more specialized internists received the questionnaire concerning the diagnostic category that fell within their own area of specialization. Without consulting the others, each physician rated each criterion item in the questionnaire as included, excluded, or not applicable, based on whether or not an item was judged to have "a significant effect on end results," or to be "of significant help in determining underlying pathology." (See for example Brook 1973, pp. 167–68.)

The chart shows the percentage of criteria which were rated identically by at least two-thirds of physicians in each group (seven or more out of 10 generalists, and five or more out of seven specialists). Using this level of consensus, each group agreed on roughly three-quarters of the criteria in the original questionnaires; pairs of groups agreed on about half of the criteria. Not shown in the chart is the observation that a vote by a two-thirds majority of either generalists or specialists to include or exclude a criterion item was never countermanded by a two-thirds majority of their counterparts. There is, then, a large core of agreement on what constitutes "adequate" care, even though differences of opinion among individuals are also very frequent. But remember that these are physicians who are connected with one medical center and who therefore share in what Brook calls the "Hopkins environment."

Chart 12–1

Percent of Proposed Explicit Criteria for the Management and Follow-up of Patients with Specified Diagnoses that Are Agreed Upon as Included, Excluded, or Not Applicable by at Least Two-Thirds of a Panel of Specialists, a Panel of Generalists, or Both Panels. Baltimore City Hospitals, Baltimore, 1971.

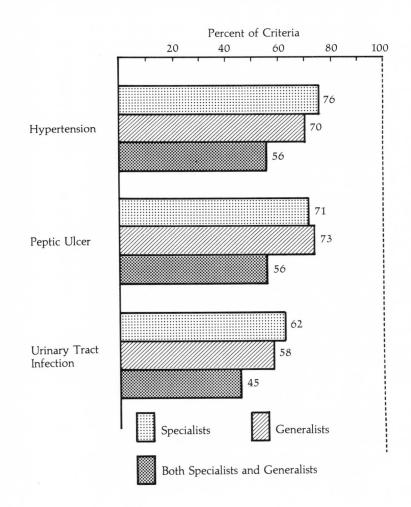

Source: Brook 1973, Tables D-34 to D-36, pp. 282-97. The percentages are based on my own counts.

Chart 12–2

This chart and several others in this section are drawn from a national study of the criteria of pediatric care sponsored by a consortium of organizations led by the American Academy of Pediatrics. As a first step, a Joint Committee on Quality Assurance, representing all participating organizations, developed lengthy lists of criteria for the health supervision of children in each of four age groups, and for the care of three diseases: tonsillopharyngitis, urinary tract infection in the female, and bronchial asthma.

Next, a panel of 452 "experts" was identified, based on nominations by the participating organizations. Each member of this panel was asked to rate each item on each list of criteria, according to its contribution to the outcome of care, as highly relevant, relevant, questionably relevant, irrelevant, and contraindicated. Each item was also rated, according to suitability for use in peer review, as essential, desirable, acceptable, or unacceptable.

The third step in the procedure was to submit the original lists of criteria (with some revisions) to a national sample of physicians who provide primary care to children: namely, pediatricians, family physicians, general practitioners, internists, and osteopathic physicians. Each physician was asked to rate the criteria following the same procedure used by the "experts."

The chart shows the comparisons between the ratings of three groups: the panel of experts, the sample of pediatricians, and the sample of all other physicians who give primary care to children. An item was considered to be agreed upon as relevant to outcome if at least 85 percent of physicians in each group rated it as "highly relevant" or "relevant." It is agreed upon to be recommended for peer review if at least 85 percent in each group rate it as "essential" or "desirable."

We see that, in general, the more highly specialized or "expert" physicians tend to endorse more criteria through consensus; that there is more agreement on the criteria for the management of illness than for health supervision; and that more criteria are agreed upon as relevant to outcome than as acceptable for peer review. These differences may reflect differences in knowledge, in the kinds of patients cared for, in the circumstances and resources of everyday practice, and in the perceived responsibility of physicians, particularly for the social and psychological aspects of health supervision.

Chart 12-2

Percent of Proposed Explicit Criteria that Are Considered by 85 Percent or More of Physicians in Specified Groups To Be Relevant to Outcome and Recommended for Peer Review, Respectively. Criteria for the Health Supervision of Infants and Children and for the Management of Three Childhood Diseases, U.S.A., circa 1975.

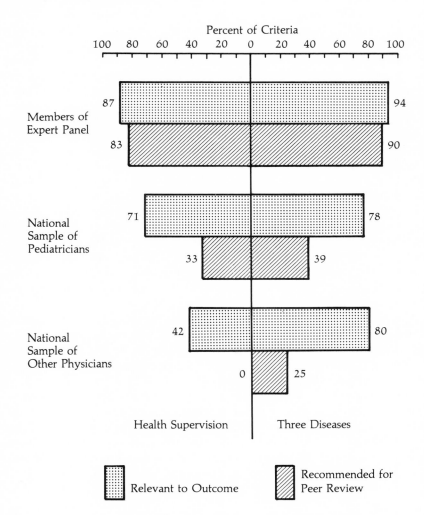

Source and Note: Thompson and Osborne 1976, Appendix B, pp. 32-38, based on my own counts. Criteria classified as contraindicated (three for health supervision and four for the management of disease) have been excluded.

Chart 12–3

This chart shows the results of another way of analyzing the data shown in the preceding chart. Here, the criteria for health supervision and the care of the three childhood diseases are combined. Furthermore, the chart shows the opinions concerning suitability for peer review, the attribute on which there is less agreement, as compared to relevance to outcome. As before, agreement that an item is "recommended" means that at least 85 percent of the physicians in each group rate the item as either "essential" or "desirable." Finally, this chart is concerned with the details of agreement and disagreement among the three groups of physicians: the expert panel, the national sample of pediatricians, and the national sample of other physicians believed to provide primary care to children.

In the upper part of the chart we see a remarkably orderly patterning of opinions into a clear hierarchy. The items endorsed by a majority of physicians at a lower level of specialization or expertise are almost always also endorsed at all remaining higher levels. Taking the opposite direction, the criterion items that are not endorsed at a higher level are also not endorsed at each successive lower level.

One consequence of this patterning is shown in the lower portion of the chart. The most "expert" physicians endorse 81 percent of the criteria by majorities of 85 percent or more. The practicing pediatricians endorse many fewer. And by the time we get down to the level of all the other physicians who provide primary care to children, only 10 percent of the items on the original lists are found to be endorsed for use in peer review.

One interpretation of the findings is that there is a group of professional leaders who are in substantial agreement on the norms of practice, but that these norms have only a limited hold on, or relevance to, other practicing physicians. As one moves further away from the leaders, in degree of specialization and circumstances of practice, the norms become less and less commanding until, at the periphery of this field, their influence is only weakly felt. But the orderliness of this normative attenuation suggests a progressively more selective application of general norms, rather than the creation of new, and contrary, norms. It is important to know what factors explain, and perhaps justify, this selectivity. (For some speculations on the subject see Volume II, pp. 298–301.)

Chart 12-3

Percent of Proposed Explicit Criteria Distributed According to Whether or Not They Are Recommended for Peer Review by at Least 85 Percent of Physicians in Specified Groups. Criteria for the Health Supervision of Infants and Children and the Management of Three Childhood Diseases, U.S.A., circa 1973.

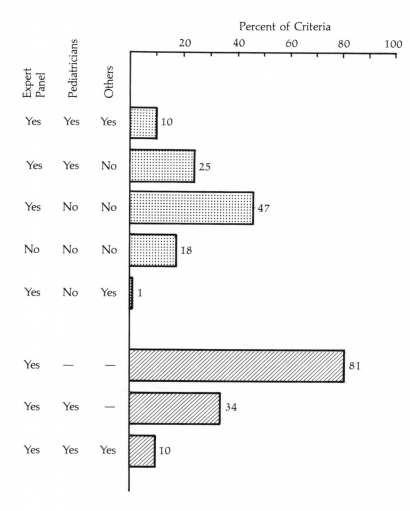

Source: Thompson and Osborne 1976, Appendix B, pp. 32-38, based on my own counts.

Chart 12–4

The findings illustrated in the preceding two charts are influenced by the arbitrary rule that consensus means agreement by at least 85 percent of physicians that a criterion item is either "relevant to outcome" or "recommended for peer review." By showing a more detailed frequency distribution of responses, this chart avoids the possible distorting effect of that rule. As in the earlier charts, a criterion item was considered to be recommended for peer review if it was rated as "essential" or "desirable" for that purpose.

This chart shows the frequency distribution of "recommended" criteria for the assessment of care for three childhood diseases, the distribution being according to the percent of physicians who rate each item as "recommended." For example, the first pair of bars at the top of the chart shows that about 17 percent of the criteria were recommended for peer review by 100 percent of the physicians on the panel of experts. By contrast, only a little over one percent of the criteria received a similarly unanimous endorsement by the nonpediatricians who provide primary care for children.

The overall pattern is one of considerable similarity in views among the members of the expert panel, and a much greater degree of dissimilarity among the members of the national sample of nonpediatricians who care for children. The data for pediatricians are omitted only to simplify the chart. Had they been included, they would have shown a degree of dispersion intermediate between that of the experts on the one hand, and the nonpediatricians on the other. The complete data are given in Volume II, Table 8-8, p. 314.

The findings reinforce the conclusion that the leaders of the profession are very much in agreement over the criteria for quality assessment of this segment of pediatric care, but that there is more and more disagreement as one moves further and further away from the leaders. This is because of less specialization and expertise, and possibly of less favorable conditions of practice as well. The findings may have been colored, however, by the influence of the expert panel on the initial revision of the criteria lists. The national sample of physicians is also faulty, since the specialty status was self-designated and the response rate was 82 percent for pediatricians, 72 percent for family physicians and only from 36 to 48 percent of the other categories. But the respondents did not differ from the nonrespondents in sex, urban/rural residence, or geographic region of the United States.

Chart 12-4

Percent Distribution of Explicit Criteria for the Management of Three Childhood Diseases, According to the Percent of Physicians in Each of Two Specified Groups Who Judged the Criteria To Be Recommended for Use in Peer Review. U.S.A., circa 1973.

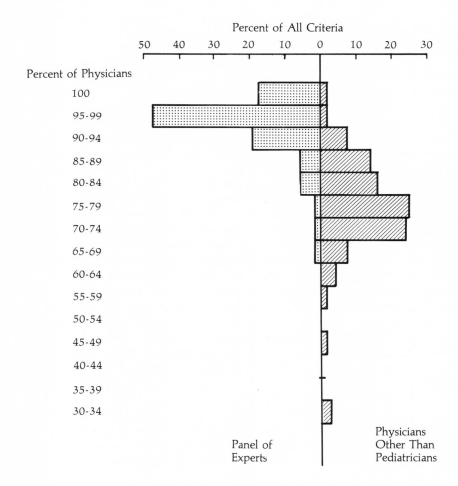

Source and Note: Thompson and Osborne 1976, Appendix B, pp. 35-38, based on my own counts. Four criteria classified as contraindicated were excluded.

Chart 12–5

This chart is drawn from a study that used a rather distinctive method to develop explicit criteria, and then tested agreement on the criteria in greater than usual detail.

The researchers began by selecting respiratory tract infection of infants as the referent for the criteria. They then prepared 125 statements, each describing a specific clinical situation and an action that might or might not be taken to deal with that situation. For example, the situation might be "fever and cough," and the relevant action "doing a throat culture."

These statements were submitted to each physician in three samples of national scope: one of family physicians, a second of general pediatricians, and a third of specialists in pediatric infectious diseases. Each physician was asked to rate each action offered in each statement by marking a seven-point scale, one end of which was labeled "absolutely necessary," and the other "completely unnecessary." A check mark in any of the first three spaces of the scale meant that the action was favored, and one in any of the last three spaces meant that the action was opposed. By checking the one space in the middle of the scale, the respondent indicated uncertainty. When 65 percent or more of the respondents in a group favored an action, and no more than 20 percent opposed it, the entire group was considered to favor that action. Similarly, when 65 percent or more of the respondents in a group opposed an action, and no more than 20 percent favored it, the group as a whole was considered to oppose the action. Other patterns of response indicated uncertainty about the action proposed.

The chart shows that all three groups agreed in favoring 52.0 percent of proposed actions and in opposing another 0.8 percent. The total, 53.0 percent, represents the consensual criteria set. The remaining 47 percent of criteria were not endorsed, using the rules described above. In 21.6 percent of cases the three groups of respondents agreed to be uncertain, and there were other responses short of consensus for the remaining 25.6 percent.

Thus, in spite of considerable disagreement, a large core of agreement emerges. What is more, Wagner et al. were able to arrange the consensual criteria into a coherent flow diagram. This represents a plan for action that at least 65 percent of physicians in each group are expected to accept, and no more than 20 percent to find some fault in.

Chart 12–5

Percent Distribution of Actions Proposed in 135 Situations Pertaining to Respiratory Tract Infections of Infants, According to the Degree of Agreement in the Majority Opinions of Three Groups of Physicians: Family Physicians, Pediatricians, and Pediatricians Who Specialize in Infectious Diseases, U.S.A., circa 1974.

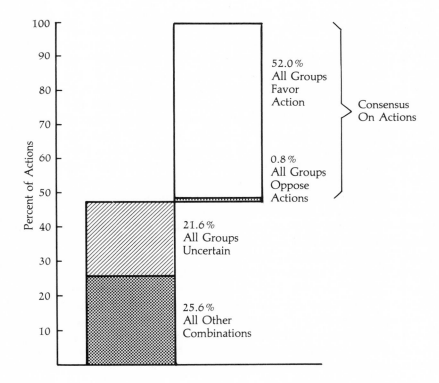

Source: Wagner et al. 1976, Table 3, p. 873.

Chart 12–6

The overall levels of agreement and disagreement portrayed in the preceding chart conceal some fascinating details. This chart, by showing only a snippet of the more detailed tabulations, begins to suggest the remarkable complexity of the interrelationships among the characteristics of the clinical situation, the action proposed, and the nature of the physicians' specializations and practices, insofar as these influence consensus within a group and agreement among groups.

The clinical descriptions are roughly arranged in order of increasing likelihood of serious lung involvement. As expected, the more serious the signs and symptoms, the more frequent the recommendation for chest X-rays. But there is, in addition, the suggestion of an interaction with the category of physicians. The most specialized physicians seem to be most likely to want an X-ray done for the least and most serious cases, whereas in the intermediate range of severity, the family physicians are most likely to recommend a chest X-ray.

Wagner et al. studied the nature and extent of disagreement in greater detail than shown here, by a method that took into account the strength of an opinion (on the seven-point scale described in connection with the preceding chart), as well as the percent of physicians who hold that opinion. Given 125 test situations, 375 comparisons are possible. There was a significant difference (at the one percent level) in 26 percent of the comparisons. As a result, the family physicians were found to be most likely to recommend action, the generalist pediatricians the least likely to do so, and the infectious disease specialists were in between, though closer to the other pediatricians than to the family physicians. In particular, the family physicians were more likely to recommend antibiotics, other drugs, and diagnostic investigations. The groups agreed most often on the more basic and stable components of clinical management: the medical history, the physical examination, and follow-up observations.

According to the investigators, "few of the 66 consensus criteria are unequivocally supported by sound data about their beneficial effects on patient outcomes. . . . Nevertheless the consensus criteria represent clear indications of the activities believed by a wide spectrum of physicians to constitute good care. The differences in opinion among physician groups provide indication of potentially important variations in clinical practice that demand resolution . . ." (Wagner et al. 1976, pp. 875–76).

Chart 12–6

Percent of Physicians in Specified Categories Who Approve of Doing a Chest X-ray When Specified Symptoms and Signs Are Present. U.S.A., circa 1974.

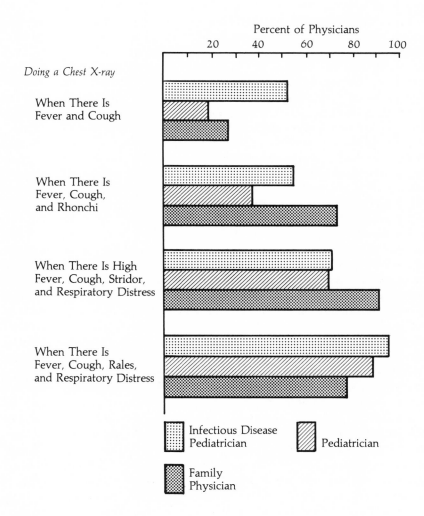

Source: Information kindly supplied by Professor Wagner to supplement Figure 3, p. 467 in Wagner et al. 1978.

Chart 12–7

Preformulated, explicit criteria and standards of the outcomes of care are used much less frequently than criteria and standards of process in quality assessment. There is, therefore, little information on the degree of agreement on expected health outcomes.

This chart is drawn from the work of Williamson, who has for many years tried to develop and propagate his method of "health accounting." This requires that physicians and other professional personnel identify important areas of weakness in their programs, as judged by a perceived failure to achieve improvements in health status that the program should be capable of achieving. An acceptable level of health outcomes is then set for each problem selected and, after the lapse of a preset time period, the degree of success in meeting the standards is determined.

Many kinds of problems and many corresponding "outcomes" lend themselves to this approach. But Williamson has also proposed a measure of health which, if used uniformly, would allow comparability among studies. This is the scale of health status shown in the chart. It is more fully described on page 126 of the source and on page 43–44 of Volume II of this series.

The standards shown in the chart come from nine organized programs of ambulatory care that selected the diagnosis and management of hypertension as one of the problems that needed attention. The standards are expectations of what percent of persons with hypertension should be in each specified level of health status after six to 12 months of care. The chart shows the lowest, highest, and median values of these percentages, pooling all nine studies. There is considerable variability, particularly for the less severe states of dysfunction. To an undetermined degree, part of the variability may reflect differences in the kinds of patients treated by each program, as well as in the resources of the programs. It is likely, however, that another part is due to uncertainty about what outcomes are reasonable to expect.

Williamson reports, very briefly, that his early studies at Baltimore City Hospitals have established the reliability of the standards of achievable performance. A repetition of standard setting by a given group several months after an initial round has shown that "although the standards set by any one panel member may vary, the team averages remained remarkably consistent" (Williamson 1978, p. 129). Staff judgments about which conditions offer significant potential for improvements in outcomes appear to be reliable and valid (Williamson et al. 1978, 1979).

Chart 12-7

Range and Median Values of Outcome Standards Expressed as the Percent of Persons with Hypertension Who Are Expected To Be in Specified Categories of Health Status after Six to 12 Months of Observation. Nine Studies of Hypertension, U.S.A., 1963–1973.

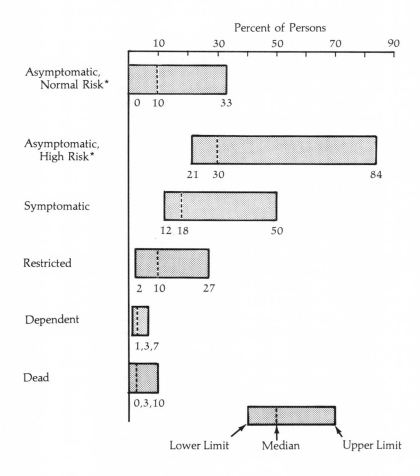

Source and Note: Williamson 1978, Table 8.2, pp. 169-73. The asterisks indicate that in two studies separate values were not available because these two categories were combined into one.

Chart 12–8

We now return to the criteria of the process of care in order to consider yet another important influence on the choice of the criteria and, therefore, on the degree of agreement about whether or not the criteria are suitable for assessing the quality of care. I refer to the likelihood that the element of care to be used as a criterion will be recorded if done or, to use a more stringent requirement, that it will be recorded even if it produced a normal finding.

The likelihood of recording was an attribute of the criteria, in addition to relevance to outcome and suitability for peer review, which was included in the study of the criteria of pediatric care led by the American Academy of Pediatrics. The respondents in the national sample of physicians who provide primary care to children were asked, for example, to classify each proposed criterion item as "perform and record," "perform but not record," and "do not perform."

The chart is based on the responses of the national sample of physicians with regard to each of the two sets of criteria: those for health supervision of infants and children, and those for three childhood diseases. It shows, as a percentage distribution, the reported propensity to record an item, assuming it has been performed. It is clear that fairly often, items are performed but not recorded, and that this is particularly true of the criteria for health supervision. For example, 4.3 percent of criteria for the management of illness are said to be recorded by less than 60 percent of the physicians who say they perform them; as many as 28.4 percent of the criteria for health supervision are said to be recorded, when performed, by less than 60 percent of physicians. This propensity not to record certain items may be part of the reason for finding them unsuitable for peer review even when their relevance to outcome is recognized.

To summarize the findings in this and some other charts based on this study, fewer criteria are recommended for peer review than are considered relevant to outcome; fewer criteria are said to be performed and recorded than are recommended; and, as we shall see soon, an even smaller number of criteria appear with any regularity in the records themselves. No wonder that the sponsors of the study concluded that "because of the lack of recording, accurate and meaningful evaluation of ambulatory child health care cannot now be accomplished by chart audit" (Osborne and Thompson 1975, p. 646).

Chart 12–8

Percent of Explicit Criteria which Specified Percentages of Physicians Say They Record When Performed. National Sample of Physicians Believed To Provide Primary Care to Children; Criteria for Health Supervision of Infants and Children and for Three Childhood Diseases; U.S.A., circa 1973.

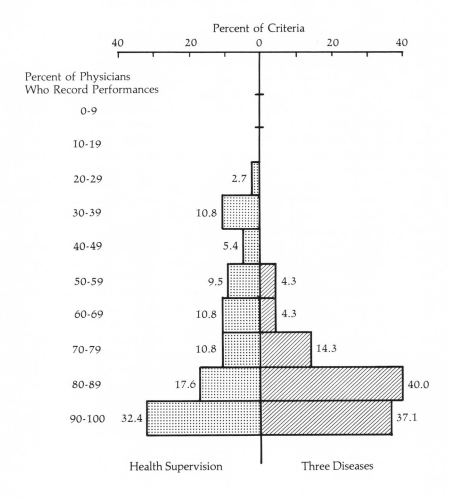

Health Supervision   Three Diseases

Source: Osborne and Thompson 1975, Appendix F, pp. 684-91, based on my counts.

Chart 12–9

The likelihood of recording was an attribute included in the choice of criteria by Hulka et al.

The first step in the process of formulating the criteria was to assemble a master list of criteria, based on earlier studies of quality, for each of four conditions in adult patients: diabetes, hypertension, dysuria (painful, frequent urination), and an annual general examination. These lists were then submitted to a sample of internists in North Carolina. Unfortunately, only 31 of 223 physicians contacted agreed to participate.

Each physician was asked to rate each criterion item in two ways. First, the item was rated as to importance in the routine care of most patients in usual office practice. This was done by marking one of seven positions on a scale which had "essential" at one end, and "completely unnecessary" at the other. Then, the physicians reported whether they would record a negative finding pertinent to each criterion, with the exception of the results of diagnostic tests. These were assumed to be always recorded.

The consensual set of criteria had to meet two conditions: (1) to be placed in one of the two positions at the "essential" end of the scale by at least 50 percent of physicians, and (2) to be reported as recorded, even if the finding were negative, by at least 65 percent. The chart shows the consequences of applying each of these two conditions. For example, 29 percent of the criteria for the medical history were eliminated because less than 50 percent of physicians considered them important enough. Another 30 percent were excluded because less than 65 percent of physicians said they would record a negative finding.

Besides the variability in these percentages among the areas of care shown in the chart, there were differences in this regard among the four medical conditions as well. For all areas of care and all conditions combined, 33 percent of criteria were eliminated on the grounds of lesser importance, and another 21 percent because, though the criterion was important, a negative finding would not be recorded often enough.

It should be noted that relevance to outcome was not an explicit requirement for the ratings of importance used in this study.

Chart 12-9

Percent of Items on a Master List of Criteria that Were Considered by a Group
of Internists To Be Essential, and that Were Considered To Be Both Essential
and Likely To Be Recorded. Specified Components of Office Care for Four
Selected Conditions, North Carolina, 1975–1977.

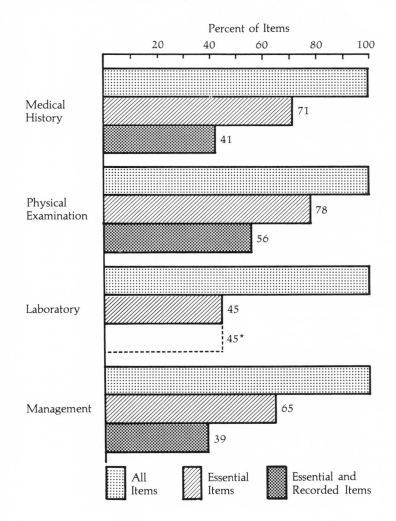

Source and Note: Hulka et al. 1979, Table 4, p. 15, and Hulka et al. 1977, the latter using my own
counts. All Laboratory tests were assumed to be recorded.

Chart 12–10

This chart shows that importance and likelihood of being recorded, the
two attributes that figure so prominently in the selection of explicit criteria, are themselves interrelated. The criteria for hypertension are used
as an example. Because the findings of laboratory tests and other diagnostic procedures were assumed to be always recorded, the corresponding criterion items have been excluded from the chart.

As described in connection with the preceding chart, Hulka et al.
asked each of the internists who consented to participate in their study
to rate the importance of each criterion item by checking one of seven
positions on a scale which had "completely unnecessary" at one end and
"essential" at the other end. The abscissa of the graph shows the percent
of physicians who rated an item as essential or next to essential.

Each physician was also asked if he would record each criterion item
even when it was associated with a negative finding. The ordinate of the
graph shows the percentage of physicians who answered in the
affirmative.

Each element in the chart represents a criterion item positioned according to the two characteristics described above: the percent of physicians who say the criterion is essential or next to essential, and the
percent of physicians who say the item would be recorded if adhered
to. If one excludes a few aberrant criteria, the arrangement of the remaining ones suggests a rather close association of the two characteristics.
The more often a criterion is considered to be essential the more often
is it reported to be recorded.

The four items that are very likely to be recorded even though they
are infrequently thought to be essential are "medication instituted before
the initial work-up completed," "leg blood pressure," "standing blood
pressure," and "lying blood pressure." Quite obviously, this is information that would be recorded if it were pertinent or obtained. The one
item which is very important but not so likely to be recorded is "explanation of disease." Its exclusion from the final consensual set is a conces-
sion to the imperfections of prevalent recording practices. The final
consensual set whose members satisfied the two conditions of essentiality and recordability is shown as a tight cluster of triangles in the
upper right-hand corner of the graph.

Chart 12-10

Proposed Explicit Criteria for the Office Care of Hypertension Distributed According to the Percent of Physicians Who Rated Each Criterion Item as Essential or Next to Essential, and According to the Percent of Physicians Who Said They Would Record Each Criterion Item. Internists in Selected Areas of North Carolina, 1975–1977.

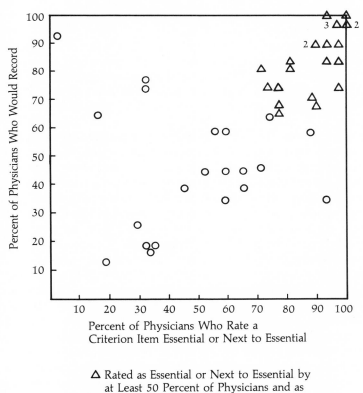

△ Rated as Essential or Next to Essential by at Least 50 Percent of Physicians and as Recorded by at Least 65 Percent

Source: Hulka et al. 1977, Appendix 11, unpaginated, based on my own counts.

Chart 12–11

The study of agreement on the criteria was only part of the broader investigation conducted by Hulka et al. Another part was a review of samples of office records, so that the actual performance of the same internists could be compared with their own ratings of the criteria, either individual by individual, or as a group.

This chart uses the criteria for the office care of hypertension to make one such comparison. As in the preceding chart, the criteria for laboratory tests and other diagnostic procedures are excluded because these criteria are assumed to be recorded in every case. To scale the remaining criteria, I multiplied for each criterion item the proportion of physicians who rated it as essential or next to essential, by the proportion of physicians who said they would record the item even if it were associated with a negative finding. This is the score shown on the abscissa of the graph. It represents, in effect, the probability that an internist in this group would find a criterion item to be both important and subject to recording.

The chart shows the scatter of the proposed criterion items according to this score and to the proportion of office records that included reasonably acceptable evidence that the criterion item had been adhered to when it was applicable. There appears to be an association between the opinions of the physicians, as reflected by their ratings of essentiality and recordability, and their performance, the latter as inferred from the medical record. But the association is not strong.

There are three possible disturbing factors. A physician may not adhere to a criterion in his practice even though it is one that he endorses. Second, a physician may practice in accord with the criterion but fail to show this in the medical record. Finally, those who abstracted the record may have failed to note existing evidence of compliance. This last reason for discrepancy was rather unimportant in this case, since a check on the reliability of abstracting showed it to be very high indeed (p. 18).

The criterion item that is very low in importance-recordability but is very often found in the medical record is "medication instituted before the initial work-up completed." Apparently this was a very frequent practice. The three consensual criteria in the lowermost tier of triangles in the chart are "instruction in regular visit schedule," history of "past renal disease," and history of "past treatment for hypertension." All are important, but apparently subject to nonrecording.

Chart 12-11

Proposed Explicit Criteria for the Office Care of Hypertension Distributed According to a Score Indicating Each Item's Importance and Likelihood of Recording, and According to the Proportion of Office Records Showing Adherence to Each Criterion Item. Internists in Selected Areas of North Carolina, 1975-1977.

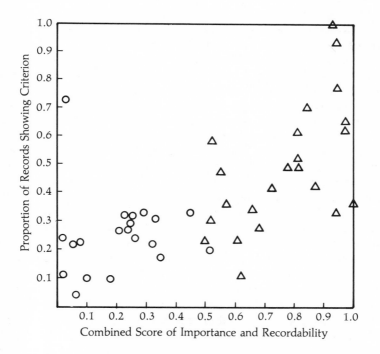

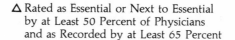

△ Rated as Essential or Next to Essential
by at Least 50 Percent of Physicians
and as Recorded by at Least 65 Percent

Source: Hulka et al. 1977, Appendix 11, unpaginated, based on my own counts and calculations.

Chart 12–12

One possible explanation for the relatively low adherence to consensus criteria, an explanation intentionally omitted from the discussion of the preceding chart, is that individual physicians are guided by their own personal criteria rather than those of the group. To test this hypothesis, Hulka et al. compiled a list of criteria for each individual physician. The list comprised all the items the physician had rated as essential or next to essential, and had said he would record. The office records of each physician were then compared with his own criteria, as well as those in the consensual set. The latter included all the items rated as essential or next to essential by at least 50 percent of the group of physicians, and as subject to recording by at least 65 percent.

The chart shows that adherence to the criteria is rather low irrespective of their source. As more germane to our immediate concern, it reveals that for the annual general examination adherence to the individual criteria is slightly higher than adherence to consensual criteria, but not significantly so. For the remaining three conditions adherence to the individual criteria is lower rather than higher, and the difference is statistically significant. In some way, which may include a reduction in the number of criteria selected, group opinion seems to refine the criteria into a somewhat more realistic set.

Hulka et al. went one step further in their comparisons. They ranked patients according to their adherence scores to individual and consensual criteria and compared the two rankings. They also ranked physicians according to the adherence scores they achieved with each of the two sets of criteria, and compared the rankings. Both sets of comparisons revealed high coefficients of correlation (pp. 26–27).

Hulka et al. also compared the ranks of their physicians, as judged by their own consensual criteria, with ranks obtained when the same physicians were judged by two other sets of criteria. One of these was developed through a national study under the auspices of the American Society of Internal Medicine (Hare and Barnoon 1973). The other was the study of ambulatory care in Hawaii by Payne et al. (1976). High correlation coefficients showed the rankings in each pair of comparisons to be quite similar.

Even though there is considerable disagreement about the criteria of care, there is a core of agreement sufficiently large to produce reasonably consistent measures of at least relative performance.

Chart 12–12

Percent of Consensus Criteria and Percent of Individual Criteria Adhered to on the Average, as Shown by the Office Records of Internists. Patients with One of Four Specified Conditions, Selected Areas of North Carolina, 1975–1977.

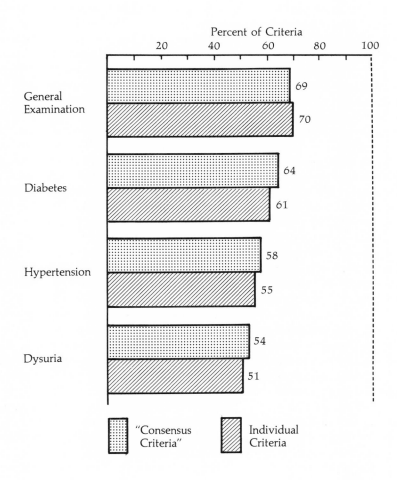

Source: Hulka et al. 1979, Table 18, p. 26.

Chart 12–13

The study of pediatric care criteria, which has figured so prominently in this section, has still more to say about the relationship between how strongly the criteria are endorsed and how often they are adhered to in actual practice. We already know that, among other things, the study sought the opinions of a representative national sample of physicians who are thought to provide primary care to infants and children. Each physician in this sample received lists of proposed criteria and was asked to rate each item on these lists according to how relevant it was to the outcome of care and how suitable it was for peer review. Each physician was also asked to say whether, as he cares for "a regular patient," he performs and records a criterion item, performs but does not record it, or does not perform it. The abscissa of the chart shows the percent of physicians in the national sample who would perform and record any given criterion item.

It was not possible, unfortunately, to test the opinions and reported practices of these physicians with their own office records. Instead, those in charge of the study sought and obtained the cooperation of selected pediatricians and family physicians in various regions of the country, hoping to obtain a reasonably true, though not a strictly representative, picture of everyday practice. To permit this picture to be drawn, each physician submitted ten cases in each of the categories covered by the criteria. The percent of cases with documented adherence to the criteria could then be computed. The ordinate of the chart shows these percentages.

The chart shows that how often physicians in one sample say they perform and record certain criteria is positively associated with how often the medical records of another sample of physicians show actual performance and recording. But the degree of association is rather weak. Furthermore, actual practice is almost always short of reported practice, often to a considerable degree.

The physicians who made their records available almost always agreed that the record did not contain the missing information. But "only 48 percent of the physicians agreed that the audit accurately portrayed the care they were delivering." The others disagreed because they claimed to be doing more than the record showed to be the case, the main reason for the discrepancy being that negative findings were not entered on the record (p. 639).

Chart 12–13

Proposed Explicit Criteria for the Management of Three Childhood Diseases
Distributed According to the Percent of Physicians Who Say They Perform
and Record Each Item, and According to the Percent of Office Records Which
Show that the Item Has Been Performed. U.S.A., circa 1973.

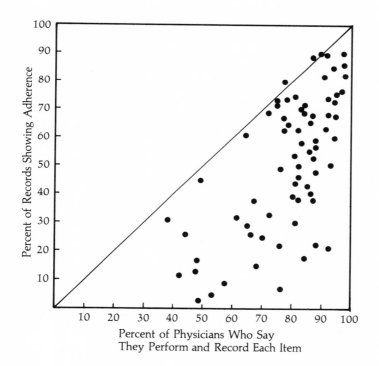

Source: Osborne and Thompson 1975, Appendix F, pp. 687-91, by my own counts.

Chart 12–14

So far in this section, we have described procedures which allow a large set of proposed criteria to be pared down into a smaller set, one more acceptable to a majority of physicians on grounds of "relevance to outcome," "essentiality," suitability for peer review, or likelihood of recording. It is possible to go another step and assign different weights to the criteria included in the endorsed set, so that the omission of the weightier items would merit heavier censure.

The several methods that have been used, or could be used, to construct differential weights are described on pages 226–83 of Volume II of this series. One such method, a simple one, was introduced by Payne et al. in their study of inpatient ambulatory care in Hawaii (1976). After a panel of experts had specified the criteria for "optimal care" for a given diagnostic category, the members of the panel were also asked to agree on a weight of importance for each item. The proposed weights ("one," "two," or "three") were acceptable most of the time, but in some instances the panel assigned weights that were less than "one" or intermediate to the other positions.

Payne et al. do not specify the basis for their weights, unless it is the contribution to "optimal care." This chart allows us to look into the meaning of the relative weights. It does so by distributing the criteria for hypertension and for dysuria submitted to the internists in North Carolina by Hulka et al. (1979) according to the percent of internists who rated each item as essential or next to essential, and according to the weights given the same items by the internists or urologists in Hawaii. The degree of overlap between the two sets is rather small. Therefore, the chart assigns a weight of zero to the criteria included in the North Carolina set alone. The items included only in the Hawaii set are, of course, not shown, but there are very few of those. Finally, due to differences of wording and some differences in the referents of the criteria, the matching of the two sets is not perfect, though it is quite close.

The chart shows that the much smaller set of criteria used in the study of ambulatory care in Hawaii is a subset of the criteria rated as essential or next to essential by at least 60 percent of internists in North Carolina. But there is no clear evidence, in this rather small number of criteria, that higher relative weights are associated with more frequent ratings of higher levels of essentiality.

Chart 12–14

Proposed Explicit Criteria for the Management of Hypertension and Dysuria Distributed According to the Percent of Internists in One Study Who Rated Them as Essential or Next to Essential, and According to the Weight of Importance Assigned to Them by Panels of Physicians in Another Study. Hawaii 1968, and Selected Areas of North Carolina, 1975-1977.

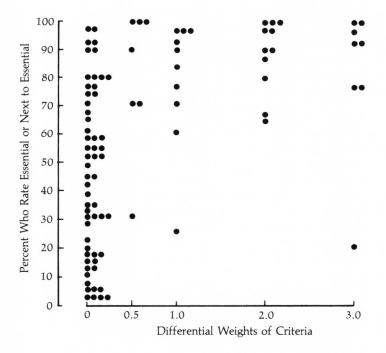

Source: Payne et al. 1976, Appendix B, pp. 132-33 and 138, and Hulka et al. 1977, Appendix 11, unpaginated, based on my counts.

Chart 12–15

The purpose of assigning different weights to the criteria included in the endorsed set is to recognize that some of the elements of care are more important than others. One consequence, as shown in this chart, is that the same areas of care acquire different degrees of importance in the management of different conditions, depending on the relative number of important items that the areas contain.

As described in connection with the preceding chart, Payne et al. asked the members of the expert panels that participated in their study of inpatient and ambulatory care in Hawaii to assign weights of "one," "two," or "three" to each item included among the recommended criteria. In most cases, the panels adopted these weights, but in some instances they assigned values smaller than "one" or intermediate between the other values suggested.

The total numerical score for each list depends on the number of criteria it contains and on the weights of importance conferred on these items. The chart shows the percentages of the total score accounted for by each of three categories of criteria: those pertinent to the medical history, to the physical examination, and to diagnostic investigations. The conditions shown are selected from a larger set, and they are arranged in order of increasing importance of the medical history as a factor in total care. Criteria for therapy were not formulated for these diagnoses. The data for the complete set of conditions are shown in Table 7–12, p. 281 of Volume II of this series.

The variability in emphasis on the three aspects of care portrayed in the chart is quite obvious. For example, the management of full-term pregnancy appears to center mainly on the physical examination and diagnostic investigations, with little importance being attached to the medical history. By contrast, the medical history is as important as the physical examination, while diagnostic investigations are much less important, in providing good care to women with breast cancer. As still another contrast, the physical examination plays no role in chronic cholecystitis; the quality of care for this condition depends first on diagnostic investigations and then on the medical history.

No claims are made for the validity of the weightings. It is possible, in fact, that the members of the panels would have reassessed their weights had they seen the consequences presented in this form. The next chart shows the reason for saying so.

Chart 12–15

Percent of Total Quality Score Assigned to Specified Components of the Process of Care for Specified Diagnostic Categories. Explicit Criteria of Inpatient Care, Hawaii, 1968.

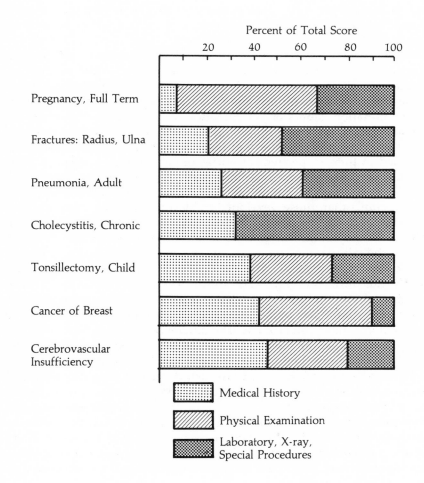

Source: Payne et al. 1976, Appendix A, pp. 93-131, based on my counts and computations.

Chart 12–16

Some years after their study of hospital and office care in Hawaii, Payne et al. did a study of the quality of care at five sites that represented different forms of organizing ambulatory care in the American Midwest. Once again, panels of physicians were asked to develop sets of criteria and to weight the individual items according to importance. But the method of weighting was different and, as this chart shows, so were the results.

Now the panelists were first asked to divide a score of 100 between diagnostic and therapeutic management according to the relative importance of the two. As a second step, the score assigned to diagnostic management was partitioned among the subcategories of history, physical examination, laboratory examination, radiological examination, and special studies. Only as a third step were the individual criterion items given weights, making sure that these added up to the scores already assigned to their respective categories or subcategories. Perhaps partly because of the new procedure, and partly because new groups of physicians served on the panels, the resulting weights were much more heterogenous than those developed in Hawaii, constrained as the latter were by the 1–2–3 scale already described. Now, it was possible to see examples of tenfold, twentyfold, or even fortyfold differences in weight among the criteria of a single condition.

Because the individual criteria and referents of the two studies match poorly, it is difficult to chart a criterion-by-criterion comparison. Instead, the chart shows the percentage distribution of the total numerical score among the component areas of care, using chronic or recurrent urinary infection in adults as an example. The differences in the pattern of weights are quite obvious, the most notable difference being the relatively large weight given to treatment in the more recent formulation.

When a few criterion items have such dominant weights, the quality of care would seem to hinge on these few items. Accordingly, one would expect that assessments of quality using the two sets of criteria would give quite different results. We do not know if this would be true in this particular instance. As described on pages 283–91 of Volume II of this series, comparisons between judgments of quality using weighted and unweighted criteria have, so far, shown remarkably little effect on relative rankings of performance.

Chart 12–16

Percent of Total Quality Score Assigned to Each of Specified Components of the Process of Care. Explicit Criteria of Ambulatory Care for Chronic or Recurrent Urinary Infection in Adults, Hawaii, 1968, and Five Midwestern Sites in the United States, 1974, Respectively.

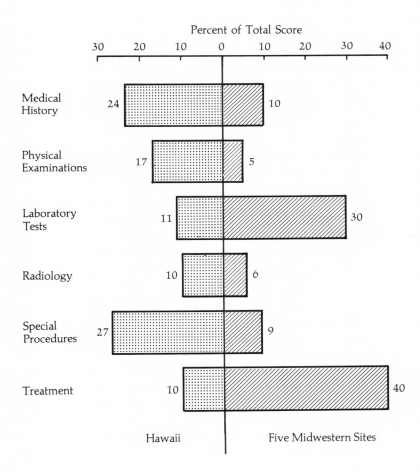

Source: Payne et al. 1976, p. 139, and Payne et al. 1978, Appendix A, p. 32 of the Appendix, based on my own counts and computations.

Chart 12–17

It would be useful to know if physicians, besides agreeing or disagreeing with each other, would be either firm or vacillating in their opinions, if these were sought from time to time.

When the Delphi technique is used to develop criteria lists, there is little change in individual opinions from one round of questioning to another. But with this procedure, the respondents know what their answers were at the preceding round (Volume II, pp. 158–59, 332–33).

This chart shows the results of a much better test of within-rater reliability. As described in connection with an earlier chart in this section, Wagner et al. offered each respondent in their study brief descriptions of 125 clinical situations and asked them to rate a diagnostic or therapeutic action proposed for each situation by checking one of seven positions on a scale which had "absolutely necessary" at one end and "completely unnecessary" at the other. The three positions closest to "absolutely necessary" were interpreted as favoring action; the three positions closest to "completely unnecessary" were interpreted as opposing action; and the one position at the center of the scale was taken to mean uncertainty.

A year later, a subset of respondents was mailed the same questionnaire, but this time the physicians were asked only to say whether the action associated with each clinical situation should be done or not. As the chart shows, the opinions are stable. The opinions that were originally stronger are more likely to be confirmed, and so are the opinions that originally favored, rather than opposed, action. The tendency to slide toward more frequent endorsement of action is also found in the category originally rated as "uncertain." Not shown in the chart is the finding that these ambiguous responses were changed, in 67.5 percent of cases, to an opinion that action should be taken; in only 32.5 percent was the change to an opinion that action should not be taken.

From such studies of consensus and reliability as have been reviewed in this section we can conclude that by selecting criteria which are strongly favored by a substantial majority of physicians we can assemble a stable, acceptable set that is also practicable. As a result of following this procedure, however, the usable criteria are a much reduced set of the lists originally submitted for approval. Obviously, this raises some questions about whether the consequent judgments of quality are sufficiently stringent.

Chart 12–17

Percent of Test Situations in which an Initial Opinion by a Physician Respondent Was Confirmed by a Second Opinion of the Same Respondent Elicited One Year Later, Ordered by Whether the First Opinion Favored or Opposed that a Specified Action Be Taken, and by the Strength of that First Opinion. U.S.A., circa 1974.

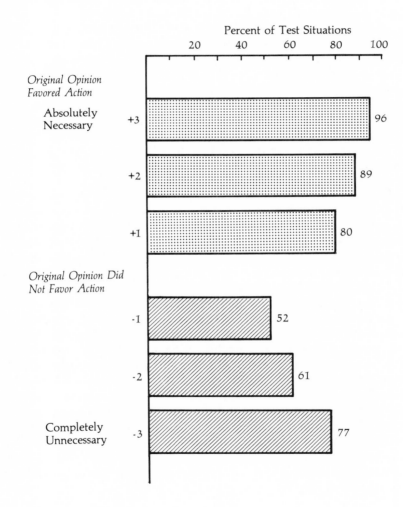

Source: Wagner et al. 1978, Table 1, p. 469.

Chart 12–18

This chart is quite unusual because it allows us to see whether or not experts can set appropriate standards for the outcomes of care.

In this study, patients with hypertension, urinary tract infection, and ulcers of the stomach or duodenum were followed up for an average of five months after their initial visit to the emergency service of the Baltimore City Hospitals. One of the methods for studying the quality of care was patterned after the method of "health accounting" advocated by Williamson, as described earlier in this chapter (Chart 12–7). As one part of testing that method, Brook asked groups of internists with expertise in each of the three conditions studied to set standards for the outcomes of care. Each physician was given a description of the kinds of patients being observed, and then was asked what proportion of patients would be expected to have experienced specified outcomes during or after an average period of five months, under each of three types of care: (1) without any therapy or follow-up, (2) with the kind of therapy and follow-up expected to be given in the emergency room, and (3) with "adequate" therapy and follow-up.

The chart shows the data for patients with urinary tract infection. On the left-hand side of the chart are the median estimates obtained from the panel of specialists at the second round of a Delphi procedure for obtaining group consensus. On the right-hand side are the outcomes actually experienced by these patients as determined by follow-up questioning and examination. It is clear that the estimates for decreased activity and continued symptoms are useless for quality assessment, since actual experience was worse than what was expected without any care. The estimate for case fatality, not shown in the chart, was precise, but deaths occur too infrequently to serve as a handy measure of outcome in studies of this kind. We are left, therefore, with the estimates for recurrent or persistent infection. The proportion of cases with a positive culture at follow-up was significantly greater than expected, but it was eight percentage points lower than that expected without any care. Since there are 29 percentage points of difference between the estimates for no therapy and adequate therapy, the observed outcome may be credited with 28 percent of the benefit achievable from care.

Of the outcome estimates for the other two conditions studied, only the blood pressure estimates for hypertension were useful as a measure of the quality of care.

Chart 12–18

Percent of Patients with Urinary Tract Infection Who, Five Months after an Initial Visit for that Episode, Were Observed To Have Experienced Specified Outcomes, as Compared to the Outcomes Envisaged by the Standards of a Group of Specialist Internists. Baltimore City Hospitals, Baltimore, 1971.

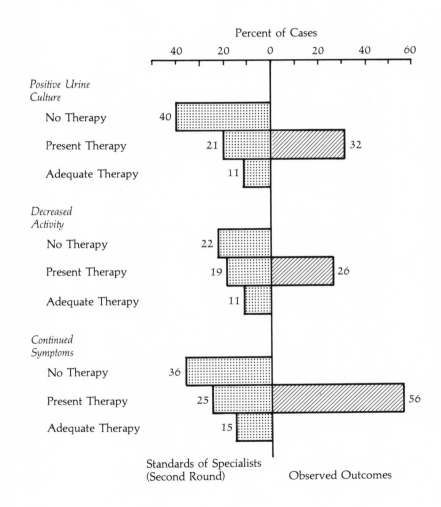

Source: Brook 1973, computed from Table 31, p. 51.

THIRTEEN

**Some Comparisons
of Methods**

THIRTEEN

We have already seen how deficient our information often is about the care provided, and how much disagreement there is about what elements of care are suitable as criteria of the quality of care. We have also seen that by selecting criteria that are particularly important to good care, especially relevant to health outcomes, and apt to be recorded, one can assemble a set of criteria which are coherent, widely acceptable, and likely to lead to reasonably reliable assessments of some of the more technical aspects of quality.

There is, nevertheless, widespread skepticism about our ability to measure quality, even within the very modest confines indicated by the adaptations described above. There are some people, of course, who would be very difficult to convince to the contrary, since it suits them to keep the concept of quality shrouded in mystery and to assert that its systematic assessment is beyond the capacities of mortal men. But even those who have an open mind on the subject, and are willing to work with less than perfect tools, are sometimes disheartened. These potential recruits to the cause of quality assessment and monitoring are troubled by disagreements among the results of different methods of measuring the quality of care, in general, and by a lack of correspondence between assessments of process and outcome, in particular.

Much of the evidence that the critics of quality assessment assemble is so flawed that it deserves little attention. But this cannot be said of the seminal work of Robert Brook (1973), who compared the results of using five different methods to assess the quality of the same care. As shown in the preceding chapter (Chart 12–18), one of these methods, based on a comparison of actual outcomes with preformulated explicit expectations of the same outcomes, may be said to have largely failed. But the other four methods, though successfully executed, produced widely divergent findings. When three judges independently assessed information about the same patients without using explicit criteria, at least one of the three judges gave a favorable verdict on the *process* of care in 23.3 percent of cases, on the *outcomes* of care in 63.2 percent of cases, and on *process and outcome combined* in 27.1 percent of cases. Moreover, in the same patients, the process of care met all the explicit criteria formulated by a group of generalist internists in only 1.4 percent of cases, and the explicit criteria of a group of more specialized internists in only 2.0 percent (Brook and Appel 1973, Table 4, p. 1327).

Seeing these wildly discrepant results, many have questioned whether these different methods can be said to measure the same thing, or to do so accurately. This section begins, therefore, with an examination of Brook's findings. The inquiry involves a comparison of judgments using implicit criteria of process with those using implicit criteria of outcomes, and a comparison of implicit judgments of process with judgments of process based on adherence to explicit criteria. We shall find, I believe, that the picture is not as bleak as it is generally painted. There is also cause for optimism in some other comparisons between the judgments of quality based on implicit and explicit criteria, as illustrated in this section.

For additional comparisons between implicit and explicit judgments of quality I shall draw on the more recent work of Novick et al. 1976, and of Hulka et al. 1979. I shall also refer to the work of Kane et al. 1981, to compare the results of using implicit and explicit criteria to determine a property that pertains to the control of both utilization and quality: the appropriate level of care for patients in nursing homes. In addition, the work of Greenfield et al. 1981, will be used to introduce the reader to the method of criteria mapping, and to show a comparison between two methods of formulating explicit criteria: the criteria map, on the one hand, and the more usual criteria lists, on the other.

Any attempt to compare the process of care to its outcomes is bound to raise issues of such complexity that no brief account can do justice to the subject. Fortunately, a very large body of literature is easily excluded because, I believe, the relationship between health status outcomes and the elements or strategies of care is primarily in the domain of the clinical sciences. Our own attention must focus on studies which offer two *judgments of quality*, one based on the process of care, and one based on its outcomes. Simply by way of illustration I have selected a few studies of this kind, hoping only to introduce the reader to some additional methods of assessing outcomes and to some of the questions that comparisons of process and outcome raise. For more on the pertinent conceptual and methodological issues the reader is referred to Volume I, Chapter 3 of this series.

Chart 13–1

The subject of this study was the care received by patients with hypertension, urinary tract infection, or ulcer of the stomach or duodenum who used the emergency services of the Baltimore City Hospitals. For each patient, Brook prepared a brief narrative which began with "background information" up to the point of diagnosis. A second paragraph described the "initial therapy and follow-up" of each case. Only the information in this second paragraph was used to judge the "medical care process," without benefit of explicit criteria, the judges being instructed only that "adequate care includes all interventions that will have a significant effect on end results and excludes those interventions likely to produce no benefit to the patient and are also clearly harmful involving definite risk to the patient's welfare" (p. 149). The chart shows the judgments of ten generalist internists, all members of the senior full-time staff, who were assigned to the task at random, so that each case was reviewed independently by each of three physicians.

As described more fully in connection with Chart 12–1, each of the same ten generalists (as well as the members of another group of more specialized internists) developed lists of explicit criteria for the same conditions, guided by a similar definition of "adequate care." The chart shows a reasonable degree of positive association between the judgments based on the two methods of assessment. Care was very infrequently judged as adequate by at least two of three generalist internists when it met only 50 percent or less of the explicit consensual criteria of the same group of generalists. When more than 50 percent of the explicit criteria were met, the case was judged as adequate by a little less than half of the majority of three judges. Brook reports a correlation coefficient of 0.481, which is significant at $p < 0.001$. Unfortunately, there is no information about the degree of correspondence between the two sets of judgments at other levels of compliance with explicit criteria, besides the observation that only 1.4 percent of the cases met all the explicit consensual criteria of the generalists, even though 23.3 percent were judged adequate by at least two out of three of the same generalists. This discrepancy, however, could simply represent two different levels of stringency in the standards of care.

Chart 13–1

Percent of Patients Whose Care Was Judged To Have Been either Adequate or Inadequate by the Implicit Criteria of at Least Two Out of Three Judges, in Each of Two Groups Classified by the Percent of Explicit Criteria Met. Patients with One of Three Diagnoses, Judged by the Implicit and Explicit Criteria of Generalist Internists, Baltimore City Hospitals, Baltimore, 1971.

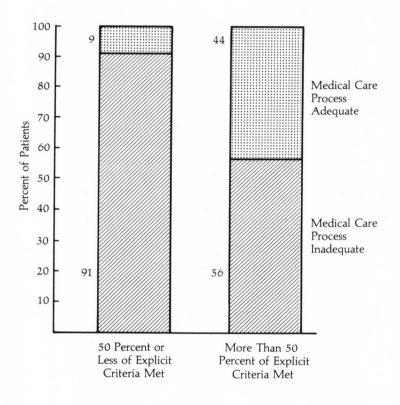

Source: Brook 1973, text on p. 50 and data in Table 5, p. 29, according to my computations.

Chart 13-2

We continue our examination of Brook's findings about the results of different methods of assessing the quality of care by comparing judgments on the process and outcomes of care using implicit criteria.

Immediately after having made a judgment on the adequacy of the process of care using implicit criteria, as described in connection with the preceding chart, each of the three generalist internists reviewing a case could read a brief description of the health outcomes which had been obtained about five months after the initiation of care. These were death, ability to perform "major activity, work or housework," the blood pressure in hypertensives, and urinalysis plus urine culture for persons with urinary tract infection (pp. 25, 151). Each physician was then asked to answer the following question: "Could the outcome obtained by this patient probably not have been improved by alteration of the medical care process, or probably have been better if the medical care process were improved?" (p. 158, with minor modifications).

Since each case was reviewed independently by each of three physicians, there were 888 verdicts on the process of care and 888 verdicts on the outcome of care in 296 patients. Of these verdicts, 25 percent judged the process of care to be adequate, and 61 percent judged the outcomes to be unimprovable. As described in the introduction to this chapter, the discrepancy between these two findings has led to questioning the reliability and validity of such quality assessments. This chart shows, however, that the two implicit judgments, one on process and the other on outcome, are positively correlated. When the process of care was judged to have been adequate, only 12 percent of judgments called the outcomes improvable; when the process was considered inadequate, the outcomes were judged to have been improvable in 48 percent of cases.

The judgment on the improvability of the outcomes of care was, of course, made with full knowledge of the antecedent process of care. It should also be remembered that the definition of "adequate" care, which the reviewers read just before judging the medical care process, dwelled heavily on the importance of the relationship between process and outcome. Both of these features may have influenced the findings. But even after making allowances for such disturbances, the results would not seem to support the view that judgments of process and outcome are unrelated. We do need to look deeper into the matter, however, if we are to understand what is meant by saying that care is inadequate, even though the outcomes are unimprovable.

Chart 13-2

Percent of Judgments that the Outcomes of Care Were Improvable or Unimprovable, when the Corresponding Judgment on the Process of Care Was that It Was Adequate or Inadequate, Respectively. Patients with One of Three Diagnoses, Judged by the Implicit Criteria of Generalist Internists, Baltimore City Hospitals, Baltimore, 1971.

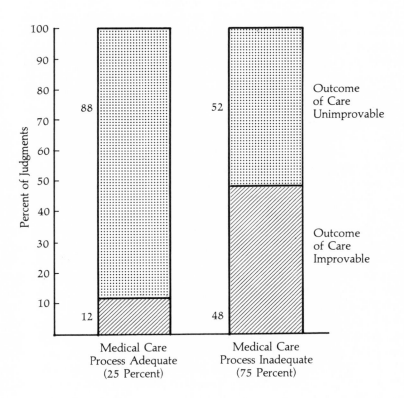

Source: Brook 1973, Table 10, p. 32.

Chart 13–3

After having judged the adequacy of the medical care process and the improvability of the outcomes of care, as described in connection with the preceding chart, each reviewer was asked to pronounce an overall judgment of quality by answering the following question: "Combining your judgments of the medical care process and the outcome data, is the quality of care received by this patient acceptable or unacceptable?" (page 158, with minor modification). This chart shows the answers.

To construct the chart, the 888 judgments, three for each case, were first classified according to how they described the adequacy of the medical care process and the improvability of outcomes. As shown in the stub of the chart, 22 percent of judgments described process and outcome, in turn, as adequate and unimprovable, three percent as adequate but improvable, 39 percent as inadequate though unimprovable, and 36 percent as inadequate and improvable.

The chart goes on to show that in the first of these categories, when the care is adequate and the outcome is unimprovable by better care, the quality of care is almost always judged to be acceptable, which is an eminently reasonable conclusion. Equally reasonable are the results shown for the last category down the chart: when the care is inadequate and the outcome improvable by better care, the quality of care is overwhelmingly judged to be unacceptable.

We must next consider the two internally inconsistent categories. As shown by the second bar from the top, when the care is adequate, the additional information that the outcomes are improvable does tend to produce a reversal to a negative judgment on the quality of care. But this category is so small that this kind of reversal is very infrequent. By contrast, the other internally inconsistent category, illustrated by the third bar of the chart, is quite large; here, the additional knowledge that the outcome is unimprovable by better care is associated with a judgment that the quality is acceptable in only a fifth of the cases. In this category, the judgment that the care is inadequate takes precedence, perhaps because the evidence on other outcomes not here represented is not yet in.

To me, these findings are evidence of reasonable judgment rather than of unreliable and invalid measurement.

Chart 13–3

Percent of Judgments, Categorized by Adequacy of Process and Improvability
of Outcome, which Correspond to Judgments that the Quality of Care is
Acceptable or Unacceptable. Care of Patients with One of Three Diagnoses,
Judged by the Implicit Criteria of Generalist Internists, Baltimore City Hospitals, Baltimore, 1971.

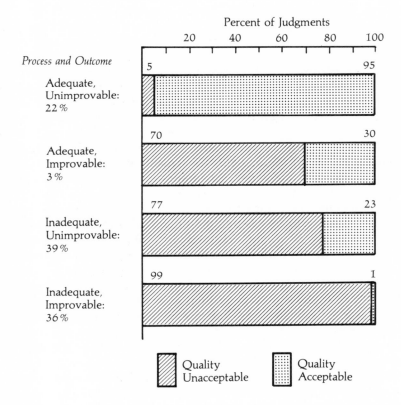

Source: Brook 1973, Table 10, p. 32.

Chart 13–4

The more recent work of Hulka et al. offers another example of a meticulous comparison between assessments of the same care using explicit and implicit criteria, respectively.

As described in the preceding chapter, which drew extensively on this work (Charts 12–9 to 12–12), lists of explicit criteria for the office care of each of four conditions were drawn up based on the opinions of each of 31 internists concerning how "essential" the items were and how likely they were to be recorded. These trimmed-down lists of "consensual" criteria were first used to abstract and assess samples of records from the practices of the same internists, the measure of quality being the percent of applicable criteria adhered to, judging by the record. Later, narrative summaries were prepared for a subsample of these records, and each summary was submitted for separate assessment by three out of a group of ten internists, most of whom had earlier participated in formulating the explicit criteria, but who were not allowed to review their own cases. Each physician was asked to assess each case without benefit of explicit criteria, guided by "how he personally would have managed or evaluated the patient." The quality of care was to be classified as "excellent," "adequate," "inadequate," or "poor," with numerical equivalents ranging from 1 to 4 (p. 53).

To construct the chart, the cases reviewed by both methods were first classified according to the degree of adherence to explicit criteria into "low," "medium," or "high." The numerical equivalents of the three implicit judgments on each case were then averaged, and the distribution of the mean values divided into quartiles designated as "excellent," "adequate," "inadequate," and "poor," respectively. The chart shows that there is a high degree of positive association between these two kinds of ratings. For all cases compared, the correlation between the percent of explicit criteria adhered to and the numerical equivalent of the implicit judgment of quality was 0.68, a statistically significant association.

The investigators conclude that either method is suitable for quality assessment of ambulatory care, but that "the most productive strategy may be a combination of the two, the explicit criteria approach being used as a screening mechanism, and the implicit review being reserved for a sample of at least the low adherence records." I shall have more to say about this widely endorsed strategy when data from other studies are examined.

Chart 13-4

Percent of Cases Classified by Degree of Adherence to Explicit Criteria of the Process of Care, which Were Judged To Have Received Care of Specified Levels of Quality when Implicit Criteria Were Used To Assess Quality. Patients with Any of Four Conditions, in the Office Practice of Selected Internists, North Carolina, 1975-1977.

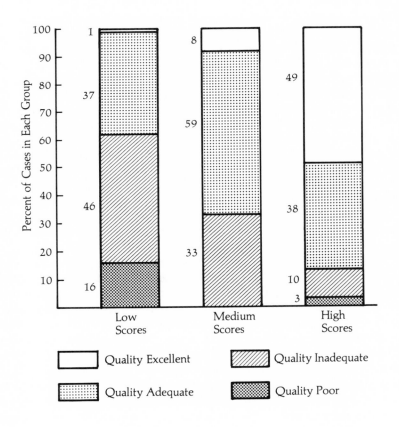

Source: Hulka et al. 1979, Table 43, p. 57.

Chart 13–5

In a study meant to test the "tracer methodology," but which was perhaps closer to the "trajectory" method described earlier in Chapter Nine of this book, Novick et al. examined the quality of care received by children with iron-deficiency. The information came from the medical records of 100 children, six months or older, reported to have a blood hemoglobin level of 11.0 gm or less per 100 ml. The "episode" of care was considered to begin with the visit during which the blood hemoglobin value was reported, and to end six months later (p. 5).

As is too often the case, the original cohort of 100 children suffered progressive attrition from step to step in the process of care. For example, in only 48 children was the presence of low hemoglobin recognized by the physician, and only 27 received treatment. (These findings can be compared with several reported in Chapter Nine of this book, and particularly with those shown in Chart 9–2.)

The quality of care received by the children with recognized anemia was assessed using explicit and implicit criteria in turn. The list of explicit criteria was made up of 22 items considered relevant to health outcomes by at least 80 percent of the medical staff who responded to a questionnaire. The review with implicit criteria was done by four pediatricians, each case being assessed independently by each of two judges. No "specific guidelines" were provided, only the care of the anemia was to be assessed, and the care was to be judged as "acceptable" or "unacceptable" in each of its parts (evaluation, diagnosis, treatment, and follow-up), and as a whole (pp. 8–9).

To construct the chart, 47 cases recognized by their physicians to have a low hemoglobin value were classified according to the "explicit criteria score," which is the percent of criteria adhered to, as shown in the record. For each of these categories, the chart shows the percent of cases which were judged, upon review by implicit criteria, to be acceptable to both judges, only to one, or to neither. It is clear that the two sets of judgments are positively associated. Kendall Rank Correlation Coefficients were computed for the care as a whole and for its subparts. The coefficients ranged from 0.37 to 0.46, all significant at $p < 0.05$ (p. 9).

The restriction of this study to a narrow circle of participant physicians may have contributed to the high degree of agreement on the explicit criteria, and to the concordance between the two sets of judgments reported above.

Chart 13–5

Percent of Children Recognized To Have Low Blood Hemoglobin, in Each of Four Categories Classified by Percent of Adherence to Explicit Criteria, Whose Care Was Found Acceptable or Unacceptable by One or Both of Two Reviewers when Judged by Implicit Criteria. Pediatric Ambulatory Clinic, Babies Hospital, Columbia-Presbyterian Medical Center, New York, May 1, 1973– April 30, 1974.

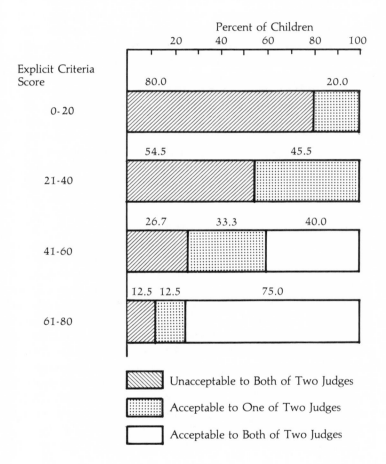

Source: Novick et al. 1976, based on additional information supplied by Dr. Novick.

Chart 13–6

Explicit criteria are difficult and costly to formulate but, once available, they can be used by nonprofessional personnel to assess care reliably and inexpensively. In many cases, however, the explicit criteria do not encompass the full variety of considerations that bear upon the management of any given patient. To make allowances for that variability, one or more expert professionals must review each case, using their own judgment, with or without the additional assistance of explicit criteria, to make a final, reasonably valid determination of the quality of care. This second method is extremely time consuming and costly. For these reasons, and because the results of assessments using explicit and implicit criteria correspond at least partially, it is usual to accomplish the monitoring of care in two steps. First, explicit criteria are used to identify cases which are likely to have been poorly managed; these cases are then submitted to "peer review," which means a full assessment, one by one.

If the judgment using implicit criteria is taken to be valid, especially when it is confirmed by two or more reviewers, the "screening efficiency" of the explicit criteria is signified by the proportion of questionable cases they correctly refer for further review, and the proportion of nonquestionable cases they correctly exclude from such review. The first is called the "sensitivity" of a test, and the second its "specificity." Generally, as one of these increases the other decreases, so that the problem is a choice of the proper balance between the two.

This chart, constructed from the data used in the preceding one, illustrates the consequences of using different levels of adherence to the explicit criteria ("explicit score") to indicate which cases require further review. For example, when only cases that fail to meet at least 20 percent of the criteria are reviewed, one sees, judging by the topmost bar on the left-hand side of the chart, that only 25 percent of the cases known to be unacceptable to both of two reviewers are included. But the corresponding bar on the right-hand side shows that the review is efficient, since 80 percent of the cases reviewed are found to be unacceptable to both judges. As the cutoff level on the range of explicit scores is raised, a larger proportion of the doubly unacceptable cases is detected, but at the cost of including progressively larger proportions of cases acceptable either to one reviewer ("mixed judgment"), or to both.

Chart 13–6

Percent that Would Be Included of All Care Known To Be Unacceptable to Both of Two Reviewers Using Implicit Criteria and the Percent Distribution of Specified Judgments Among Reviewed Cases, when Specified Levels of the Explicit Score Are Used To Select Cases for Further Review. Children with Low Blood Hemoglobin, Pediatric Ambulatory Clinic, Babies Hospital, Columbia-Presbyterian Medical Center, New York, May 1, 1973–April 30, 1974.

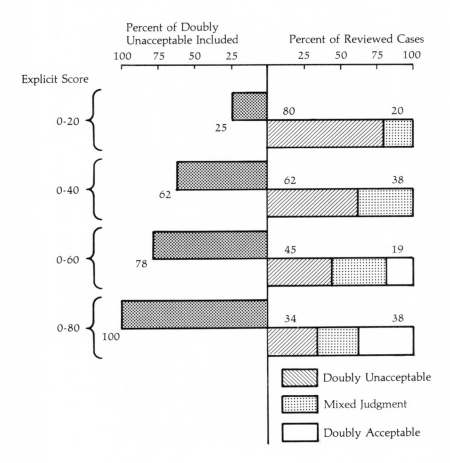

Source: Novick et al. 1976, based on additional information supplied by Dr. Novick.

Chart 13–7

Besides illustrating the use of "level of care" criteria, this chart offers another example of the considerations that enter a determination of the "screening efficiency" of explicit criteria, as judged by the correspondence between their dictates and the presumably more valid judgments based on professional review using implicit criteria.

The professional judgments are those of several teams, each made up of a physician and a nurse, who reviewed the care of patients in long-term institutions, mainly based on information in the record, but supplemented by questioning nurses and, if necessary, visiting the patients themselves. Some of the same information was then reassessed using certain explicit criteria. These were rather simple descriptions of (1) whether or not the patient's condition was unstable or worsening, (2) the number of the patient's functional limitations, (3) the number of nursing procedures in force, (4) the number of rehabilitative procedures used, and (5) the number of medications taken. This information was combined in several ways to arrive at six decision rules according to each of which one could classify a patient as needing skilled care or not. The chart shows how the decisions indicated by each of a selection of these rules would correspond to the presumably more valid professional judgments based on implicit criteria.

Beginning at the top of the chart, we see that Rule Six is very "sensitive," since it would correctly include 95 percent of the cases professional review had determined to require skilled care. It would, however, also incorrectly include a large proportion of the cases judged by professional review not to need it. This percentage is the complement of the property called "specificity," which for Rule Six is quite low: 33 percent. The percent of all cases correctly identified by Rule Six to either require or not require skilled care is 41 percent, as indicated by the corresponding bar on the right-hand side of the chart. As one goes down the chart, the decision rules become successively less "sensitive" and more "specific." The last of the four rules shown leads to the most accurate decisions, even though it correctly identifies only 71 percent of those requiring care. It may not be, however, the best rule to adopt. That depends on which of the two errors is more costly and dangerous to health: that of placing a person who requires skilled care in an institution that does not provide it, or of placing one who does not require skilled care in an institution that does provide it.

Chart 13–7

Percent of Patients Who, Compared to a Judgment Using Implicit Criteria,
Would Be Correctly or Incorrectly Excluded or Included, by Specified Rules
Using Explicit Criteria, among Those Needing Skilled Care. Federally Funded
Patients in Long-term Care Facilities, Baltimore Professional Standards Review
Organization (PSRO), Maryland, February–June 1977.

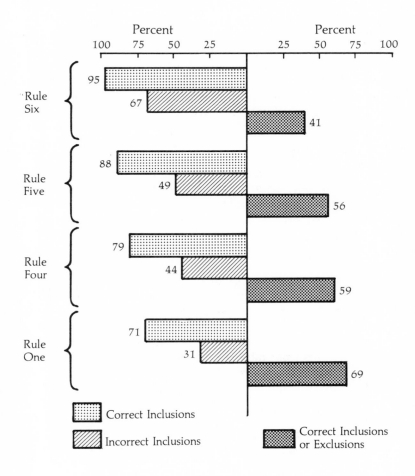

Source and Note: Kane et al. 1981, Table 1, p. 6. The phenomena to which the percentages on the
abscissas refer are identified in the text.

Chart 13–8

The contribution of a set of patient characteristics, individually or in combination, to the probability that skilled care is needed can also be determined more precisely by a logistic regression, assuming one has a valid determination of that need. Kane et al. used the information they had obtained (as described in connection with the preceding chart) on half of their patients to develop four logistic equations; the information on the other half was used to test the equations.

Given the characteristics of any one patient, the logistic equation yields the probability that the patient would be judged by professional review to need skilled care. By arraying a set of patients according to these probabilities, it is possible to determine the consequences of using successively higher levels of the probability as a threshold, or cutoff level, for deciding which patients would be likely truly to need skilled nursing care, as judged by professional review, and which not. The chart shows the results for the two most different logistic equations: A and D. For any given threshold, the ordinate of the chart gives the percent of those cases known by professional review to need skilled care that would be correctly identified. This is the "sensitivity," or "true positive," ratio of the scale at that threshold. Simultaneously, the abscissa shows the percent of cases known not to require skilled care which would be incorrectly identified as needing such care when that threshold is used. This is the "false positive ratio," the complement of the "specificity" of the scale at that threshold.

The curve shown was fitted by inspection to the successive probability thresholds derived from Equation A. Such a curve, one that shows the true positive and false positive yields of a measurement scale at successive cutoff levels of that scale, is called a receiver operating characteristic curve, or ROC curve. It represents the overall power of a test to discriminate true positives from false positives, and can be used to select the most efficient cutoff level, provided that one knows the proportion of true positives in the population being screened, and can also specify the consequences of finding and missing true positives and negatives.

The chart shows that the two logistic equations yield information of about equal discriminating power since they fall on, or close to, the same curve. This is also true of the much simpler "empirical decision rules" illustrated in the preceding chart.

Chart 13–8

Receiver Operating Characteristic Curve Portraying the Ability of Specified Types of Explicit Criteria to Discriminate between Patients Who Do or Do Not Require Skilled Care, as Determined by Professional Review Using Implicit Criteria. Federally Funded Patients in Long-term Care Facilities, Baltimore Professional Standards Review Organization (PSRO), Maryland, February–June 1977.

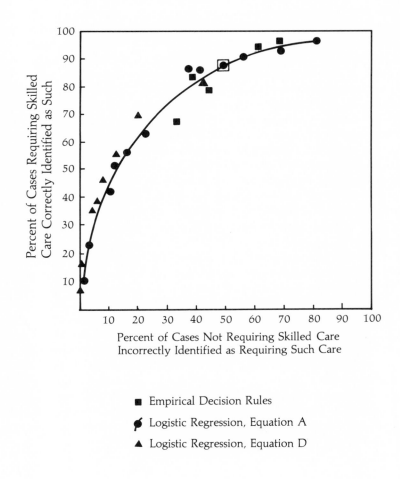

Percent of Cases Not Requiring Skilled Care
Incorrectly Identified as Requiring Such Care

■ Empirical Decision Rules

∮ Logistic Regression, Equation A

▲ Logistic Regression, Equation D

Source: Kane et al. 1981, Table 7, p. 13, including my own computations.

Chart 13–9

We now move on to a comparison of two different forms of explicit criteria: the criteria map and the criteria list. To accomplish the comparison, the investigators studied a sample of patients, 30 years old or older, who came to one of two emergency departments complaining of chest pain. The medical records were used to assess the care received.

The first method of assessment used one of four lists that specified the items of information, from the medical history, physical examination, and diagnostic tests, that were deemed necessary to arrive at a decision to admit or not admit the patient to the hospital. The items on the lists were weighted differentially, and the quality of care was measured by the "list score," which is the weighted percent of items complied with. The second method of assessment used a "criteria map" for chest pain. The map takes the form of a branching logic tree. It first classifies patients according to characteristics determined when they come for care. These characteristics may indicate the need for further investigations which the map specifies, and the findings of these investigations may indicate a second set of appropriate actions which are also specified, and so on, until the map indicates the need either to admit the patient to the hospital or to send him home. In this case, the map included estimates of the probabilities that patients with specified characteristics and findings would be sick enough to require hospital care. These probabilities are the "map scores" which were compared to the "list scores" already described.

The appropriateness of the decision to discharge the patient was verified by checking the patient's condition within the following week or two. The decision to admit was assessed by knowing what happened during the hospital stay. In this way all patients were classified as having had or not having had "admissible disease" when first seen.

The right-hand side of the chart shows that the criteria map scores were successful in indicating the presence of "admissible disease": as the scores rise, the percentage with "admissible disease" increases, the association being highly significant statistically. The relationship with criteria-list scores, shown on the left-hand side of the chart, is also significant, but in the opposite direction. The cases that are least fully investigated in the emergency department are the ones most likely to have "admissible disease." The consequences of this disparity are shown in the next chart.

Chart 13-9

Percent of Patients with Disease Severe Enough to Require Admission to the Hospital, among Patients Classified by Scores Derived from a Criteria Map or Applicable Criteria Lists, Respectively. Adult Patients with Chest Pain at Two Emergency Departments, Los Angeles, California, April–August 1977, and January–April 1978.

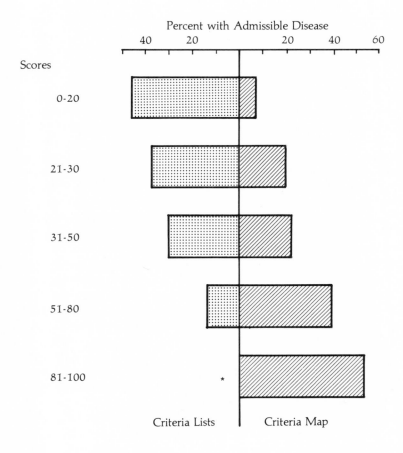

Source and Note: Greenfield et al. 1981, based on my measurements from earlier and larger versions of Figures 4-7, pp. 263-65, and on my computations. The asterisk indicates that no cases earned a criteria-list score higher than 80.

Chart 13–10

The second step in the investigation portrayed in the preceding chart was to determine the ability of the criteria to distinguish patients who should be sent home from those who should be admitted to the hospital.

The investigators expected that as the criteria-map scores became larger, the decision to admit the patient to the hospital would be more likely to be correct, and the decision to send the patient home to be incorrect. They also reasoned that higher criteria-list scores would mean a more thorough investigation of the patient in the emergency department and, therefore, a greater likelihood of a correct decision either to admit or not. But the predictive power of either scale would not be perfect: at any cutoff level of the scale, some patients would be correctly and others erroneously classified.

The chart shows the findings for patients admitted to the hospital. The question pertaining to "screening efficiency" may be posed as follows: If the hospitalized cases are arrayed according to (1) the criteria-map score and (2) the criteria-list score, and successive cutoff levels (or "operating positions") are selected to review cases because they are presumed to have been inappropriately admitted, what percent of inappropriate admissions would one correctly include in the review, and what percent of appropriate admissions would one review unnecessarily? The chart provides the answer for "operating positions" at ten-point intervals of each scale, and shows the receiver operating characteristic (ROC) curve that may be plotted as a result.

The shape of the ROC curve for the criteria-map scale, convex upward and to the left, suggests that the scale is reasonably discriminating. The information it offers "permits a user to select a rational cut-point, explicitly acknowledging the tradeoffs between failure to review a case of inappropriate disposition and needless review of appropriate disposition" (Greenfield et al. 1982, p. 29). The ROC curve generated by the selected "operating positions" on the criteria-list scale is either very close to, or somewhat worse than, the discrimination one would obtain by random sampling, which is represented by the diagonal on the chart. This inferior performance may be explained by the indirect and complex relationship between the list score and the accuracy of the decision to admit. On the one hand, more thorough investigation should lead to better decisions, but on the other hand, when a patient is obviously quite sick, it is reasonable to hospitalize without completing the ordinarily prescribed investigations.

Chart 13-10

Receiver Operating Characteristic (ROC) Curves Showing, Respectively, the
Percent of Inappropriate Admissions and the Percent of Appropriate Admis-
sions that Would Be Reviewed Using Each of Specified Operating Positions on
Scales of Criteria-Map Scores and Criteria-List Scores. Adult Patients with Chest
Pain Admitted to the Hospital from Two Emergency Departments, Los
Angeles, California, April–August 1977, and January–April 1978.

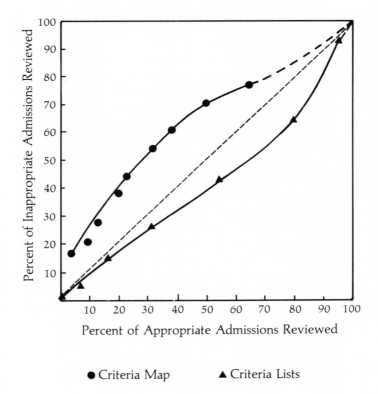

Source: Greenfield et al. 1981, based on my measurements from earlier and larger versions of
Figures 4–7, pp. 263-65, and on my computations.

Chart 13–11

With this chart we take another step in our comparison of assessment methods, this time to look at the degree of agreement between judgments of quality based on outcomes and those based on process. Neither the study from which the chart was drawn nor the kind of comparison it presents are new to us. The antecedents and the implementation of the "problem status" method were described in connection with Chart 8–10, and a comparison of outcome and process was illustrated in Chart 8–11. This chart and the next will pick up the thread of a narrative already begun.

We now have a group of children with otitis media, upper respiratory tract infection, sore throat, and conjunctivitis. The standards specify that within a month of receiving care all should have recovered fully: none having any symptoms, limitation of activity, or anxiety referable to these illnesses. In fact, 87 percent achieved this happy state, but in the remaining 13 percent the outcome was "substandard" because it failed to fully achieve one or more of the objectives mentioned above.

The quality of care provided to these patients was determined by professional review of the medical record without prior knowledge of the "problem status outcome." The reviewing physicians were guided by explicit criteria that specified, for each illness, the diagnostic and therapeutic activities which should be performed and recorded in every case. But the reviewers went beyond that; they also used their own judgments "to identify any errors in diagnosis or management that may have adversely affected the outcome" (p. 9).

The chart, by demonstrating an absence of a relationship between outcome and process, should delight the iconoclast. Had I wanted a different conclusion, I could have chosen to show another segment of this larger study, one in which the outcomes of caring for three acute conditions in adults were very strongly related to judgments of quality made in the way described above (pp. 25–30). I chose the negative findings partly to have them stand for all such reports in the literature, but mainly to use them as a step leading to the findings shown in the next chart.

Chart 13–11

Percent of Children with Acceptable or Substandard Outcomes Whose Care Was Judged by Professional Review Using a Combination of Explicit and Implicit Criteria to Have Specified Deficiencies or None. Columbia Medical Plan, Columbia, Maryland, May 22–June 13, 1974.

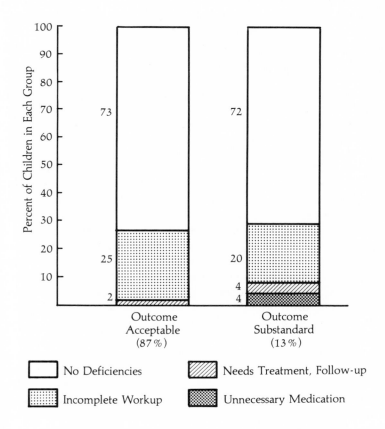

Source: Mushlin and Appel 1980, Table 4-8, p. 31 and text on p. 30.

Chart 13–12

Unlike the study illustrated in the preceding chart, this investigation included all children with problems, the standards of expected outcome were set individually by each child's physician, and the deadline for checking on the outcomes was moved forward to ten days following the initiation of care. At this time, the parents were questioned by telephone, not only about the child's "problem status," but also about things like the time spent at the clinic and with the physician, instructions received, knowledge acquired, compliance with recommendations, and satisfaction with the care received.

All children who failed to achieve any one of the outcomes forecast by their physicians, and a sample of those who achieved them all, were called back for reexamination by a pediatrician not connected with the health plan. The medical records of the children were assessed using implicit criteria, and care was classified as acceptable or substandard. The care received was also classified as improvable or not based on all the information amassed, including the parents' reports, the findings on reexamination, and the chart audit.

The chart shows that 77 percent of the children were judged to have attained acceptable "problem status outcomes," while 23 percent failed to do so. The findings of the chart audit were very infrequently unfavorable, and failed to distinguish between cases with acceptable or substandard outcomes. By contrast, more complete information, particularly about the interpersonal aspects of care and compliance with the regimen, showed the process of care to be improvable in 56 percent of cases with substandard outcomes, as compared to only seven percent of those with acceptable outcomes. Moreover, in 72 percent of cases with substandard outcomes but unimprovable care, the child was only taking longer to recover than expected by the physician, an error of the method that might have been corrected by better forecasts, a change in the time of observation, or another telephone call a little later. In the remaining cases, a complication of the current illness, or a new illness, had intervened.

Of the deficiencies in care revealed by this study, 42 percent were attributed to the practitioners, 50 percent to the patients and their families, and eight percent to the health plan. By reviewing the 23 percent of all cases with substandard outcomes, one would identify 70 percent of the cases with such deficiencies: a creditable level of "screening efficiency."

Chart 13–12

Percent of Children with Acceptable or Substandard Outcomes Whose Care Was Judged To Be Substandard by Chart Audit and Improvable Based on More Complete Information. Columbia Medical Plan, Columbia, Maryland, October 1975.

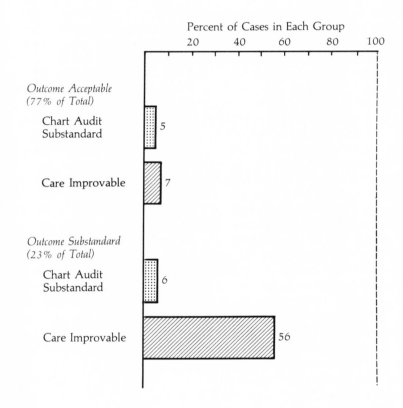

Source: Mushlin and Appel 1980, Table 4-15, p. 38, with minor recomputations.

Chart 13–13

This chart provides more finely detailed information about the relationship between two quantitative measures of quality, one based on explicit
criteria of process and the other on explicit criteria of outcome. The
subjects of the first study were women, between 15 and 50 years of age,
who came to the emergency departments of a voluntary and municipal
hospital complaining of symptoms indicating urinary tract infection, but
who had no other serious complicating disease. The subjects of the second study were patients of both sexes, between the ages of 19 and 55,
treated for asthma not complicated by chronic obstructive pulmonary
disease at the emergency services of the same voluntary hospital and of
a municipal hospital that replaced the one studied earlier.

The process of care was assessed on the basis of information in the
medical record, using a list of weighted explicit criteria. The outcomes
of care were assessed on the basis of information obtained by telephone,
using a list of weighted explicit criteria pertaining to three objectives:
(1) satisfaction with the physician and the clinic; (2) feeling better; and
(3) knowing about the diagnosis, the treatment, and the arrangements
for follow-up. The about 50 percent of patients who could be reached at
home seemed similar to those who could not be contacted.

The chart shows a significant relationship between process and outcome scores for both conditions, even though the assessment of process
was based entirely on adherence to criteria of technical care, and the
assessment of outcome was based preponderantly on the clients' satisfaction and knowledge. The coefficient of the correlation between the
process and outcome scores for urinary tract infection was 0.379 ($p <$
0.02), and for asthma it was 0.350 ($p < 0.005$). The chart does not show
the outcomes that patients with asthma reported seven days after the
initiation of care. The fact that these were not significantly related to
process highlights the need to select the appropriate time interval for
assessing the outcomes of care in each instance.

The chart suggests that, at least for asthma, the relationship between
process and outcome is curvilinear, so that beyond a certain point, further improvements in process do not contribute to the outcomes measured. But that does not necessarily mean that other, unmeasured
outcomes are not favorably influenced.

Chart 13–13

Mean Outcome Scores for Patients with Asthma and Urinary Tract Infection, Respectively, Classified According to a Physician Performance Index Based on Adherence to Explicit Criteria of Process. Emergency Services of Two Hospitals, North Bronx, New York. Adult Women with Urinary Tract Infection, circa 1975, and Adults with Asthma, 1978.

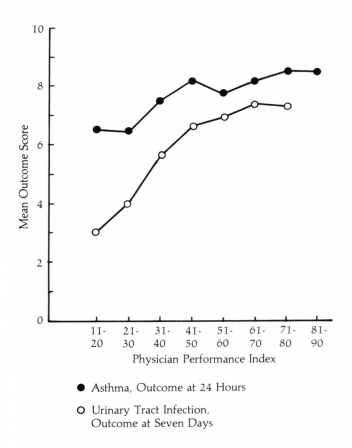

Physician Performance Index

● Asthma, Outcome at 24 Hours

○ Urinary Tract Infection,
Outcome at Seven Days

Source: Mates and Sidel 1981, Figure 2, p. 690. Reprinted by permission, American Public Health Association. Also see Rubenstein et al. 1977.

Chart 13–14

The final chart in this chapter offers a rare glimpse of a subject about which we know next to nothing: the extent to which experts and clients agree about the quality of the same care.

The data come from the first of two studies of hospital care received by members of a Teamsters Union local and their families who lived in and around New York City. The care assessed is that of patients with one of eight diagnoses selected to represent obstetrics and gynecology, general surgery, and medicine (p. 8). The complete medical record of each case was reviewed by an expert skilled in such audits. Each reviewer was simply asked: "Would you have handled this particular case in this fashion and if not, why?" (p. 16). Accordingly, the reviewers designated the management of each case as "excellent," "good," "fair," or "poor." During a household interview about the use of health services and their costs, each patient was also asked to say whether the care received during the sampled hospital admission was "best," "reasonably good," or "not good" (p. 42).

The chart shows that there is some correspondence between the two separate opinions of the quality of the same care, one an expert's and one the patient's. When the patients saw their care as "best," the experts judged the care to be "fair" or "poor" in 38 percent of cases; when the patients judged their care as "not good," the experts concurred by finding the care to have been "fair" or "poor" in 82 percent. But the correspondence is not close.

By other manipulations of the data we see that these patients had a much more favorable view of their care than was warranted. Of the cases judged by the experts to have been less than "good," the patients found only 20 percent to be less than the "best," and a mere five percent to be "not good." When the care was judged by experts to have been "excellent" or "good," it was almost never called "not good" by patients, such a discrepancy occurring in only 0.8 percent of cases. Thus, patient judgment was highly "specific," though rather "insensitive."

Though this study does not tell us what made patients believe that their care was less than the "best," we may conclude that, to a very large degree, patients judge quality on grounds very different from the technical considerations that preoccupy the expert reviewer of medical records. We have only just begun to act on the conviction that the quality of health care is not exclusively in the professionals' domain.

Chart 13-14

Percent Distribution of Hospital Admissions According to Expert Judgments of the Quality of Care Based on Implicit Criteria, in Each of Specified Categories Classified According to the Patients' Opinions of the Quality of Care. Hospital Admissions of Families of Members of a Teamsters Union Local, for Selected Diagnoses, New York Metropolitan Area and Environs, 1975.

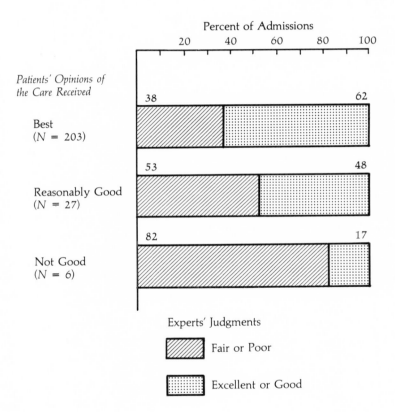

Source: Ehrlich et al., 1962 , Table 30, p. 79.

Epilogue

EPILOGUE

Introduction

Any book that requires an epilogue may be suspected of having been dilatory and inconclusive. In this case, the very nature of the subject matter may have made it so; for I have attempted to arrest, as it were, a bird in midflight, hoping thereby to understand its origins, its destination, and the dazzling mystery of its performance. Where the quality of care is concerned, though we know something about these matters, there is much, much more that we are ignorant of. "For now we see," as did the Apostle, only "through a glass, darkly" (1 Cor. 13:12). Almost everything we say, therefore, is provisional, hedged with reservations, tinged with doubt. And yet, while we search for a more perfect truth, we must act, in good faith, upon what we now think we know.

The Definition of Quality

We may begin with some fundamental postulates. We cannot assess quality until we have decided with what meanings to invest the concept. A clear definition of quality is the foundation upon which everything else is built.

These *Explorations* have adopted the view that quality comprises those attributes of the process of care that contribute to its desired outcomes. The assessment of quality varies, therefore, depending on the outcomes sought, the valuations placed on the outcomes, and the appropriateness of the means used to attain them. These considerations, in their turn, are modified by whether the assessment is made on behalf of individual patients or the community at large, whether the preferences of individuals are explicitly sought and taken into account, and whether monetary cost is included in assessing the means employed.

Because many of these issues are conceptual, almost philosophical, in nature, and because they are only now beginning to be made explicit, there is little empirical information that is directly pertinent to them. By a review of the available literature, as illustrated in the first chapter of this book, we find that clients and practitioners have somewhat different views of what makes a good physician or a good clinic, and of what the properties of good care are. There is, nevertheless, a core of attributes upon which most seem to agree. And the area of agreement would no doubt grow wider if clients and practitioners were to listen to each other.

From such an exchange we would perhaps come away convinced that personal attention and technical competence are the inseparable pair of attributes upon which all else depends, except for the disturbing presence of monetary cost.

Quality and Monetary Cost

From the data assembled in Chapter Two we see that there are different styles of clinical management; some are more costly than others, but not necessarily more efficacious. By reducing redundant care one lowers costs without damaging quality; by eliminating harmful care one lowers costs while quality is actually improved. So far, there should be no disagreement on how monetary cost and quality relate to one another, though it has been remarkably difficult to specify what should be considered to be redundant care. The bewildering, almost insuperable, difficulty comes about when one has to weigh the additional benefits against the additional costs, as care becomes progressively more elaborate and costly. While the balancing of costs and benefits is, fundamentally, an ethical issue, it is becoming clear that quality assessment is not complete unless the relation between costs and benefits has been elucidated.

The Strategies and Criteria of Care

Understanding and documenting the relation between quality and costs is part of a larger enterprise whose findings determine how the definition of quality is translated into more specific criteria and standards. Insofar as technical care is concerned, these criteria derive from the scientific bases of clinical practice. This is the science that tells us how the procedures of care contribute to specified outcomes. At any given time, the assessment of technical quality is totally contingent on the clinical sciences; whatever certainty or ambiguity characterizes the latter will also, necessarily, be reflected in the former.

Technical care is best characterized as a strategy that defines the stepwise progression of diagnosis and therapy as these are governed by specified decision rules. The specification of optimal strategies, with or without attention to monetary cost, is the responsibility of the clinical sciences. Quality assessment is primarily concerned with whether or not the strategies that are already known to be optimal have been applied.

Because the notion of strategies is so important to quality assessment, I have provided, mainly in Chapter Ten, some examples of how strategies are specified, and how they are tested by decision analysis (Charts 2–1; 10–4, 10–5), epidemiological investigation (10–1 through 10–3, 10–6), or clinical trial (10–7). Their direct application to quality assessment is illustrated in Chapter 13 by the work of Greenfield and his associates (13–9, 13–10). It should be remembered, however, that all the criteria of technical care, whatever their nature or format, are more or less faithful representations of underlying strategies of care that are, themselves, more or less rigorously tested, and more or less clearly perceived.

Choice of an Approach to Assessment

Having in hand a clear definition of quality, and the necessary knowledge that ties means to consequences, we can proceed to the assessment itself. Here we have a range of choices which I have grouped under the three headings of "process," "outcome," and "structure."

The relative merits of assessing process as compared to outcome have been much debated, often under rather dubious assumptions. Having dealt with the subject in great detail in Volume I of these *Explorations* (Donabedian 1980), I will spare the reader yet another lengthy disquisition. It is enough to say that process and outcome are members of a symmetrical pair; that neither is inherently more valid than the other, since validity resides in the bond that ties them; that the choice of one in preference to the other is mainly based on practical considerations such as the availability, costliness, accuracy, and timeliness of information; and that where possible there is safety and persuasiveness in obtaining information about both. There are, nevertheless, enough differences between the methods of assessing process and outcome to justify classifying these methods, as was done in this book, as belonging primarily under one or the other of the two approaches, provided the presence of combined or hybrid forms is also recognized.

The Assessment of Process

Assessments of process seem to fall into two general classes that correspond to what are usually known as "utilization review" and "quality assessment" respectively. I have observed this distinction by devoting a chapter to "The Justification of Resource Use" (Chapter Three) and another to "The Justification of Surgery" (Chapter Four). One should recognize, however, that the distinction between utilization review and quality assessment rests on a presumed separation between quantity and quality that can sometimes be made on reasonable grounds, but which is often difficult or impossible to justify.

There can be two kinds of judgments on the process of care. One is based on the extent to which the care provided is expected to attain the greatest improvement in health that the science of health care makes possible, irrespective of monetary cost. The other judgment is whether or not the least costly means have been used to seek the largest expected benefits in health care. If one could devise a new nomenclature, the procedures used to arrive at the first of these judgments would be called "effectiveness review" or "effectiveness assessment," and those that lead to the second judgment would be called "efficiency review" or "efficiency assessment." Strictly speaking, "utilization review" would then be identified with "efficiency review," insofar as efficiency or inefficiency are attributable to the judgments of the practitioners whose performance is being assessed. It would not, as often happens now, include considerations of whether or not the use of services is harmful to health.

Pursuant to this analysis, quality assessment would always include "effectiveness assessment" or "review" to the extent that variations in that effectiveness or ineffectiveness are brought about by variations in clinical judgment or skill. Whether it would include "efficiency assessment" or "review" would depend on whether monetary cost is or is not considered to be a component in the definition of quality, as I have explained elsewhere (Donabedian 1980, pp. 7–16; Donabedian et al. 1982).

Assessments of resource use in particular, and of the process of care in general, can rest on evidence of many kinds, leading to different degrees of certainty. In some cases a procedure is so clearly obsolete or so rarely indicated that its mere occurrence deserves investigation (3–1 through 3–3). More often, there is an even weaker presumption of error based on evidence that some element of care (which is often appropriate) is used more frequently or less often than one might expect (2–3 through 2–5, 2–8; 4–1 through 4–13, 4–15 through 4–17). The presumption is strengthened if the discrepancies persist after corrections are made for population attributes that might justify them; the presumption is still further strengthened if an association with a higher incidence of adverse outcomes is observed (4–2, 4–3, 4–10). Greater certainty that an error has occurred, and a deeper understanding of the nature and causation of error, require a more detailed examination of the process of care, an examination that calls for implicit or explicit criteria and standards of good care.

Assessments of the process of care can also vary in their timing. Sometimes they are "prospective," being made after a service has been recommended, but before it is actually delivered. The purpose is to prevent injudicious use. At other times they are "concurrent," being instituted during the course of care. The purpose is to intervene so as to minimize the consequences of past error and prevent the occurrence of future error. Most often, the assessments of process are "retrospective," being based on the records of past care. The purpose of retrospective assessments is to prevent future error through a variety of interventions that may include education and changes in how the system of care is designed and run.

We have seen illustrations of all these variants of process assessment in the chapters that constitute Part II of this book. Surgical procedures offer a particularly interesting example of the way in which epidemiological observations contribute to an understanding of the quality of health care (4–1 through 4–18). Second surgical opinion programs are an illustration of "prospective" intervention (4–24 through 4–31). "Concurrent" monitoring and intervention are illustrated by their most celebrated exemplar, that of assessing the appropriateness of hospital stay (3–13 through 3–18). Particular pains were taken to show how an understanding of the properties of inappropriate hospital admission and of stays is needed to design a monitoring procedure, and how that design, in its turn, influences the costs and benefits of monitoring.

The Assessment of Outcomes

The assessment of process can be supplemented, or to some degree replaced, by the assessment of outcomes. I have perceived outcomes to be primarily states of health or ill health. But the outcomes suitable for assessing quality can include knowledge, attitudes, and behaviors that have the potential either to ameliorate, or cause a deterioration in, future health. The satisfaction of the client with past or present care is partly an outcome of that care. Satisfaction is also a judgment by the client on aspects of the quality of care that the client is particularly capable of appreciating, as well as an attribute that is conducive to better care in the future.

The outcomes that have a bearing on quality assessment are changes that can be attributed to health care in the immediate or more distant past. This relation leads to several consequences which are represented in Part III of this book, where the studies of outcome are classified and reviewed.

The requirement that outcomes be readily attributable to prior care narrows the choice to phenomena that are relevant to the feasible goals of that care and are sensitive to variations in its quality. Since many factors other than health care can also influence outcomes independently of, or by interaction with, prior health care, it is important that the influence of such factors should be relatively small and, in addition, be well understood so that it can be allowed for in the collection and analysis of data. (See, for example, 7–4 through 7–6, 7–11.) Such considerations, plus the availability of data, have influenced the choice of the outcome measures illustrated in Chapter Seven. These include maternal mortality (7–2), infant mortality and its subparts (7–1 through 7–3), case fatality (7–4, 7–5, 7–9), postoperative mortality and morbidity (7–6 through 7–8, 7–10), and preventable morbidity (7–12). Neither crude mortality nor overall longevity are sensitive or specific enough as measures of quality. But longevity following particular types of care for specific conditions is a measure of great potential usefulness, especially if attributes of the quality of life are added to the record of mere survival (7–11).

Because the relationship between process and outcome is a change in the probability of certain outcomes being observed, a large number of observations is needed to order to establish the relationship. Moreover, it is important, as shown in Chapter Seven, to adjust for the effect of factors (other than variations in health care) which may also have influenced the outcomes observed. In some instances it is not feasible to make such adjustments, either because the factors are not clearly understood or the information needed about known factors is not available. When, as is often true in clinical practice, the cases to be assessed are few in number, statistical findings are too subject to sampling variation to be conclusive. And, of course, statistical analyses are inapplicable to the assessment of individual cases.

The methods of outcome assessment depicted and described in Chapter Eight are a response to one or more of these considerations. These methods have a common feature: the resort to an assessment of process whenever the outcomes are unsatisfactory. In other words, adverse outcomes are only taken as presumptive evidence of poor quality; the definitive judgment rests on the assessment of the process of care.

Beyond this key feature, the methods differ in several ways. In some, the occurrence of an unacceptable outcome in any one case is sufficient to prompt review. The adverse event may be, as in the studies conducted under the aegis of the New York Academy of Medicine, either a maternal death (8–1 through 8–4) or the death of an infant (8–5 through 8–7). It may also be, as in the work of Mushlin and Appel, a goal either set for each individual patient by his physician, or for a group of similar patients by a committee of physicians who define the achievable standard which *every* patient in the group should attain (8–10, 8–11; 13–11, 13–12). In still another method, devised by Williamson, the standard of achievement is set for groups of patients, rather than individuals, and it is expressed as a probability of the occurrence of any one of a wide range of outcomes (8–9; 12–7, 12–18). Because this probability is almost always much below 100 percent, the failure of any one patient to attain the expected outcomes does not trigger a review. The process of care is reviewed only when the observed occurrence of prespecified outcomes is significantly outside a preselected acceptable range.

Outcomes always follow the care to which they are attributed. The methods that use outcomes to pass a judgment on the quality of antecedent care are, therefore, always "retrospective." But this truth notwithstanding, the classification adopted for Chapter Eight does recognize the peculiar significance of specifying the expected outcomes prior to the assessment of care by considering the methods that use this approach as "prospective" in orientation (8–9 through 8–11). Besides setting this category apart from the "retrospective" methods of outcome assessment that do not set such expectations in advance (8–1 through 8–8), this distinction alerts us to the difficulties of formulating valid criteria of outcome—a difficulty that is illustrated in Chapter Twelve of this book (12–7, 12–18).

The methods that depend on the observation of outcomes to trigger an assessment of process may be seen as combining two approaches to assessment. There are a number of other methods that present this ambiguity. These methods, besides combining the assessment of process and outcome, also seem more oriented to evaluating the performance of systems of care than of individual practitioners or groups of practitioners. Partly because they have these features, but mainly for convenience, these methods have been grouped in Chapter Nine of this book, being described there as the "staging concept," the "trajectory," and the "tracer method."

The "staging" method introduced by Gonnella and Goran (1975) may be used to classify cases into clinically homogeneous groups, so that their further progress can be more readily attributed to differences in health care. The more distinctive contribution of this approach, however, is the use of the stage at which the disease first comes to notice (for example, when the patient is admitted to the hospital) as a presumptive indicator of the effectiveness of the system of care responsible for care prior to this event (9–8).

Brook and Stevenson (1970) are responsible for calling renewed attention to a method that I have called the "trajectory." This method consists of selecting a cohort of patients and following their progression through a system of health care so as to note how successfully they attain specified landmarks in the process of care, and with what changes in health status (9–1 through 9–5). The "tracer method" introduced by Kessner et al. (1973) can be seen to use a collection of such trajectories, except that the selection of the "tracers" whose trajectories are to be delineated are rigorously systematized by a "matrix" which defines the features of the health care system concerning which information is being sought (9–6,

9–7). All these trajectories, irrespective of their number or method of selection, can either be constructed "retrospectively" using the records of past care, or "prospectively" by starting in the present and obtaining information about events as they unfold.

The Assessment of Structure

The potential contribution of "structure" to quality assessment is recognized only indirectly in this book. It is revealed through information about the relation between the quality of process or outcome on the one hand, and the attributes of practitioners and organizations on the other. The elucidation of these relations is part of the science of health care organization, insofar as such a science can be said to exist. In turn, whatever we learn about the relation will permit us, in the future, to use the structural attributes, with varying degrees of confidence, as more or less rough indicators of the expected quality of the process and outcomes of care.

The contribution of structural attributes to quality has, of course, implications far beyond the construction of devices to measure quality. A knowledge of that contribution helps us map what might be called the "epidemiology of quality," which is its distribution among the providers of care on the one hand, and among its potential recipients on the other. Since, in essence, this constitutes the main body of substantive findings which quality assessments produce, I shall return to the subject after this brief summary of the methods of quality assessment and monitoring is completed.

Selection of the Care To Be Assessed

Having chosen "structure," "process," or "outcome" as the primary "approach" to assessment, it is next necessary to select the care to be assessed, to specify the criteria and standards of assessment, and to obtain the necessary information.

The choice of the care to be assessed is dictated by the circumstances and purposes of the assessment. It is determined, first, by the nature of organizational responsibility. Since this responsibility is often confined to a single site (such as the hospital) or a category of practitioners (such as physicians), it is rare to find assessments of the process of care that comprehend all phases of an episode, including care at a succession of sites by a variety of practitioners. This limitation is amply documented in this book by virtue of its having dealt almost exclusively with the care provided by physicians either in hospitals or in ambulatory care settings, though there are occasional examples of assessments that attempted to combine ambulatory and hospital care—as in the studies conducted by Payne et al. in Hawaii (6–13 through 6–22), to assess care in other than these two settings—as in the study of nursing homes by Kane et al. (13–7, 13–8), and to evaluate the performance of practitioners other than physicians—as in the studies of pharmaceutical services (2–9) and of the care provided by nurses in the hospital (5–8) or in the patient's home (6–6).

The selection of the categories of sites and practitioners is only the first step in the identification of the care to be assessed. Next, one needs to select the specific sites, the specific practitioners, the specific sequences of care, and the specific populations served. In all these choices, organizational responsibility and feasibility are almost always the determining factors. The findings, as we have seen, are consequently anecdotal and illustrative, rather than representative and generalizable.

There are, of course, some exceptions. We have seen examples of representative sampling of physicians (as in the studies of general practice by Peterson et al. and by Clute), of hospitals (as in the work of Payne et al.), of hospital admissions (as in the work of Morehead et al.), and of maternal and infant deaths (as in the studies at the New York Academy of Medicine). But in each of these instances, the sampling is deficient in ways that seriously limit the inferences that can be drawn. The general practitioners studied by Peterson et al. or by Clute (5–1 to 5–7; 11–1) do not represent their fellow students in medical school. Payne et al. sampled admissions, not physicians, and they confined their sample to a subset of diagnoses which do not necessarily represent all others (6–13 through 6–22; 12–15). Similarly, the care provided to mothers or infants who die (8–1 through 8–8) cannot be said to represent the care of those who do not. And all these studies, as well as all the others cited in this book, are shaped and constrained by the circumstances of their time and place. It takes a sustained effort of creative, but disciplined, imagination to weave their findings into a persuasively coherent whole.

In most studies of quality, the segments of care chosen for assessment are highly selected. Conditions are included for a variety of reasons: because they are common; because it is suspected that deficiencies in care are frequent and consequential, but remediable; because the criteria and standards of care are reasonably clear and agreed upon; because the necessary information is more likely to be available in the medical record or elsewhere; because successful care is not highly dependent on patient cooperation. As a result of these requirements, one finds a remarkable repetitiousness in the conditions chosen for study, a repetitiousness that the reader will have already noted.

This selectivity in the choice of conditions for assessment limits our ability to generalize, but it also helps us to compare studies more easily. Moreover, selectivity is not only permissible, but also desirable, when the only purpose is to monitor care in order to detect and correct significant deficiencies. But even when monitoring, rather than research, is the objective, there may be room for a modest program of representative sampling; the purpose is to make sure that no important weaknesses have been overlooked.

Insofar as the selection of conditions for study is concerned, the "tracer" method advocated by Kessner et al. (9–6) offers a reasonable compromise between probability sampling and unsystematic selection. The "tracer matrix" specifies the dimensions of the health care system concerning which information is to be sought. By a judicious selection of conditions (each called a "tracer") it is possible to obtain information about each cell of the matrix. The yet unsubstantiated assumption is that there is a high degree of correlation between the quality of care for each tracer and the quality of care for all other conditions for which that tracer is a stand-in (9–6, 9–7).

The Criteria and Standards of Assessment

There is a relationship between the method of selecting conditions for assessment and the nature of the criteria and standards by which the quality of care is to be judged. Through a representative sampling of all care one garners a wide assortment of cases which defies our capacity to provide preformulated explicit criteria. Hence the resort either to fully implicit criteria—as in the work of Morehead et al. (3–21; 6–1 through 6–4), or to implicit criteria that are guided by a preformulated framework—as in the work of Peterson et al. (5–1 through 5–7; 11–1) and Rosenfeld (6–5). Similarly, there is a clear affinity between preformulated explicit criteria and the highly selective choice of conditions to be assessed.

The explicit criteria and standards of quality assessment and monitoring are the concrete, specific instruments by which the more general conceptions of quality are translated to actual measuring devices which, in turn, lead to judgments on the quality of care. For that reason, the formulation and testing of criteria has received much attention in this book and elsewhere (Donabedian 1982).

Chapter Twelve of this book documents the remarkable variability of opinions about what the criteria and standards for any given condition should be, especially among categories of physicians rather removed from a more expert, and perhaps more coherent, group of professional leaders. Yet, lest this dissension lead to despair, we also find that it is possible, first by excluding the requirements that are less important, and then those which the medical record is less likely to document, to arrive at smaller subsets of criteria which enjoy wide support. This progressive winnowing no doubt affects the judgments of quality that result from the use of the criteria, perhaps making the judgments less stringent, and less reflective of the aspirations espoused by professional leaders, but not shared by the rank and file. However, given the agreed-upon core of criteria, there is no reason to believe that lack of compliance is due, to any great degree, to a disparity between the criteria and standards espoused by an individual practitioner as compared to those endorsed by a majority of his peers (12–12).

The comparative advantages and disadvantages of implicit and explicit criteria have been much debated (Donabedian 1982, pp. 53–59). Implicit criteria enjoy the advantage of an almost infinite adaptability to the particular features of individual cases. Their disadvantages are that they lead to valid, reliable judgments only when applied by highly expert, meticulous judges. They are, therefore, very costly to use. By comparison, explicit criteria are difficult and costly in their initial formulation, but once agreed upon they can be readily used, at low cost, with highly replicable results. Their main disadvantage is their inability to foresee and adapt to the variability in the manifestations of the conditions to which they are meant to apply. When the criteria are designed to encompass much of this variability, they tend to include redundancies that are claimed to encourage wasteful care. When, by contrast, the criteria are pared down to the essentials that apply to all cases, the standards of quality which they represent may have become too improverished as a result.

These considerations have moved us in two directions. On the one hand, the lists of explicit criteria can be made more flexible by the introduction of branchings that specify different contingencies. The criteria maps developed and tested by Greenfield et al. (13–9, 13–10) are the culmination of this line of development. On the other hand, it is recognized that short lists of explicit criteria can be used primarily as a screening device to identify the cases that merit more detailed scrutiny by a method that uses implicit criteria, with or without supplementation by more elaborately formulated explicit criteria. The design of a two-step system such as this requires an understanding of the "screening efficiency" of the explicit criteria, the efficiency depending on the proportion of questionable cases identified (sensitivity, or true-positive ratio) and the proportion of nonquestionable cases subjected to unnecessary review (false-positive ratio). Chapter Thirteen provides several examples that illustrate this important principle in the design of systems to monitor the appropriate use of resources and the quality of care (13–6 through 13–8). The principle is also illustrated in Chapter Three, where we see how the selection of the precise postadmission day on which the hospital stay is to be recertified influences both the number of cases reviewed and the "yield" from the procedure (3–15 through 3–18). The more general principle that the costs of monitoring procedures should be justified by the benefits that they produce is well illustrated by the cost-benefit analysis of second surgical opinion programs as shown in Chapter Four (4–29).

The Sources of Information

Having decided what "approach" to assessment to use, what segments of care to assess, and what criteria to use in the assessment, the next step in the progression is to obtain the necessary information. But besides occupying a critically important position in this sequence, knowledge of the availability of information influences, preemptively as it were, the antecedent steps as well; it casts its shadow even on the definition of quality adopted to guide the assessment.

So critical is the choice of the source of information that I have classified studies of quality partly on these grounds, distinguishing studies based on the direct observation of process (Chapter Five) from those based on the documentation of process in the medical record (Chapter Six). As the examples in Chapter Six show, the medical record itself can be used in a variety of ways. In the study of hospital care by Morehead et al. it was used in full, including the nursing notes, as a basis for judgments that derived from fully implicit criteria (3–21; 6–1 through 6–4). Brook prepared abstracts of the record which were then assessed using criteria that were sometimes implicit and at other times explicit (12–1, 12–18; 13–1 through 13–3). The work of Lembcke (4–23) inaugurates a method which was later developed and used by other investigators whom I see as belonging to the "Michigan School." According to this method, with a list of explicit criteria in hand, one searches the record for evidence of compliance, abstracting only the specifically relevant information. (See, for example, 3–7 through 3–12; 6–13 through 6–26.)

There are, of course, other sources of information as well. Claims for reimbursement submitted to governmental agencies and other third-party payers contain pertinent information, particularly on charges and resource use. (See, for example, 2–4; 3–1 through 3–6.) Records of vital statistics tell us about births, deaths, and certain conditions subject to reporting. (See, for example, 8–1 through 8–7.) It is possible—sometimes necessary—to obtain information from practitioners and their clients, either by interview or by mailed questionnaire. (See, for example, 11–9.) In some cases, particularly when the detailed outcomes of care are to be verified, it may be necessary to actually examine a sample of patients.

The direct observation of practice, besides being extremely costly, has been questioned for its potential influence on the behavior of those being observed. The few pieces of information assembled in Chapter 11 of this book (11–5 through 11–7) are insufficient to resolve the question.

Though reliability and validity are matters of critical importance no matter what the source of information is, it is the medical record that has attracted the greatest amount of the most bitter criticism. We find by an examination of the findings depicted in Chapter Eleven that the medical record is, indeed, often incomplete, particularly with regard to the personal interaction between practitioner and patient. There is also reason to doubt the accuracy of the clinical and laboratory data enshrined in the record as if they were beyond reproach (11–10 through 11–12). Nevertheless, one also finds that many items of more technical information are reasonably well recorded (11–2 through 11–4); that there is a correlation, though a small one, between the quality of recording and of observed practice (11–6); and that there is a correlation, also small, between judgments based on items of information which are almost invariably recorded and other items of information which the physician has more discretion to record or not (11–8). There is reason, therefore, for cautious optimism. At the same time, it is important to improve medical recording, having in mind the requirements of quality assessment as well as the uses of the record as a legal document and an indispensable tool in clinical management and research.

Comparisons of Methods of Assessment

The failings of the medical record are only one reason for the widespread skepticism about our ability to assess the quality of care with any accuracy. A more fundamental reason is a deep seated mistrust of our ability to specify the criteria and standards of good care.

The evidence assembled in Chapter Thirteen lends partial support to these doubts, but it also shows that there is much cause for optimism. We see, for example, that judgments of process based on implicit criteria are at least moderately correlated with judgments based on explicit criteria (13–1, 13–4, 13–5). Accordingly, it seems possible to devise an efficient method of monitoring care that uses explicit criteria to screen cases which are then reviewed by a method that includes the use of implicit criteria (13–6 through 13–8).

The relations between process and outcome, though less easily observed, are also demonstrable, provided appropriate precautions are taken. We have seen, for example, that it is possible to construct a "criteria map" that accurately predicts the presence of disease worthy of admitting patients with chest pain to the hospital (13–9). Implicit judgments of process have shown a reasonable association with implicit judgments on the outcomes of care (13–2, 13–3). Judgments of quality based on explicit criteria of outcome have also been shown to be associated with judgments on the quality of process, provided appropriate outcomes are observed at the appropriate times, and one includes in judging the process of care elements that signify patient cooperation and satisfaction (8–10; 13–11 though 13–13).

All this suggests that, though our methods for assessing the quality of care leave much room for improvement, there is good reason to celebrate what has been accomplished, even as we strive to do better in the future. But before we end on this defiantly hopeful note, we need to review briefly what the many studies that we have encountered in this book seem to say about the factors that influence the level and distribution of quality. As I have already pointed out, the findings of these studies imply the relationships between structure on the one hand, and either process or outcomes on the other. And taken together, these findings reveal what I would like to call "the epidemiology of quality."

The Epidemiology of Quality

The epidemiology of quality is peculiar in having two sets of populations: one of providers, and another of clients. I shall briefly describe some of the information illustrated in this book about the distribution of quality in each of these populations, citing a selection of relevant charts as I proceed. But before I go on, I would like to make two comments: one on procedure, and the other on substance.

With respect to the procedure I intend to follow, I would like to emphasize that I shall limit myself to some of what is visually illustrated in the charts assembled in this book. By using the subject index of the book the reader will be able to find additional information in the charts themselves as well as in the text. The text will alert the reader to the deficiencies of method that compromise the validity and generalizability of the relations I shall describe.

With regard to substance, it is important to realize that we have no national studies of quality from which one could obtain a true picture of the level and distribution of quality, either here or abroad. For that reason, and also to obtain a picture of temporal trends in quality, we must depend on reports of mortality, morbidity, longevity, and use of service—reports that are, at best, extremely difficult to interpret. What we do have is a rather large assemblage of studies, using methods that vary in accuracy and stringency, to assess diverse aspects of the quality of care, provided by selected practitioners, to circumscribed populations, at different periods. The studies conducted by Payne et al. (1976) in Hawaii are perhaps the closest we come to investigations of the quality of care in a large, reasonably representative population in its natural habitat; but that study is limited in its representativeness, as we have seen, by many features of its design and implementation.

The upshot of all this is that there is little we can say about the levels of quality in the United States, besides noting that almost invariably performance seems to fall far short of the criteria used to judge the quality of care. And since one expects that as science progresses the criteria and standards become correspondingly more stringent, there is little to be learned about secular trends from comparisons of current studies with those in the past, even if on other grounds the comparison might seem appropriate. For the same reasons, what I am about to say concerning the factors that influence quality should also be treated with caution, even though in this case we can be somewhat more assured of the general applicability of the observed associations, particularly when they are repeatedly observed and also seem to be reasonable in the light of what we know about the health care system in general.

With all these limitations in mind, we begin by noting that the distribution of behaviors that directly or indirectly connote quality reveals an astounding degree of variability among geographic areas, practitioners, and institutions. Particular attention has been paid in recent years to the poorly understood variations in the incidence of surgical procedures among small areas within the United States (4–2 through 4–8), within other countries (4–11), and also among countries (4–9, 4–10). There is also considerable variation among practitioners and institutions in any given, rather circumscribed, geographic area and, even, among practitioners within a given institution. Adherence to the implicit or explicit criteria of good care has been observed to vary among general practitioners (5–1 through 5–7) and internists (6–28) practicing in an area. The same is true for physicians in a set of associated group practices (6–7 through 6–12). There are wide variations in the cost of care provided by physicians in a group practice (2–2), and by physicians and other practitioners in a university-affiliated clinic (2–10). The number and cost of diagnostic procedures vary considerably among physicians who practice in a geographic locale (2–4), a hospital (2–8), or a group practice (2–3). The propensity to remove normal tissue in primary appendectomies is astoundingly variable among physicians in a hospital, and also among the staffs of different hospitals, each taken as a whole (4–20). Hospitals and ambulatory care institutions are known to vary with regard to other aspects of quality as well. For example, hospitals have been observed to differ greatly in the proportion of unjustified hysterectomies performed in them (4–22), in the incidence of postoperative fatality (7–6 through 7–8), in the occurrence of preventable maternal mortality (8–3), and in the adherence of their staffs to the implicit or explicit criteria of appropriate use and quality (3–21; 6–3, 6–5, 6–19). The quality of care provided by organized ambulatory care settings has been observed to be similarly variable (6–24, 6–31).

Greatly variable though the practice of health care may be, the variability is far from random. Questionable practices, on the contrary, are known to be highly concentrated or localized. It has been observed, for example, that relatively small proportions of physicians account for a relatively large share of questionable drugs (3–1) and injections (3–4). The concentration of tonsillectomies (4–16) and of other surgery (4–17) in relatively few hands raises the suspicion that those who are responsible for most of the operations may be doing too many, whereas those who are doing too few are not able to maintain their surgical skills.

Variability and localization are the twin necessities of epidemiology. What remains is to identify the attributes with which appropriate use and quality are associated. Insofar as physicians are concerned, the key attributes (beyond the possible influence of personality traits, a subject concerning which I have no information) are apparently training, experience, and specialization.

The effect of training is illustrated repeatedly in this book. General practice has been observed to be of higher quality among physicians who were better students (5–3; 6–8), who were educated in certain categories of medical schools (6–8), and who had longer periods of certain kinds of training (5–4; 6–7), there being a mutually reinforcing effect when two or more of these attributes coexist (5–5; 6–8). Generalists taken as a group, however, are usually found to maintain a lower standard of practice when compared to their more highly specialized colleagues, at least when judged by criteria that usually correspond more closely to the opinions of specialists.

Specialists appear to perform better than generalists in many aspects of ambulatory and inpatient care. Specialists use X-ray examinations more appropriately (2–5), give fewer questionable injections (3–5), use the hospital more appropriately (3–21; 6–13), more often comply with the implicit or explicit criteria of hospital care (6–2, 6–13 through 6–15) and of ambulatory care (6–25, 6–26), and are responsible for fewer "preventable" perinatal deaths (8–6). There is evidence, moreover, that the effect of specialization is contingent upon a specialist's restricting his "domain" of practice to the cases that fall strictly within the corresponding area of specialization (6–13, 6–15, 6–25). Furthermore, organizations that, *as a whole,* are more specialized in their functions appear to provide better care (6–31).

Training and specialization are, of course, intimately related to experience. There are two additional components to experience: years in practice, and volume of similar cases treated or nearly identical procedures performed each year. Concerning the second of these two (the volume of care), there is evidence that larger hospitals provide better care (6–19). But institutional size is an attribute with several connotations: experience with larger volumes of similar cases, either by individual practitioners or by the hospital's staff as a whole, is only one of these. It is interesting to find, therefore, that fatality following more complex surgical procedures is lower in hospitals where more of these procedures are performed (7–10), and that "preventable" maternal deaths are judged to occur less often in hospitals where a large number of deliveries take place (8–3). A contrary observation, perhaps attributable to adverse factors associated with hospital size, is a positive association of the annual number of births with neonatal and maternal mortality in a national sample of hospitals (7–2).

The effect of the experience that accrues with a longer duration of practice seems to be obscured by the obsolescence of medical knowledge that apparently occurs at the same time. As a result, advanced age seems almost always to be associated with lower levels of performance. Although it is not clear whether it is good or bad to do so, older physicians use fewer laboratory tests and roentgenograms (2–4). Other observations, more clearly indicative of quality, have shown that older physicians with more years in practice use X-ray procedures less appropriately (2–5); more often use questionable injections (3–6); perform less appropriately as general practitioners in a community (5–3, 5–6), as family physicians in group practice (6–9), as physicians in a variety of ambulatory care settings (6–25); and provide hospital care which is less likely to conform to preformulated explicit criteria than is care provided by physicians in their intermediate years of practice (6–17).

Besides being influenced by the personal attributes already detailed (education, training, specialization, experience, and age), the performance of physicians is also influenced by the conditions in their own practices and in the organizations or institutions where they work. For example, general practitioners seem to do better work when they have a larger variety of certain kinds of equipment (5–7) in their offices. Family practitioners in group practice are judged to perform better when they see more of their patients by appointment, have a full-time assistant, or use a medical record with a larger format (6–12). Physicians who are very busy may begin to provide less complete care (as judged by the records they keep) when the number of patients seen each hour becomes too large (6–25). As physicians become busier, their office records show evidence of less compliance with criteria for history taking and physical examination while, at the same time, there is greater compliance with criteria for laboratory tests (6–27); this suggests that the latter could be a substitute for the former.

There is also evidence, not always fully convincing, that financial incentives may influence practice. It appears that physicians who own X-ray equipment are more likely to use it, and to do so less appropriately (2–5); that more surgery is performed when surgeons are less able or willing to make charges additional to those approved by an insurer (4–18); that appendectomies are probably less often justified when the hospital stay is financed by Blue Cross (4–21); and that patients who have help in paying for their hospital care experience overstays more often and understays less often than do patients who pay the entire bill themselves (3–20).

Participation in an organized group, or work in another kind of institution, can be expected to alter radically the terms and conditions of practice, bringing about corresponding changes in the quality of technical care. It has been observed, for example, that the quality of ambulatory care for children is better in hospital outpatient departments than in office practice, at least as judged by entries in the medical record (6–26). Disappointingly, a study in Hawaii suggests that physicians in multispecialty groups do not provide ambulatory care that is indisputably better than that provided by solo practitioners (6–23). The physicians in such groups do, however, clearly use the hospital more appropriately, and provide better hospital care, than do physicians in solo practice (6–14). But this association between belonging to a group practice and the nature of hospital care was entirely explained by the fact that the groups employed specialists who restricted their practice to the domains of their respective specialties (6–18).

It would be interesting and important to know if group practice exerts an effect on quality through mechanisms additional to the mere selection of the physicians who participate in the group, important though that is. Evidence for more subtle forms of influence may be inferred from observations that the quality of care provided by family physicians in a set of associated group practices was better when the physicians had a longer affiliation with the group, gave more of their time to the group, and spent more time in the facility owned by the group (6–11). The importance of an active hospital affiliation is confirmed by the observation that the quality of ambulatory care was better when the physicians had such an appointment, when the appointment was at a higher rank, and when more hospital visits were made (6–10).

There is some evidence about the association between access of patients to an organized practice and the outcomes of care. The incidence of first attacks of rheumatic fever has been observed to be lowered after the establishment of a comprehensive-care center in a low-income area (7–12). Enrollees in one prepaid group practice plan received more prenatal care and experienced a lower rate of neonatal mortality than a sample of the general population, the advantage being greater for blacks than whites (7–1). But a more recent study in another community shows that the enrollees of a prepaid group practice received less prenatal care but had an equal level of neonatal morality, leading the investigators to suggest a higher degree of "efficiency" in the attainment of a given outcome (7–3).

Of all the organizations that provide health care, hospitals are perhaps the most likely to control the quality of care provided in them. The attributes of hospitals, alone or in association with the characteristics of the physicians who work in them, can be expected, therefore, to have a large influence on the quality of care. I have already alluded to the possible effects of hospital size. More important by far appears to be the teaching function of the hospital, particularly when that function is signaled and reinforced by a close affiliation with a medical school. Teaching hospitals are more often appropriately used (3–21). Appendectomies in teaching hospitals more often appear to be justified (4–21). The care provided in teaching hospitals more often conforms to implicit and explicit criteria of quality, at least as shown by the medical record (6–3, 6–19, 6–30). Case fatality is lower in teaching hospitals in England and Wales (7–4), and preventable perinatal deaths were lower in teaching hospitals in New York City as compared to their voluntary or municipal counterparts that had no teaching functions (8–7).

Hospitals no doubt influence quality partly through the facilities and equipment they provide, and partly through selecting the physicians and other personnel who are permitted to work in them. There appears to be, however, yet another effect, one mediated through organizational controls. In any event, there is an interaction between the characteristics of hospitals and the attributes of the physicians who practice in them. The formal qualifications of individual physicians seem less important indicators of quality in hospitals affiliated with a university than in one that is not. By contrast, the less able the hospital and its medical staff are to control the practice of medicine in the hospital, the more likely is the care received by patients to depend on the qualifications of individual physicians (6–4). Irrespective of university affiliation, the quality of care seems to be best in the hands of highly trained physicians in tightly organized hospitals, and worst in the hands of less highly trained physicians in hospitals with looser forms of organization (6–20).

So far, we have been concerned with the distribution of quality among providers. Much less is known about its distribution among clients, though this should be a matter of the greatest importance to public policy.

Differences in the quality of care provided to different categories of persons may arise in one of two ways. Different people may have different degrees of access to different kinds of practitioners and institutions. This is a form of social differentiation which we seem willing to tolerate, even when we regard it as unfortunate. We are less able to contemplate the second possibility: that patients with similar needs for technical care will be treated differently when seen by the same practitioner, or cared for in the same institution, unless the difference is only in the amenities of care. This reluctance may partly explain our unwillingness or inability even to study the subject, with the result that there is very little known about it. More is known about a third factor that influences the quality of care, namely the ability or willingness of clients to participate in influencing the recommendations of the physician and in carrying them out. But this book does not include studies of patient participation and compliance, beyond an occasional reference to the subject.

The variability in the quantity and quality of care that was noted in the preceding description of the distribution of care among providers must have its counterpart among the people who use these providers. We can expect to see, therefore, corresponding differences among those who reside in different geographic areas, or who are clients of different hospitals and practitioners. The clients of any given set of practitioners can also be expected to vary a great deal in the quality of care they receive (6–29).

As to the association between client attributes and the quality of care received, there are snippets of information about the effects of place of residence, age, sex, race, occupation, having insurance, and indexes of socioeconomic status.

It is reasonable to expect that rural residents experience the adverse consequences of reduced access to care, and particularly to care by more highly specialized physicians and those in the larger, university-affiliated hospitals. For example, the improper use of an antibiotic has been shown to be more frequent in rural areas, even when the physicians' specialty status has been taken into account, at least to some extent (3–2). Surgical procedures are less often performed for residents of less highly urbanized areas (4–12). But if the possibility of unnecessary intervention is considered, being less subject to surgery may not necessarily be a bad thing. At least one study has noted an association of urban residence with more frequent appendectomies, and higher fatality from appendicitis (4–3).

The evidence concerning the possible effect of age and sex is fragmentary and inconclusive. There appears to have been no consistent association between the age of the patient and the quality of hospital care in Hawaii (6–21). On the other hand, the quality of nursing services in a selected group of urban hospitals has been observed to be somewhat better for younger males, as compared to younger females, and better for older females, as compared to older males (5–8). In one study abroad, females were found to be more subject to appendectomy and the surgery more often yielded normal tissue, but this could be explained by the greater difficulty of diagnosing appendicitis in females (4–13).

Comparisons based on differences in race are equally sparse and inconclusive. There was no association between ethnic origin and the quality of hospital care in Hawaii (6–22); but Hawaii could be atypical in this regard. Other studies have found that surgical operations are fewer among nonwhites (4–12); that nonwhites may be receiving nursing care of lower quality (5–8); and that when surgery is done, it is more often performed by the resident staff than by surgeons with more experience or higher qualifications (4–14). One cannot conclude, of course, that the care provided by resident staff is necessarily inferior. In one study, house staff were found to perform quite well (6–2); in another study their performance was reported to be rather poor (8–6).

Occupational differences are interesting partly because occupation is an important indicator of socioeconomic status (as is, unfortunately, ethnic origin), and partly because it has been suggested that use of services by physicians and members of their families may be used as a standard of care (Bunker and Brown 1974). It has been noted, for example, that the wives of physicians are much more likely to have had a hysterectomy than are women in general (4–15). This may also mean, however, that the wives of physicians are more exposed to unnecessary surgery. Hysterectomies are known to be very frequently proposed and performed when not completely justified (4–22 to 4–24). A study in the German city of Hannover shows that white-collar workers have more appendectomies, but that the tissue removed is less often acutely inflamed (4–13). Much more to the point is the observation that persons connected with medicine or nursing may experience higher risk because of the much greater readiness to subject them to appendectomies that prove to have been unjustified (10–3).

These observations suggest that greater access to care may have adverse as well as beneficial consequences. This principle appears to apply when coverage by private health insurance or by a governmental program improves the ability to pay for care. It has been observed that such coverage decreases underuse of the hospital, but at the same time increases overuse (3–20). Appendectomies for patients who have their hospital stays financed by Blue Cross appear to yield normal or questionable tissue in a higher proportion of cases (4–21).

In some studies, the outcomes of care have been used to tell us something about the influence of social and economic factors on the quality of care and its consequences. For example, mothers assigned to lower socioeconomic categories on the basis of average house rents have been shown to experience higher rates of "preventable" maternal mortality, the difference being largely attributable to failure of the expectant mother to obtain suitable care (8–4). The proportion of perinatal deaths considered to be "preventable" is larger when the birth takes place in a municipal hospital rather than a voluntary one, or the mother and child are cared for in a ward rather than the private service of a hospital (8–7). When the organization of care is improved, there may be an associated improvement in prenatal care and a reduction in neonatal mortality, the relative improvements being greater for those who are ordinarily disadvantaged. But the disadvantage is not completely effaced (7–1). Even approximately equal access to reasonably equal care does not necessarily result in equal enjoyment of health.

That does not mean, of course, that we must abandon hope; it only means that we must try harder, and on a wider front. It is my dearest wish that this book, and any other professional contributions I may have made, would serve this higher purpose: the advent of a more caring, more just society.

Bibliography

American Child Health Association. *Physical Defects: The Pathway to Correction.* New York: American Child Health Association, 1934. 171 pp.

American College of Obstetricians and Gynecologists, Committee on Maternal Health. *National Study of Maternity Care: Survey of Obstetric Practice and Associated Services in Hospitals in the United States.* Chicago: American College of Obstetricians and Gynecologists, 1970. 154 pp.

American Medical Association, Council on Drugs. *American Medical Association Drug Evaluations 1971.* Chicago: American Medical Association, 1971. 675 pp. plus New Drugs Section, Appendix and indexes.

Averill, Richard F., and McMahon, Laurence F., Jr. "A Cost Benefit Analysis of Continued Stay Certification." *Medical Care* 15 (February 1977):158–73.

Barr, Daniel M. "The Patients' Problem: Concept, Method, and Use in Health Services Research." Master's thesis, Johns Hopkins University, 1974.

Barr, Daniel M.; Mushlin, Alvin I.; and Seltser, B. J. "Patient Problem Status as a Measure of Outcome in Health Service." Baltimore: Health Services Research and Development Center, Johns Hopkins University, 1973. Mimeo.

Bombardier, Claire; Fuchs, Victor R.; Lillard, Lee A.; and Warner, Kenneth E. "Socioeconomic Factors Affecting the Utilization of Surgical Operations." *New England Journal of Medicine* 297 (September 29, 1977):699–705.

Brook, Robert H. *Quality of Care Assessment: A Comparison of Five Methods of Peer Review.* Washington, D.C.: U.S. Department of Health, Education, and Welfare, Public Health Service, Health Resources Administration, Bureau of Health Services Research and Evaluation, July 1973. 343 pp. (DHEW Publication No. HRA–74–3100.)

Brook, Robert H., and Appel, Francis A. "Quality-of-Care Assessment: Choosing a Method for Peer Review." *New England Journal of Medicine* 288 (June 21, 1973):1323–29.

Brook, Robert H., and Stevenson, Robert L., Jr. "Effectiveness of Patient Care in an Emergency Room." *New England Journal of Medicine* 283 (October 22, 1970):904–07.

Brook, Robert H., and Williams, Kathleen N. "Evaluation of the New Mexico Peer Review System, 1971 to 1973." *Supplement to Medical Care* 14 (December 1976):1–122.

Bunker, John P. "Surgical Manpower: A Comparison of Operations and Surgeons in the United States and in England and Wales." *New England Journal of Medicine* 282 (January 15, 1970):135–44.

Bunker, John P., and Brown, Byron Wm., Jr. "The Physician-Patient as an Informed Consumer of Surgical Services." *New England Journal of Medicine* 290 (May 9, 1974):1051–55.

Bunker, John P.; Forrest, William H., Jr.; Mosteller, Frederick; and Vandam, Leroy D.; eds. *The National Halothane Study: A Study of the Possible Association between Halothane Anesthesia and Postoperative Hepatic Necrosis.* Report of the Subcommittee on the National Halothane Study of the Committee on Anesthesia, National Academy of Sciences, National Research Council. Bethesda, Md.: National Institutes of Health, National Institute of General Medical Sciences, 1969. 418 pp. (U.S. Government Printing Office, 0–334–553.)

Burgess, A. "Outcome of Care of Patients with Myocardial Infarct." Lecture presented to the American Heart Association, New Orleans, March 1970.

Bynder, Herbert. "Doctors as Patients: A Study of the Medical Care of Physicians and Their Families." *Medical Care* 6 (March-April 1968):157–67.

Cartwright, Ann. *Patients and Their Doctors: A Study of General Practice.* New York: Atherton Press, 1967. 295 pp.

Childs, Alfred W., and Hunter, E. Diane. "Non-Medical Factors Influencing Use of Diagnostic X-ray by Physicians." *Medical Care* 10 (July-August 1972):323–35.

Clute, Kenneth F. *The General Practitioner: A Study of Medical Education and Practice in Ontario and Nova Scotia.* Toronto: University of Toronto Press, 1963. 566 pp.

Commission on Professional and Hospital Activities. *Hemoglobin.* Professional Activities Study Report 36. Ann Arbor, Mich.: Commission on Professional and Hospital Activities, August 25, 1959. 12 pp. [1959a in text]

————. *Reliability of Laboratory Determinations.* Professional Activities Study Report 37. Ann Arbor, Mich.: Commission on Professional and Hospital Activities, November 10, 1959. 8 pp. [1959b in text]

Corder, Michael P.; Lachenbruch, Peter A.; Lindle, Samuel G.; Sisson, Joseph H.; Johnson, Paul S.; and Kosier, James T. "A Financial Analysis of Hodgkin Lymphoma Staging." *American Journal of Public Health* 71 (April 1981):376–80.

Daily, Edwin F., and Morehead, Mildred A. "A Method of Evaluating and Improving the Quality of Medical Care." *American Journal of Public Health* (July 1956): 848–54.

de Dombal, F. T.; Leaper, D. J.; Staniland, J. R.; McCann, A. P.; and Horrocks, Jane C. "Computer-aided Diagnosis of Acute Abdominal Pain." *British Medical Journal* 2 (April 1, 1972):9–13.

Demlo, Linda K., and Campbell, Paul M. "Improving Hospital Discharge Data: Lessons from the National Hospital Discharge Survey." *Medical Care* 19 (October 1981):1030–40.

Donabedian, Avedis. *A Guide to Medical Care Administration, Volume II: Medical Care Appraisal—Quality and Utilization.* New York (now Washington, D.C.): American Public Health Association, 1969. 176 pp. (Plus an annotated selected bibliography prepared by Alice J. Anderson.) [1969a in text]

————. "An Evaluation of Prepaid Group Practice." *Inquiry* 6 (September 1969):3–27. [1969b in text]

————. *Aspect of Medical Care Administration: Specifying Requirements for Health Care.* Cambridge: Harvard University Press, for the Commonwealth Fund, 1973. 649 pp.

————. *Benefits in Medical Care Programs.* Cambridge: Harvard University Press, 1976. 436 pp.

————. *Explorations in Quality Assessment and Monitoring, Volume I: The Definition of Quality and Approaches to its Assessment.* Ann Arbor, Mich.: Health Administration Press, 1980. 163 pp.

————. *Explorations in Quality Assessment and Monitoring, Volume II: The Criteria and Standards of Quality.* Ann Arbor, Mich.: Health Administration Press, 1982. 504 pp.

————. "Quality, Cost, and Clinical Decisions." *The Annals of the American Academy of Political and Social Science* 468 (July 1983):196–204.

Donabedian, Avedis; Wheeler, John R. C.; and Wyszewianski, Leon. "Quality, Cost, and Health: An Integrative Model." *Medical Care* 20 (October 1982):975–92.

Doyle, James C. "Unnecessary Hysterectomies: Study of 6,248 Operations in Thirty-Five Hospitals During 1948." *Journal of the American Medical Association* 51 (January 31, 1953):360–65.

Egbert, Lawrence D., and Rothman, Ilene L. "Relation Between the Race and Economic Status of Patients and Who Performs Their Surgery." *New England Journal of Medicine* 297 (July 14, 1977):90–91.

Ehrlich, June; Morehead, Mildred A.; and Trussell, Ray E. *The Quantity, Quality and Costs of Medical and Hospital Care Secured by a Sample of Teamster Families in the New York Area.* New York: School of Public Health and Administrative Medicine, Columbia University, 1962. 83 pp.

Eisenberg, John M., and Nicklin, David. "Use of Diagnostic Services by Physicians in Community Practice." *Medical Care* 19 (March 1981):297–309.

Evans, Lloyd R., and Bybee, John R. "Evaluation of Student Skills in Physical Diagnosis." *Journal of Medical Education* 40 (February 1965):199–204.

Fine, Jacob, and Morehead, Mildred A. "Study of Peer Review of Inhospital Patient Care." *New York State Journal of Medicine* 71 (August 15, 1971):1963–73.

Finkel, Madelon Lubin; McCarthy, Eugene G.; and Miller, Dan. "Podiatric Surgery: The Need for a Second Opinion." *Medical Care* 20 (August 1982):862–70.

Fitzpatrick, Thomas B.; Riedel, Donald C.; and Payne, Beverly C. "The Effectiveness of Hospital Use," "Criteria and Data Collection," "Appropriateness of Admission and Length of Stay," and "The Physician Interview." Chapters 24–27, pp. 449–509. In Walter J. McNerney and Study Staff, *Hospital and Medical Economics: A Study of Population, Services, Costs, Methods of Payment, and Controls.* Volume I. Chicago: Hospital Research and Educational Trust, 1962. 716 pp.

Flood, Ann Barry, and Scott, W. Richard. "Professional Power and Professional Effectiveness: The Power of the Surgical Staff and the Quality of Surgical Care in Hospitals." *Journal of Health and Social Behavior* 19 (September 1978):240–54.

Flood, Ann Barry; Ewy, Wayne; Scott, W. Richard; Forrest, William H., Jr.; and Brown, Byron William, Jr. "The Relationship Between Intensity and Duration of Medical Services and Outcomes for Hospitalized Patients." *Medical Care* 17 (November 1979):1088–1102.

Flood, Ann Barry; Scott, W. Richard; Ewy, Wayne; and Forrest, William H., Jr. "Effectiveness in Professional Organizations: The Impact of Surgeons and Surgical Staff Organizations on the Quality of Care in Hospitals." *Health Services Research* 17 (Winter 1982):341–66.

Freeborn, Donald K.; Baer, Daniel; Greenlick, Merwyn R.; and Bailey, Jeffry W. "Determinants of Medical Care Utilization: Physicians' Use of Laboratory Services." *American Journal of Public Health* 62 (June 1972):846–53.

Freidson, Eliot. *Patients' Views of Medical Practice.* New York: Russell Sage Foundation, 1961. 268 pp.

Gittelsohn, Alan M., and Wennberg, John E. "On the Incidence of Tonsillectomy and Other Common Surgical Procedures." Chapter 7, pp. 91–106. In John P. Bunker, Benjamin A. Barnes, and Frederick Mosteller, eds., *Costs, Risks, and Benefits of Surgery.* New York: Oxford University Press, 1977. 401 pp.

Gonnella, Joseph S., ed. *Clinical Criteria for Disease Staging.* Santa Barbara, Calif.: SysteMetrics, Inc. 1982. 617 pp.

Gonnella, Joseph S., and Goran, Michael J. "Quality of Patient Care—A Measurement of Change: The Staging Concept." *Medical Care* 13 (June 1975):467–73.

Gonnella, Joseph S.; Goran, Michael J.; Williamson, John W.; and Cotsonas, Nicholas J., Jr. "Evaluation of Patient Care: An Approach." *Journal of the American Medical Association* 214 (December 14, 1970):2040–43.

Gonnella, Joseph S.; Louis, Daniel Z.; McCord, John J.; Spirka, Craig S.; and Cattani, Jacqueline A. "Controlled Study: Comparison of Disease Stages at Hospital Admission Between Comprehensive Health Center (CHC) Enrollees and Non-CHC Participants." *Quality Review Bulletin* 3 (October 1977):15–18.

Goodrich, Charles H.; Olendzki, Margaret C.; and Reader, George G. *Welfare Medical Care: An Experiment.* Cambridge: Harvard University Press, 1970. 343 pp.

Gordis, Leon. "Effectiveness of Comprehensive-Care Programs in Preventing Rheumatic Fever." *New England Journal of Medicine* 289 (August 16, 1973):331–35.

Gordis, Leon, and Markowitz, Milton. "Evaluation of the Effectiveness of Comprehensive and Continuous Pediatric Care." *Pediatrics* 48 (November 1971):766–76.

Goss, Mary E. W., and Reed, Joseph I. "Evaluating the Quality of Hospital Care Through Severity-Adjusted Death Rates: Some Pitfalls." *Medical Care* 12 (March 1974):202–13.

Graham, John B., and Paloucek, Frank P. "Where Should Cancer of the Cervix Be Treated? A Preliminary Report." *American Journal of Obstetrics and Gynecology* 87 (October 1963):405–09.

Greegor, David H. "Detection of Silent Cancer in Routine Examination." *Ca: A Cancer Journal for Clinicians* 19 (November-December 1969):330–37.

Greenfield, Sheldon; Cretin, Shan; Worthman, Linda G.; and Dorey, Frederick. "The Use of an ROC Curve to Express Quality of Care Results." *Medical Decision Making* 2 (Spring 1982):23–31.

Greenfield, Sheldon; Cretin, Shan; Worthman, Linda G.; Dorey, Frederick J.; Solomon, Nancy E.; and Goldberg, George A. "Comparison of a Criteria Map to a Criteria List in Quality-of-Care Assessment for Patients with Chest Pain: The Relation of Each to Outcome." *Medical Care* 19 (March 1981):255–72.

Greenfield, Sheldon; Lewis, Charles E.; Kaplan, Sherrie H.; and Davidson,

Mayer B. "Peer Review by Criteria Mapping: Criteria for Diabetes Mellitus: The Use of Decision-Making in Chart Audit." *Annals of Internal Medicine* 83 (December 1975):761–70.

Griffith, John R.; Restuccia, Joseph D.; Tedeschi, Philip J.; Wilson, Peter A.; and Zuckerman, Howard S. "Measuring Community Hospital Services in Michigan." *Health Services Research* 16 (Summer 1981):135–60.

Grimm, Richard H., Jr.; Shimoni, Kitty; Harlan, William R., Jr.; and Estes, E. Harvey, Jr. "Evaluation of Patient-Care Protocol Use by Various Providers." *New England Journal of Medicine* 292 (March 6, 1975):507–11.

Grover, Maleah, and Greenberg, Tony. "Quality of Care Given to First Time Birth Control Patients at a Free Clinic." *American Journal of Public Health* 66 (October 1976):986–87.

Hare, Robert L., and Barnoon, Shlomo. *Medical Care Appraisal and Quality Assurance in the Office Practice of Internal Medicine.* San Francisco: American Society of Internal Medicine, 1973. 432 pp.

Howie, John G. R. "Death from Appendicitis and Appendicectomy: An Epidemiological Survey." *Lancet* 2 (December 17, 1966):1334–37.

————. "The Place of Appendicectomy in the Treatment of Young Adult Patients with Possible Appendicitis." *Lancet* 1 (June 22, 1968):1365–67.

Hulka, Barbara S.; Romm, Fredric J.; and Parkerson, George R., Jr. *Physician Non-Adherence to Self-Formulated Process Criteria.* Draft of Final Report, HRA 230–75–0186. Chapel Hill, N.C.: School of Public Health, University of North Carolina, October 31, 1977. 177 pp. plus 13 appendixes which are not consecutively paginated.

Hulka, Barbara S.; Romm, Fredric J.; Parkerson, George R., Jr.; Russell, Ian T.; Clapp, Nancy E.; and Johnson, Frances S. "Peer Review in Ambulatory Care: Use of Explicit Criteria and Implicit Judgments." *Supplement to Medical Care* 17 (March 1979):1–73.

Jackson, Richard A., and Smith, Mickey C. "Relations Between Price and Quality in Community Pharmacy." *Medical Care* 12 (January 1974):32–9.

Janzen, Erica. "Quality Nursing Care Assurance: Initial Survey." Paper presented at the American Public Health Association Annual Meeting, New Orleans, October 23, 1974. 16 pp. plus tables and figures.

Kane, Robert L.; Rubinstein, Laurence Z.; Brook, Robert H.; VanRyzin, John; Masthay, Patricia; Schoenrich, Edyth; and Harrell, Bert. "Utilization Review in Nursing Homes: Making Implicit Level-of-Care Judgments Explicit." *Medical Care* 19 (January 1981):3–13.

Kessner, David M.; Kalk, Carolyn E.; and Singer, James. "Assessing Health Quality—The Case for Tracers." *New England Journal of Medicine* 288 (January 25, 1973):189–94.

Kessner, David M.; Snow, Carolyn Kalk; and Singer, James. *Assessment of Medical Care for Children.* Vol. 3 of *Contrasts in Health Status.* Washington, D.C.: Institute of Medicine, National Academy of Sciences, 1974. 231 pp.

Kilpatrick, G[eorge] S. "Observer Error in Medicine." *Journal of Medical Education* 38 (January 1963):38–43.

Klarman, Herbert E. "Effect of Prepaid Group Practice on Hospital Use." *Public Health Reports* 78 (November 1963):955–65.

Knobel, R[oland] J. "Placement of Foreign-Trained Physicians in U.S. Medical Residencies." *Medical Care* 11 (May-June 1973):224–39.

Kohl, Schuyler G. *Perinatal Mortality in New York City: Responsible Factors*. A Study by the Subcommittee on Neonatal Mortality, Committee on Public Health Relations, New York Academy of Medicine. Cambridge: Harvard University Press, for the Commonwealth Fund, 1955. 109 pp.

Koran, Lorrin M. "The Reliability of Clinical Methods, Data and Judgments." *New England Journal of Medicine* 293 (September 25 and October 2, 1975):642–46 and 695–701.

Kroeger, Hilda H.; Altman, Isidore; Clark, Dean A.; Johnson, Allen C.; and Sheps, Cecil G. "The Office Practice of Internists. I: The Feasibility of Evaluating Quality of Care." *Journal of the American Medical Association* 193 (August 2, 1965):371–76.

Lemcke, Paul A. "Measuring the Quality of Medical Care Through Vital Statistics Based on Hospital Service Areas: 1. Comparative Study of Appendectomy Rates." *American Journal of Public Health* 42 (March 1952):276–86.

——————. "Medical Auditing by Scientific Methods: Illustrated by Major Female Pelvic Surgery." *Journal of the American Medical Association* 162 (October 13, 1956):646–55, plus Appendixes A and B supplied by the author.

Lewis, Charles E. "Variations in the Incidence of Surgery." *New England Journal of Medicine* 281 (October 16, 1969):880–84.

Lichtner, Sigrid, and Pflanz, Manfred. "Appendectomy in the Federal Republic of Germany: Epidemiology and Medical Care Patterns." *Medical Care* 9 (July-August 1971):311–30.

Lipworth, L.; Lee, J. A. H.; and Morris, J. N. "Case-Fatality in Teaching and Non-Teaching Hospitals 1956–59." *Medical Care* 1 (April-June 1963):71–6.

Lohr, Kathleen N.; Brook, Robert H.; and Kaufman, Michael A. "Quality of Care in the New Mexico Medicaid Program (1971–1975)." *Supplement to Medical Care* 18 (January 1980):1–129.

Luft, Harold S. "Assessing the Evidence on HMO Performance." *Health and Society: Milbank Memorial Fund Quarterly* 58 (Fall 1980):501–36. [1980a in text]

——————. "The Relation Between Surgical Volume and Mortality: An Exploration of Causal Factors and Alternative Models." *Medical Care* 18 (September 1980):940–59. [1980b in text]

Luft, Harold S.; Bunker, John P.; and Enthoven, Alain C. "Should Operations Be Regionalized? The Empirical Relation Between Surgical Volume and Mortality." *New England Journal of Medicine* 301 (December 20, 1979):1364–69.

Lyle, Carl B.; Citron, David S.; Sugg, William C.; and Williams, O. Dale. "Cost of Medical Care in a Practice of Internal Medicine: A Study in a Group of Seven Internists." *Annals of Internal Medicine* 81 (July 1974):1–6.

Lyons, Thomas F., and Payne, Beverly C. "The Quality of Physicians' Health-Care Performance: A Comparison Against Optimal Criteria for Treatment of the Elderly and Younger Adults in Community Hospitals." *Journal of the American Medical Association* 227 (February 25, 1974):925–28. [1974a in text]

_____. "The Relationship of Physicians' Medical Recording Performance to Their Medical Care Performance." *Medical Care* 12 (August 1974):714–20. [1974b in text]

_____. "Quality of Physicians' Office-Care Performance: Different for Elderly Than for Younger Adults?" *Journal of the American Medical Association* 229 (September 16, 1974):1621–22. [1974c in text]

McCarthy, Eugene G., and Finkel, Madelon Lubin. "Surgical Utilization in the U.S.A." *Medical Care* 18 (September 1980):883–92. [1980a in text]

_____. "Second Consultant Opinion for Elective Gynecologic Surgery." *Obstetrics and Gynecology* 56 (October 1980):403–10. [1980b in text]

McCarthy, Eugene G.; Finkel, Madelon Lubin; and Ruchlin, Hirsch S. *Second Opinion Elective Surgery.* Boston: Auburn House Publishing, 1981. 193 pp.

McNerney, Walter J., and Study Staff. *Hospital and Medical Economics: A Study of Population, Services, Costs, Methods of Payment, and Controls.* 2 vols. Chicago: Hospital Research and Educational Trust, 1962, 1492 pp.

Makover, Henry B. "The Quality of Medical Care." *American Journal of Public Health* 41 (July 1951):824–32.

Maloney, Milton C.; Trussell, Ray E.; and Elinson, Jack. "Physicians Choose Medical Care: A Sociometric Approach to Quality Appraisal." *American Journal of Public Health* 50 (November 1960):1678–86.

Mann, Joseph D.; Woodson, G. Stanley; Hoffman, Robert G.; and Martinek, Robert G. "The Relation Between Reported Values for Hemoglobin and the Transfusion Rate in a General Hospital." *American Journal of Clinical Pathology* 22 (September 1959):225–32.

Martin, Samuel P.; Donaldson, Magruder C.; London, David; Peterson, Osler L.; and Colton, Theodore. "Inputs into Coronary Care During 30 Years: A Cost Effectiveness Study." *Annals of Internal Medicine* 81 (September 1974):289–93.

Martin, Suzanne Grisez; Shwartz, Michael; Cooper, Deborah D'Arpa; McKusick, Anne E.; Thorne, John H.; and Whalen, Bernadette J. *The Effect of a Mandatory Second Opinion Program on Medicaid Surgery Rates: An Analysis of the Massachusetts Consultation Program for Elective Surgery.* Boston: School of Management, Boston University, January 1980. 204 pp.

Martin, Suzanne Grisez; Shwartz, Michael; Whalen, Bernadette J.; D'Arpa, Deborah; Ljung, Greta M.; Thorne, John Holden; and McKusick, Anne E. "Impact of a Mandatory Second-Opinion Program on Medicaid Surgery Rates." *Medical Care* 20 (January 1982):21–45.

Mates, Susan, and Sidel, Victor W. "Quality Assessment by Process and Outcome Methods: Evaluation of Emergency Room Care of Asthmatic Adults." *American Journal of Public Health* 71 (July 1981):687–93.

Miles, David L. "Multiple Prescriptions and Drug Appropriateness." *Health Services Research* 12 (Spring 1977):3–10.

Miller, Norman F. "Hysterectomy: Therapeutic Necessity or Surgical Racket?" *American Journal of Obstetrics and Gynecology* 51 (June 1946):804–10.

Morehead, Mildred A. *Quality of Medical Care Provided by Family Physicians as Related to Their Education, Training and Methods of Practice.* New York: Health Insurance Plan of Greater New York, May 1958. 86 pp.

————. "The Medical Audit as an Operational Tool." *American Journal of Public Health* 57 (September 1967):1643–56.

————. "Evaluating Quality of Medical Care in the Neighborhood Health Center Program of the Office of Economic Opportunity." *Medical Care* 8 (March-April 1970):118–31.

Morehead, Mildred A., and Donaldson, Rose. "Quality of Clinical Management of Disease in Comprehensive Neighborhood Health Centers." *Medical Care* 12 (April 1974):301–15.

Morehead, Mildred A.; Donaldson, Rose S.; and Seravalli, Mary R. "Comparisons between OEO Neighborhood Health Centers and Other Health Care Providers of Ratings of the Quality of Health Care." *American Journal of Public Health* 61 (July 1971):1294–1306.

Morehead, Mildred A.; Donaldson, Rose S.; et al. *A Study of the Quality of Hospital Care Secured by a Sample of Teamster Family Members in New York City.* New York: School of Public Health and Administrative Medicine, Columbia University, 1964. 98 pp.

Mushlin, Alvin I., and Appel, Francis A. "Testing an Outcome-Based Quality Assurance Strategy in Primary Care." *Supplement to Medical Care* 18 (May 1980):1–100.

National Center for Health Statistics. *Surgical Operations in Short-Stay Hospitals: United States, 1975.* Vital and Health Statistics, Series 13, No. 34. Hyattsville, Md.: U.S. Department of Health, Education, and Welfare, April 1978. 68 pp.

————. *Utilization of Short-Stay Hospitals: Annual Summary of the United States, 1977.* Vital and Health Statistics, Series 13, No. 41. Hyattsville, Md.: U.S. Department of Health, Education, and Welfare, March 1979. 62 pp.

————. *Utilization of Short-Stay Hospitals: Annual Summary for the United States, 1980.* Vital and Health Statistics, Series 13, No. 64. Hyattsville, Md.: U.S. Department of Health and Human Services, March 1982. 60 pp.

Neuhauser, Duncan, and Lewicki, Ann M. "What Do We Gain from the Sixth Stool Guaiac?" *New England Journal of Medicine* 293 (July 31, 1975):226–28.

Neutra, Raymond. "Indications for the Surgical Treatment of Suspected Acute Appendicitis: A Cost-Effectiveness Approach." Chapter 18, pp. 277–307. In John P. Bunker, Benjamin A. Barnes and Frederick Mosteller, eds., *Costs, Risks, and Benefits of Surgery.* New York: Oxford University Press, 1977. 401 pp.

New York Academy of Medicine, Committee on Public Health Relations. *Maternal Mortality in New York City: A Study of All Puerperal Deaths 1930–1932.* New York: Oxford University Press, for the Commonwealth Fund, 1933. 290 pp.

Nickerson, Rita J.; Colton, Theodore; Peterson, Osler L.; Bloom, Bernard S.; and Hauck, Walter W., Jr. "Doctors Who Perform Operations: A Study on In-Hospital Surgery in Four Diverse Geographic Areas." *New England Journal of Medicine* 295 (October 21 and October 28, 1976):921–26 and 982–89.

Novick, Lloyd F.; Dickinson, Karen; Asnes, Russell; Lan, S-P May; and Lowenstein, Regina. "Assessment of Ambulatory Care: Application of the Tracer Methodology." *Medical Care* 14 (January 1976):1–12.

Nutting, Paul A.; Shorr, Gregory I.; and Burkhalter, Barton R. "Assessing the Performance of Medical Care Systems: A Method and Its Application." *Medical Care* 19 (March 1981):281–96.

Oakley, J. R.; Hayes-Allen, M.; McWeeny, Patricia M.; and Emery, J. L. "Possibly Avoidable Deaths in Hospital in the Age-Group One Week to Two Years." *Lancet* 1 (April 10, 1976):770–72.

Osborne, Charles E., and Thompson, Hugh C. "Criteria for Evaluation of Ambulatory Child Health Care by Chart Audit: Development and Testing of a Methodology." *Supplement to Pediatrics* 56 (October 1975):625–92.

Payne, Beverly C.; Lyons, Thomas F.; Dwarshius, Louis; Kolton, Marilyn; and Morris, William. *The Quality of Medical Care: Evaluation and Improvement.* Chicago: Hospital Research and Educational Trust, 1976. 157 pp.

Payne, Beverly C.; Lyons, Thomas F.; Neuhaus, Evelyn; Kolton, Marilyn; and Dwarshius, Louis. *Method for Evaluating and Improving Ambulatory Care.* Ann Arbor, Mich.: Health Services Research Center, 1978. 195 pp. plus nonpaginated Appendixes A to F. (Report of Research Project RO1-HS-01583.)

Peterson, Osler L.; Andrews, Leon P.; Spain, Robert S.; and Greenberg, Bernard G. "An Analytical Study of North Carolina General Practice, 1953–1954." *Journal of Medical Education* 31, Part 2 (December 1956):1–165.

Phaneuf, Maria C. "Analysis of a Nursing Audit." *Nursing Outlook* 16 (January 1968):57–60.

—————. *The Nursing Audit.* 2d ed. New York: Appleton-Century-Crofts, 1976. 205 pp.

Piachaud, D., and Weddell, J. M. "The Economics of Treating Varicose Veins." *International Journal of Epidemiology* 1 (Autumn 1972):287–94.

Poland, Eleanor, and Lembcke, Paul A. *Delineation of Hospital Service Districts, a Fundamental Requirement in Hospital Planning.* Publication No. 135. Kansas City, Mo.: Community Studies, Inc., January 1962. 117 pp. plus appendixes.

Price, Philip B.; Taylor, Calvin W.; Nelson, David E.; Lewis, Evan G.; Loughmiller, Grover C.; Mathiesen, Ronald; Murray, Stephen L.; and Maxwell, J. Gary. *Measurement and Predictors of Physician Performance: Two Decades of Intermittently Sustained Research.* Salt Lake City: University of Utah Press, 1972. 164 pp.

Quick, Jonathan D.; Greenlick, Merwyn R.; and Roghmann, Klaus J. "Prenatal Care and Pregnancy Outcome in an HMO and General Population: A Multivariate Cohort Analysis." *American Journal of Public Health* 71 (April 1981):381–90.

Ray, Wayne A.; Federspiel, Charles F.; and Schaffner, William. "Prescribing of Chloramphenicol in Ambulatory Practice: An Epidemiologic Study Among Tennessee Medicaid Recipients." *Annals of Internal Medicine* 84 (March 1976):266–70.

—————. "The Mal-Prescribing of Liquid Tetracycline Preparations." *American Journal of Public Health* 67 (August 1977):762–63.

Restuccia, Joseph D., and Holloway, Don C. "Barriers to Appropriate Utilization of an Acute Facility." *Medical Care* 14 (July 1976):559–73.

Rhee, Sang-O. "Relative Influence of Specialty Status, Organization of Office Care and Organization of Hospital Care on the Quality of Medical Care: A Multivariate Analysis." Ph.D. diss., University of Michigan, 1975. 235 pp.

—————. "Factors Determining the Quality of Physician Performance in Patient Care." *Medical Care* 14 (September 1976):733–50.

—————. "U.S. Medical Graduates versus Foreign Medical Graduates: Are There Performance Differences in Practice?" *Medical Care* 15 (July 1977):568–77.

Rhee, Sang-O; Luke, Roice D.; Lyons, Thomas F.; and Payne, Beverly C. "Domain of Practice and the Quality of Physician Performance." *Medical Care* 19 (January 1981):14–23.

Rhee, Sang-O; Lyons, Thomas F.; and Payne, Beverly C. "Patient Race and Physician Performances: Quality of Medical Care, Hospital Admissions and Hospital Stays." *Medical Care* 17 (July 1979):737–47.

Riedel, Donald C., and Fitzpatrick, Thomas B. *Patterns of Patient Care: A Study of Hospital Use in Six Diagnoses*. Research Series No. 4. Ann Arbor, Mich.: Bureau of Hospital Administration, Graduate School of Business Administration, University of Michigan, 1964. 292 pp.

Riedel, Ruth Lyn, and Riedel, Donald C. *Practice and Performance: An Assessment of Ambulatory Care*. Ann Arbor, Mich.: Health Administration Press, 1979. 306 pp.

Roemer, Milton I., and Friedman, Jay W. *Doctors in Hospitals: Medical Staff Organization and Hospital Performance*. Baltimore: Johns Hopkins University Press, 1971. 322 pp.

Roemer, Milton I., and Shonick, William. "HMO Performance: The Recent Evidence." *Health and Society: Milbank Memorial Fund Quarterly* 51 (Summer 1973):271–317.

Roemer, Milton I.; Moustafa, A. Taher; and Hopkins, Carl E. "A Proposed Hospital Quality Index: Hospital Death Rates Adjusted for Case Severity." *Health Services Research* 3 (Summer 1968):96–118.

Romm, Fredric J., and Putnam, Samuel M. "The Validity of the Medical Record." *Medical Care* 19 (March 1981):310–15.

Rosenfeld, Leonard S. "Quality of Medical Care in Hospitals." *American Journal of Public Health* 47 (July 1957):856–65.

Rubenstein, Lisa; Mates, Susan; and Sidel, Victor W. "Quality-of-Care Assessment by Process and Outcome Scoring: Use of Weighted Algorithmic Assessment Criteria for Evaluation of Emergency Room Care of Women with Symptoms of Urinary Tract Infection." *Annals of Internal Medicine* 86 (May 1977):617–25.

Rutstein, David D.; Berenberg, William; Chalmers, Thomas C.; Child, Charles G., III; Fishman, Alfred P.; and Perrin, Edward B. "Measuring the Quality of Medical Care: A Clinical Method." *New England Journal of Medicine* 294 (March 11, 1976):582–88.

Sanazaro, Paul J., and Williamson, John W. "A Classification of Physician Performance in Internal Medicine." *Journal of Medical Education* 43 (March 1968):389–97.

Schmidt, Edward C.; Schall, David W.; and Morrison, Charles C. "Computerized Problem-Oriented Medical Record for Ambulatory Practice." *Medical Care* 12 (April 1974):316–27.

Schroeder, Steven A.; Kenders, Kathryn; Cooper, James K.; and Piemme, Thomas E. "Use of Laboratory Tests and Pharmaceuticals: Variation Among Physicians and Effect of Cost Audit on Subsequent Use." *Journal of the American Medical Association* 225 (August 20, 1973):969–73.

Schroeder, Steven A.; Schliftman, Alan; and Piemme, Thomas E. "Variation Among Physicians in Use of Laboratory Tests: Relation to Quality of Care." *Medical Care* 12 (August 1974):709–13.

Scott, W. Richard; Flood, Ann Barry; and Ewy, Wayne. "Organizational Determinants of Services, Quality and Cost of Care in Hospitals." *Health and Society: Milbank Memorial Fund Quarterly* 57 (Spring 1979):234–64.

Scott, W. Richard; Forrest, William H., Jr.; and Brown, Byron Wm., Jr. "Hospital Structure and Postoperative Mortality and Morbidity." Chapter 5, pp. 72–89. In Stephen M. Shortell and Montague Brown, eds., *Organizational Research in Hospitals*. Chicago: Blue Cross Association, 1976. 112 pp.

Shapiro, Sam; Jacobziner, Harold; Densen, Paul M.; and Weiner, Louis. "Further Observations on Prematurity and Perinatal Mortality in a General Population and in the Population of a Prepaid Group Practice Medical Care Plan." *American Journal of Public Health* 50 (September 1960):1304–17.

Shapiro, Sam; Weiner, Louis; and Densen, Paul M. "Comparison of Prematurity and Perinatal Mortality in a General Population and in the Population of a Prepaid Group Practice, Medical Care Plan." *American Journal of Public Health* 48 (February 1958):170–87.

Shorr, Gregory I., and Nutting, Paul A. "A Population-Based Assessment of the Continuity of Ambulatory Care." *Medical Care* 15 (June 1977):455–64.

Smith, David Barton, and Metzner, Charles A. "Differential Perceptions of Health Care Quality in a Prepaid Group Practice." *Medical Care* 8 (July-August 1970):264–75.

Sparling, J. Frederick. "Measuring Medical Care Quality: A Comparative Study." *Hospitals* 36 (March 16 and April 1, 1962):62–68 and 56–57, 60–61.

Staff of the Stanford Center for Health Care Research. *Study of Institutional Differences in Postoperative Mortality*. Report Prepared for the National Center for Health Services Research. Springfield, Va.: U.S. Department of Commerce, National Technical Information Service, December 15, 1974. 771 pp. (Publication No. PB-250-940.)

Staniland, J. R.; Dichtburn, Janet; and de Dombal, F. T. "Clinical Presentation of Acute Abdomen: Study of 600 Patients." *British Medical Journal* 3 (August 12, 1972):393–98.

Starfield, Barbara, and Scheff, David. "Effectiveness of Pediatric Care: The Relationship between Process and Outcome." *Pediatrics* 49 (April 1972):547–52.

Starfield, Barbara; Steinwachs, Donald; Morris, Ira; Bause, George; Siebert, Stephen; and Westin, Craig. "Concordance Between Medical Records and Observations Regarding Information on Coordination of Care." *Medical Care* 17 (July 1979):758–66. [1979a in text]

————. "Presence of Observers at Patient-Practitioner Interactions: Impact on Coordination of Care and Methodologic Implications." *American Journal of Public Health* 69 (October 1979):1021–25. [1979b in text]

Stockwell, Heather, and Vayda, Eugene. "Variations in Surgery in Ontario." *Medical Care* 17 (April 1979):390–96.

Sussman, Marvin B.; Caplan, Eleanor K.; Haug, Marie R.; and Stern, Marjorie R. *The Walking Patient: A Study in Outpatient Care.* Cleveland: The Press of Western Reserve University, 1967. 260 pp.

Thompson, Hugh C., and Osborne, Charles E. "Quality Assurance of Ambulatory Child Health Care: Opinions of Practicing Physicians About Proposed Criteria." *Medical Care* 14 (January 1976):22–38.

United Steelworkers of America, Public Relations Department. *Special Study on the Medical Care Program for Steelworkers and Their Families.* Report by the Insurance, Pension and Unemployment Benefits Department. Pittsburgh: The Department, September 1960. 108 pp.

Vayda, Eugene. "A Comparison of Surgical Rates in Canada and in England and Wales." *New England Journal of Medicine* 289 (December 6, 1973):1224–29.

Wagner, Edward H.; Greenberg, Robert A.; Imrey, Peter B.; Williams, Carolyn A.; Wolf, Susanne H.; and Ibrahim, Michel A. "Influence of Training and Experience on Selecting Criteria to Evaluate Medical Care." *New England Journal of Medicine* 294 (April 15, 1976):871–76.

Wagner, Edward H.; Williams, Carolyn A.; Greenberg, Robert; Kleinbaum, David; Wolf, Susanne; and Ibrahim, Michel A. "A Method for Selecting Criteria to Evaluate Medical Care." *American Journal of Public Health* 68 (May 1978):464–70.

Wandelt, Mabel A., and Ager, Joel. *Quality of Patient Care Scale.* Detroit: College of Nursing, Wayne State University, 1970. (A more recent edition has been published by Appleton-Century-Crofts, New York, 1974. 84 pp.)

Weed, Lawrence L. *Medical Records, Medical Education, and Patient Care.* Chicago: Year-Book Medical Publishers, Inc., 1971. 297 pp.

Weeks, H. Ashley. "Tightness of Organization Related to Patterns of Patient Care." Bureau of Public Health Economics, School of Public Health, University of Michigan, n.d.

Wennberg, John, and Gittelsohn, Alan. "Small Area Variations in Health Care Delivery." *Science* 182 (December 14, 1973):1102–08.

White, John J.; Satillana, Miguel; and Haller, J. Alex, Jr. "Intensive In-hospital Observation: A Safe Way to Decrease Unnecessary Appendectomy." *American Surgeon* 41 (December 1975):793–98.

Williamson, John W. *Assesssing and Improving Health Care Outcomes: The Health Accounting Approach to Quality Assurance.* Cambridge, Mass.: Ballinger Publishing Company, 1978. 327 pp.

Williamson, John W.; Braswell, Harriet R.; and Horn, Susan D. "Validity of Medical Staff Judgments in Establishing Quality Assurance Priorities." *Medical Care* 17 (April 1979):331–46.

Williamson, John W.; Braswell, Harriet R.; Horn, Susan D.; and Lohmeyer, Susan. "Priority Setting in Quality Assurance: Reliability of Staff Judgments in Medical Institutions." *Medical Care* 16 (November 1978):931–40.

Wright, Diana Dryer; Kane, Robert L.; Snell, George F.; and Woolley, F. Ross. "Costs and Outcomes for Different Primary Care Providers." *Journal of the American Medical Association* 238 (July 4, 1977):46–50.

Zimmer, James G. "Length of Stay and Hospital Bed Misutilization." *Medical Care* 12 (May 1974):453–62.

Zuckerman, Alan E.; Starfield, Barbara; Hochreiter, Clare; and Kovasznay, Beatrice. "Validating the Content of Pediatric Outpatient Medical Records by Means of Tape-Recording Doctor-Patient Encounters." *Pediatrics* 56 (September 1975):407–11.

Author Index

Subject Index

explicit criteria contribution, 380;
physicians, reported by, 14
England, 129, 301, 345
England and Wales, 9, 117-19, 265
Epidemiology: abdominal pain, acute,
333-35; appendicitis, 342; observations, limitations of, 280; quality,
of, 54, 227-29, 463-71; studies, contribution to assessment, 331, 342;
surgical care, of, 115-27, 135
Episodes of care: definition of, 428;
quality of care, 211-29
Equality of distribution: measurement
of, 131
Experiment, natural: appendicitis, 342
Explicit criteria. *See* Criteria, explicit
Eyeglasses: correction, accuracy of,
323

Family practice (*see also* General practice); ambulatory care, 45, 55,
199-209, 382, 385-91, 395; antibiotic
use, 55; appointment systems,
209; cost-quality relationship, 45;
criteria, agreement on, 389-91;
criteria, endorsement of, 382,
385-87; diagnostic procedures, use
of, 391; faculty, medical school, 45;
foreign graduates, 201; geographic
variation, 55; group practice, prepaid, 199-209; hospital visit
volume, 205; house staff, 45; inpatient care, 205; internists, 198;
medical record, size of, 209; medical records, quality of, 395; office
practice attributes, 209; outcomes of
care, 45; performance, 199-209;
physician attribute effect, 55,
199-207; physician attributes, desirable, 9; practice setting, type of,
207; practice, styles of, 207-9; prescribing patterns, 55; process of
care, 45, 55, 199-209, 383-91, 395;
recording criteria, if performed,
395; resource use, 55; x-ray proce-

dures, use of, 391
Fatality. *See* Case fatality rate;
Mortality
Filipinos, 229
Financial incentives: ambulatory
care, 29; equipment ownership
effect, 35; group practice, 29; inpatient care, 29; physician-induced
demand, 135, 141; physicians
care, 29, 34; referral patterns, 34;
surgical care, 135, 141; x-ray procedures, use of, 34
Follow-up care: ambulatory care,
313-15, 319, 325, 357; anemia, 315,
325; compliance effect, 313, 319,
325; continuity of care effect, 318;
criteria for (*see* Criteria, explicit,
follow-up care; Specification of
criteria, follow-up care); diagnostic
findings, follow-up on, 313-15,
319; gastrointestinal symptoms,
313; house staff, 242, 313-15; hypertension, 319; Indians, 319, 325;
pediatric care, 315, 357; prenatal
care, 325; process of care, 243,
313-15, 319, 325, 357, 381; quality
of, 243, 313-15, 319, 325; recording
of, 357; urinary tract disease, 325
Foot surgery, 147-48, 155
Foreign medical school graduates. *See*
Physicians, foreign graduates
Fractures, 71, 227, 409
Function status: daily activities, limitations, 305-6; index, 44; outcomes
of care, 305-6

Gallbladder disease, 71-73, 119, 227,
327, 409
Gallbladder surgery, 271. *See also*
Cholecystectomy
Gastrointestinal symptoms, 313
General practice (*see also* Family practice); ambulatory care, 55-57,
167-79, 230, 237, 301, 353, 382,
385-87, 395; antibiotic use, 55; cost-

About the Author

Dr. Avedis Donabedian maintains a longtime association with The University of Michigan where he is presently the Nathan Sinai Distinguished Professor of Public Health. Dr. Donabedian, who received his M.D. from the American University of Beirut and M.P.H. from the Harvard School of Public Health, taught previously at the American University of Beirut, at the Harvard School of Public Health and at New York Medical College. Dr. Donabedian was elected a member of The Institute of Medicine, National Academy of Sciences in 1971 and an honorary fellow of the American College of Hospital Administrators in 1982. He is the author of numerous papers and several books pertinent to the organization and administration of personal health care services in general, and quality assessment and monitoring in particular. Books he has written include *Aspects of Medical Care Administration: Specifying Requirements for Health Care*, and *Benefits in Medical Care Programs*. This is the third volume of his *Explorations in Quality Assessment and Monitoring*. Volume I, *The Definition of Quality and Approaches to its Assessment*, was published by Health Administration Press in 1980. Volume II, *The Criteria and Standards of Quality*, was published by Health Administration Press in 1982. Dr. Donabedian's previous publications have won the Dean Conley Award of the American College of Hospital Administrators in 1969, the Norman A. Welch Award of the National Association of Blue Shield Plans in 1976, and the Elizur Wright Award of the American Risk and Insurance Association in 1978.